QUALITY ASSURANCE IN HEALTH CARE

Edited by
Richard H. Egdahl, M.D., Ph.D.
and
Paul M. Gertman, M.D.

Aspen Systems Corporation
Germantown, Maryland

1976

Library of Congress Catalog Card Number: 76-15770
ISBN:0-912862-23-8

Printed in the United States of America

TABLE OF CONTENTS

Editors

Paul M. Gertman, M.D.
CHIEF, HEALTH CARE RESEARCH SECTION
DIVISION OF MEDICINE
BOSTON UNIVERSITY SCHOOL OF MEDICINE

Richard H. Egdahl, M.D., Ph.D.
ACADEMIC VICE PRESIDENT FOR
    HEALTH AFFAIRS
BOSTON UNIVERSITY
DIRECTOR
BOSTON UNIVERSITY MEDICAL CENTER

Contributors

George J. Annas, J.D., M.P.H.
DIRECTOR, CENTER FOR LAW AND HEALTH
    SCIENCES
BOSTON UNIVERSITY SCHOOL OF LAW
BOSTON, MASSACHUSETTS

Allyson Davies Avery, M.P.H.
HEALTH SERVICES RESEARCHER
RAND CORPORATION
SANTA MONICA, CALIFORNIA

Robert Brook, M.D.
SENIOR RESEARCHER, HEALTH SERVICES
RAND CORPORATION
SANTA MONICA, CALIFORNIA

Rick Carlson, J.D.
HEALTH CONSULTANT
MILL VALLEY, CALIFORNIA

Steven Epstein, J.D.
PARTNER, EPSTEIN & BECKER
WASHINGTON, D. C.

Michael J. Goran, M.D.
DIRECTOR, BUREAU OF QUALITY ASSURANCE
HEALTH SERVICES ADMINISTRATION
DEPARTMENT OF HEALTH, EDUCATION,
    AND WELFARE
ROCKVILLE, MARYLAND

Gregory T. Halbert, J.D.
RESEARCH ASSOCIATE IN HEALTH LAW
BOSTON UNIVERSITY PROGRAM ON PUBLIC
    POLICY FOR QUALITY HEALTH CARE
BOSTON, MASSACHUSETTS

David Kinzer
PRESIDENT, MASSACHUSETTS HOSPITAL
    ASSOCIATION
BURLINGTON, MASSACHUSETTS

William Knaus, M.D.
PROFESSIONAL STAFF MEMBER, OFFICE OF
    THE ASSISTANT SECRETARY, PLANNING
    AND EVALUATION
DEPARTMENT OF HEALTH, EDUCATION,
    AND WELFARE
WASHINGTON, D. C.

Sol Levine, Ph.D.
PROFESSOR OF SOCIOLOGY AND COMMUNITY
    MEDICINE, UNIVERSITY PROFESSOR
BOSTON UNIVERSITY

Daniel W. Pettengill, F.A.A.
VICE PRESIDENT, GROUP DIVISION
AETNA LIFE INSURANCE COMPANY
HARTFORD, CONNECTICUT

Charles Phelps, Ph.D.
SENIOR RESEARCH ECONOMIST
RAND CORPORATION
SANTA MONICA, CALIFORNIA

Kenneth Platt, M.D.
GENERAL SURGEON, WESTMINISTER MEDICAL
    CLINIC
DENVER, COLORADO

James S. Roberts, M.D.
DIRECTOR, DIVISION OF PEER REVIEW
BUREAU OF QUALITY ASSURANCE
HEALTH SERVICES ADMINISTRATION
DEPARTMENT OF HEALTH, EDUCATION,
    AND WELFARE
WASHINGTON, D.C.

John Rodak, S.M.
CHIEF, PROVIDERS STANDARDS BRANCH
DIVISION OF PROVIDER STANDARDS AND
    CERTIFICATION
BUREAU OF QUALITY ASSURANCE
HEALTH SERVICES ADMINISTRATION
DEPARTMENT OF HEALTH, EDUCATION,
    AND WELFARE
WASHINGTON, D.C.

Cynthia H. Taft, B.A.
RESEARCH ASSOCIATE IN HEALTH PLANNING
BOSTON UNIVERSITY PROGRAM ON PUBLIC
    POLICY FOR QUALITY HEALTH CARE
BOSTON, MASSACHUSETTS

Claude Welch, M.D.
GENERAL SURGEON, MASSACHUSETTS
    GENERAL HOSPITAL
BOSTON, MASSACHUSETTS

Kathleen N. Williams, M.A.
GRADUATE FELLOW
RAND GRADUATE INSTITUTE
SANTA MONICA, CALIFORNIA

Other Participants in November, 1975 Conference on "Quality Assurance in Hospitals"

Gregory J. Ahart, J.D.
DIRECTOR, MANPOWER AND WELFARE
    DIVISION
GOVERNMENT ACCOUNTING OFFICE
WASHINGTON, D.C.

Carl Baker, M.D.
ASSOCIATE DIRECTOR FOR SCIENTIFIC AFFAIRS
HEALTH RESOURCES ADMINISTRATION
DEPARTMENT OF HEALTH, EDUCATION,
    AND WELFARE
ROCKVILLE, MARYLAND

Melvin Blumenthal
SPECIAL PROGRAM ADVISOR
BUREAU OF HEALTH INSURANCE
SOCIAL SECURITY ADMINISTRATION
BALTIMORE, MARYLAND

E. Langdon Burwell, M.D.
INTERNIST
FALMOUTH, MASSACHUSETTS

James Cooper, M.D.
DIRECTOR, HEALTH CARE SYSTEMS

OFFICE OF POLICY DEVELOPMENT AND
PLANNING
DEPARTMENT OF HEALTH, EDUCATION,
AND WELFARE
ROCKVILLE, MARYLAND

David Cusic, M.P.H.

PROGRAM OFFICER, ROBERT WOOD JOHNSON
FOUNDATION
PRINCETON, NEW JERSEY

Karen Davis, Ph.D.

SENIOR FELLOW, BROOKINGS INSTITUTION
WASHINGTON, D.C.

Jonathan Fielding, M.D.

COMMISSIONER, MASSACHUSETTS
DEPARTMENT OF PUBLIC HEALTH
BOSTON, MASSACHUSETTS

C. Rollins Hanlon, M.D.

DIRECTOR, AMERICAN COLLEGE OF
SURGEONS
CHICAGO, ILLINOIS

Arthur E. Hess

FORMER ACTING DEPUTY COMMISSIONER
SOCIAL SECURITY ADMINISTRATION
DEPARTMENT OF HEALTH, EDUCATION,

AND WELFARE
BALTIMORE, MARYLAND

Erwin Hytner

PROFESSIONAL STAFF MEMBER
HOUSE COMMITTEE ON WAYS AND MEANS
SUBCOMMITTEE ON HEALTH
U. S. HOUSE OF REPRESENTATIVES
WASHINGTON, D. C.

J. Alexander McMahon, J.D.

PRESIDENT, AMERICAN HOSPITAL
ASSOCIATION
CHICAGO, ILLINOIS

Charles Sanders, M.D.

GENERAL DIRECTOR, MASSACHUSETTS
GENERAL HOSPITAL
BOSTON, MASSACHUSETTS

Bernard Tresnowski, M.P.H.A.

SENIOR VICE PRESIDENT, FEDERAL PROGRAM
ON HEALTH CARE SERVICE
BLUE CROSS ASSOCIATION OF AMERICA
CHICAGO, ILLINOIS

Sidney Wolfe, M.D.

DIRECTOR, HEALTH RESEARCH GROUP
WASHINGTON, D. C.

Staff Members—Boston University Program on Public Policy for Quality Health Care

Program Director:

Richard H. Egdahl, M.D., Ph.D.
ACADEMIC VICE PRESIDENT FOR HEALTH AFFAIRS
BOSTON UNIVERSITY
DIRECTOR
BOSTON UNIVERSITY MEDICAL CENTER

Senior Advisers:

George J. Annas, J.D., M.P.H.
DIRECTOR, CENTER FOR LAW AND HEALTH
SCIENCES
BOSTON UNIVERSITY SCHOOL OF LAW

Paul M. Gertman, M.D.
CHIEF, HEALTH CARE RESEARCH SECTION
DIVISION OF MEDICINE
BOSTON UNIVERSITY SCHOOL OF MEDICINE

Sol Levine, Ph.D.
PROFESSOR OF SOCIOLOGY AND COMMUNITY
MEDICINE,
AND UNIVERSITY PROFESSOR
BOSTON UNIVERSITY

Research Associates:

John Blum, J.D., M.P.H.
HEALTH LAW

Donald R. Giller, M.S.
HEALTH COMMUNICATIONS

Gregory T. Halbert, J.D.
HEALTH LAW

Alan Monheit, Ph.D.
HEALTH ECONOMICS

Cynthia Taft, B.A.
HEALTH PLANNING

Regina A. Robbins, B.A.
ADMINISTRATIVE ASSISTANT

Preface

This volume of challenging essays is one of the products of a seminar on Quality Assurance in Hospitals held in November 1975 in Boston. The meeting was the first in a series of semiannual conferences conducted by the Boston University Program on Public Policy for Quality Health Care, a project supported by the Robert Wood Johnson Foundation of Princeton, New Jersey. The goal of the meetings was to provide a forum for cogent, in-depth discussion by individuals from the public and private sectors who have major involvement in health policy issues affecting the quality of health care. The topic of this first conference was selected because of the controversy surrounding the development of Professional Standards Review Organizations and their relationship to other quality assurance activities.

The thirty-three individuals who participated in the November seminar represented a wide range of viewpoints on quality assurance in health care. To provide the participants with a common ground for discussion and debate, fourteen background papers were prepared under the aegis of the Program on Public Policy for Quality Health Care and distributed in advance of the meeting; these papers compose the core of this volume. Prepared by acknowledged authorities on each respective topic, the papers represent a valuable compendium of current thought about the broad field of quality assurance in health institutions.

The November meeting was devoted to open discussion aimed at clarifying differences of opinion and exposing participants to meaningful debate on the policy alternatives. The recommendations that flowed from the conference discussions were refined by the program staff and published in April 1976 as *Quality Assurance in Hospitals: Policy Alternatives.** The monograph con-

---

*Copies can be obtained by writing the Boston University Program on Public Policy, 720 Harrison Avenue, Suite 203, Boston, Massachusetts 02118. Please enclose $1.00 per copy for shipping and handling.

tains a discussion of policy alternatives in quality assurance, as well as synopses of the conference discussions. The policy recommendations emanating from the November conference are also in Chapter 15 of this volume.

The Program on Public Policy for Quality Health Care is planning future meetings on the relationship of continuing medical education, hospital rate setting, and health planning to the quality of health care. It is our hope that these meetings, and the background papers and policy monographs associated with them, will represent an important contribution toward greater quality in the delivery of health services.

RICHARD H. EGDAHL, M.D., Ph.D.

Boston
May 17, 1976

Introduction

A decade ago there was almost no public discussion of the quality of care in American hospitals, except for occasional "best in the world" rhetoric. Today, assurance of that quality has become one of the central health policy issues of the 1970s—so controversial, in fact, that it often has eclipsed the health profession's concerns over national health insurance.

A massive and unprecedented governmental regulatory effort, the Professional Standards Review Organization (PSRO) program, has been launched to develop a nationwide system of hospital quality assurance, organized from the smallest local hospitals to regional, state, and federal levels. Even in the early stages of this program, the direct and indirect costs in public monies probably have reached a level of several hundred million dollars. This sum may exceed all public expenditures on research to conquer heart disease, the leading cause of death in the United States. Viewed from another perspective, however, this expense probably represents less than one percent of out nation's expenditures for hospital care. If the current quality assurance efforts are expanded to include nonhospital institutional care and ambulatory care and to encompass care reimbursed by private health insurance as well as governmental programs, annual expenditures for quality assurance in health care may well reach a billion dollars.

Although most individuals and groups concerned with the delivery of health care support the overall goals of the PSRO program and believe that systematic efforts are vitally important to improve the efficiency and quality of hospital services, there has been increasing concern over both the substance and the organization of the PSRO program and similar quality assurance efforts.

To delineate the nature of the current problems in national quality assurance efforts and to identify potential policy actions that might be taken to deal with these problems, the Boston University Program on Public Policy for Quality Health Care convened a small conference of experts and authorities in the field in November 1975. The conference was organized around the following five distinct, but interrelated, topics:

(1) Current Current Quality Assurance Mechanisms: Need for Redirection?

(2) Inpatient Inpatient Quality Assurance Activities: Coordination of Federal, State, and Private Roles

(3) Quality Quality Assessment Information: Management of Data and the Question of Public Access

(4) Professional Professional Licensure and Hospital Delineation of Clinical Privileges: Relationship to Quality Assurance

(5) Financing Financing Mechanisms and Costs in Quality Assurance Activities

For each session, a set of background papers was prepared and distributed prior to the conference; these were briefly reviewed by a moderator and formed the basis for the ensuing discussion.* Eleven of the participants and three senior Boston University staff members were asked to prepare these background papers. Each was asked to identify a policy problem related to his assigned subject, critically analyze the issues surrounding that subject, and suggest potential action. The authors were encouraged to be critical—even provocative—in the way they dealt with their subject, and to organize their ideas as they wished.

The papers varied in style, approach, and length; but virtually all participants found them extremely stimulating. That the papers represented a unique body of written material on current quality assurance problems and policy options from some of the leading experts in the field was agreed to by the conference members. It is worth reviewing for the reader the rationale for the topic areas and subjects selected, and some of the major points presented in each part of the book.

One of the problems facing conferences on controversial health policy issues is a tendency to become enmeshed in debates over details of programs and minor points of current controversy. Thus, the goal of the first part is to place the current debate in a broader perspective. Robert Brook and his associates at the Rand Corporation present a view of where quality assurance efforts should go in the remainder of the century, and how we should proceed to get there. They suggest that the next five years be regarded as a "transitional" period of organizational development and research, during which time few visible effects of the PSRO program should be expected.

---

* The conference proceedings and recommendations have been published recently in a Boston University policy monograph entitled *Quality Assurance in Hospitals: Policy Alternatives.* The recommendations also appear in this volume as Chapter 15.

Additionally, the authors define a four-step, long term research strategy, which would facilitate the effectiveness of quality assurance efforts. Sol Levine and Cynthia Taft of Boston University in Chapter 2 attempt to assess why the federal government has had difficulties in correcting quality of care problems despite numerous regulatory and special program efforts. The critique emphasizes the tendency of federal policy makers to ignore the lack of consensus among interest groups affected by these programs; they utilize the PSRO problems to illustrate how policies should be developed and implemented in the future.

Part II explores the issue of coordination of interest and activity between three of these major interest groups, with contributions from a senior health official, a medical society and foundation president, and a state hospital association president. As background, Michael Goran, director of the Bureau of Quality Assurance, and his colleagues not only review the PSRO program but attempt also to place it within the spectrum of the broad range of activities that the federal government is undertaking in regulating in health institutions. Looking toward the future role of federal efforts in quality assurance under national health insurance, the authors emphasize the need to coordinate the patchwork of current statutory and regulatory government actions in quality assurance and to support extensive research and evaluation. Kenneth Platt, former president of the Colorado Foundation for Medical Care, sets the current quality assurance efforts in an historical and philosophical context. He stresses his belief that much of the impetus for these programs has grown from a concern over the rapid rise in health care costs and a general public disillusionment not only with medicine but also with a broad range of social institutions. Platt's paper highlights the tensions between the dual objectives of the PSRO program for quality assurance and cost control, the problems this has produced, and the danger of developing two separate levels of quality assurance—one for beneficiaries of federal health insurance programs and another for the private sector. David Kinzer, president of the Massachusetts Hospital Association, attempts to describe the major forces interacting on the PSRO scene, with principal attention to the views of the interest groups. He then explores the dilemma hospitals face when PSROs remove authority from hospital trustees; yet, simultaneously, the courts hold those persons increasingly liable for the quality of care. Additionally, Kinzer notes the lack of coordination between the PSROs' cost containment features and the multitude of other private, state, and federal efforts to control the rising costs of hospital care. The description of the current quality assurance efforts, the interests of different parties, and the priorities for coordination from these three different perspectives serve to illuminate the current problems and future potential of hospital quality assurance.

No issue better illustrates the current controversies besetting the PSRO program than the question of how data systems are to be developed, who will control them, and who will have access to what types of information. In Part III James Baker, vice president of the Cullinane Corporation, presents a down to earth perspective on the PSRO data management problem by an "outsider"—an expert from the field of large scale financial data management. His practical review of the needs of and the options open to most PSROs tends to deflate some of the Orwellian nightmares about a vast medical data computer network. He suggests that many groups will not need computers at all in their initial stages, and that even at a later time probably should be satisfied with minicomputers.

The subject of confidentiality and access to other quality assurance data produced the strongest debate at the conference; the reasons for this are contained in the latter two chapter of this part. George Annas, director of the Boston University Center for Law and Health Sciences, presents a scholarly brief, with extensive legal citations, for the patients' rights of access to *almost all* data about the quality of care given by health providers. In opposition, Steven Epstein, a Washington health lawyer, argues the case for limited disclosure of provider information, emphasizing the potential harm that might be done through misinterpretation of "raw" data. Though not resolving the data controversy, these views are a valuable guide to important issues.

Two of the key links in systems of hospital quality assurance have been the public licensure of health professionals and the delineation of physicians' hospital privileges; these form the topic for Part IV. Claude Welch, general surgeon at Massachusetts General Hospital, analyzes the development of licensure and specialty certification and the reasons why these have been and, in his view, should remain a mainstay of national quality assurance efforts. The legal bases for the current powers of the medical profession to regulate the quality of care delivered by its members—through state licensure, specialty board certification, and limitation of hospital privileges—are thoroughly delineated by Gregory Halbert of Boston University. The third chapter, however, presents a forceful case *against* maintenance of the current type of licensure and credentialing system. Its author, Rick Carlson, first attacks the premise that today's medical care system improves health. He then reviews some negative evidence on the impact of medical licensure and certification on quality of care, such as the lack of disciplinary action by state boards and the inhibiting effects on the mobility and distribution of health professionals. Finally, Carlson suggests some major changes in the system, including the relaxation of licensing standards and the introduction of lay control of licensure boards. The opposing views taken in these papers are not today's area of major controversy in quality assurance, but they might be tomorrow's.

Part V is devoted to the cost and financing mechanisms of hospital quality assurance programs, a subject of pressing concern to many involved with the PSRO program. As background for these discussions, William Knaus, a physician on the staff of the Department of Health, Education, and Welfare's Office of Assistant Secretary for Planning and Evaluation, reviews both the current status and future options of PSRO financing. Further, he shows how these options are really tied to the underlying debate of whether Congress or the executive branch will dominate national PSRO policy. The case for expansion of the PSRO hosptial quality assurance program to cover all patients through cooperative financing from the private sector is presented by Daniel Pettengill, vice president of Aetna Life Insurance Company. He argues for financing these programs through routine hospital charges and warns that unless expansion of the review mandate occurs, we will develop a "two-class" system of hospital care. The concluding viewpoint in this volume, by Rand health economist Charles Phelps, is a delineation of a basic cost/benefit methodology for evaluating quality assurance programs. This first conceptual attempt to develop a key policy tool explores many of the hidden costs that potentially exist in the PSRO program, which go beyond line items in a federal budget.

These fourteen contributions contain a wealth of ideas, insights, and recommendations for action. For all those interested in improving the quality of health care in our nation's hospitals, we hope they prove enlightening and useful.

Paul M. Gertman, M.D.
Boston
May 5, 1976

Part I

Current Quality Assurance Mechanisms: Need For Redirection?

Chapter 1

Quality Assurance in the 20th Century: Will It Lead to Improved Health in the 21st?[1]

Robert H. Brook,
Kathleen N. Williams,
and
Allyson Davies Avery

DATELINE 1999—Washington Post—Amidst emotional debate and despite strong pressure brought by the AAMC against the proposed bill, Congress today passed a law which requires a physician to wear, at all times, a sign stating "I am dangerous to your health—beware." At the same time, Congress has approved payment for medical services rendered by experts in faithhealing, parapsychology, biofeedback, and acupuncture. The reason for this not-so-subtle hostility to "traditional" medical care can be traced to efforts to assess quality of care which began in the 1970s. After the academicians finally became convinced that they should be involved in this activity, they proceeded vigorously to set process criteria which they thought would improve quality of care and health of people.

An example of a criteria set for a disease, which back in the 1970s was called a common cold and today is called "type 62 antigen immunologically determined discharge from the upper turbinate of the left nostril," is as follows: Each person who presents with a nasal discharge has a fiber optic scope inserted into each turbinate from which a biopsy of the epithelium and a culture are obtained. The biopsy material is immediately fixed and placed under the electron microscope (standard equipment in each doctor's office) to determine what viral particle is present in what cells. Meanwhile, the material obtained for culture is immediately inserted into 75 different test tubes containing tissue culture cells obtainable only from a bald eagle. To ensure 100 percent compliance, the patient is chained to a seat in the office for 24 hours until the results from all tests have been received, at which point the patient is told the diagnosis and given a bill for $10,000. As a parting gesture (the only hold-over from more traditional practice), the patient is told to stay in bed, take aspirin, and, if he can find his mother, have her make him a bowl of chicken soup. After discounting for inflation, the cost for treating the common cold in 1970 dollars is $1000.

Because of similar criteria established for other conditions, the percentage of the gross national product (GNP) spent on medical care has risen from 7

3

percent in 1970 to over 50 percent in 1999. This actually has decreased the health of most people, since the average citizen can no longer afford to buy adequate food; moreover, most of America, in the name of medical care, has turned into a slum. After many years of inaction, however, the Congress has been forced to act; the President, even though he is a former professor of medicine, is expected to sign the bill, since the likelihood of anarchy is real.

INTRODUCTION

Quality assurance has arrived. No longer is it pursued solely by researchers, but instead is mandated by two federal laws and by one professional body—the Joint Commission on the Accreditation of Hospitals. In just a few years, the amount of money spent on quality assurance activities has grown from a few million or so to a hundred million dollars. If these activities become fully operational in the 1980s, they are likely to consume 2 to 5 percent of the dollar spent on personal medical care services—or about 2 to 5 billion dollars per year. The issue at hand is whether this expenditure of funds will increase health levels by improving the quality of care provided, or whether it will decrease health by transferring money from providing *new* medical services to quality assurance efforts that lead to nonproductive activities in the medical care field. Our purpose here is to address this issue and to suggest courses of action along both research and policy lines that could be pursued to maximize the possibility that quality assurance activities will improve health. (The larger policy issue is the relative effectiveness of the medical care system *vis-à-vis* other social systems, such as public health, education, and housing, in improving health and is not discussed here.)

This chapter discusses two. The first topic concerns itself both with describing what is known about quality assessment and assurance and with deriving research recommendations about how to extend this knowledge. The second, building in part on those recommendations, describes how a quality assurance system for the 1980s and beyond, that would improve the health of the nation, might be developed. Issues identified in the first section—especially those concerning the measurement of quality—are discussed in more detail than those identified in the second, since failure to adequately resolve the former will lead to erroneous solutions of the latter. Details about specific studies are, in general, not reported below. For readers interested in this aspect of quality assessment and assurance, other documents are available which fulfill those needs.[2-9]

At the outset, the seven terms that will recur frequently in this discussion—quality assessment, quality assurance, structure, process, outcome, efficacy, and effectiveness—must be defined. Quality assessment involves measuring the level of quality provided at some point in time; it connotes no effort to change or improve that level of care. Quality assurance has been used in the literature to mean both measuring the level of care provided *and,* when necessary, improving it. Thus, quality assessment is the first step in quality assurance.

Structure, process, and outcome refer to three different variables that can be used to assess or measure quality of care. Structural measurements are concerned with the descriptive, innate characteristics of facilities or providers (e.g., the soundness of a building, whether a poison chart is posted in an emergency room, or the age and board certification status of the physician). Process measures are, in a sense, simply those measures that evaluate what a provider does to and for a patient (e.g., ordering a cardiogram for a patient with chest pain). They can also mean how well a person is moved through the medical care system, either in a "macro" sense (e.g., from first symptom to seeking care to obtaining care) or in a "micro" sense (e.g., from arrival to departure at an emergency room or outpatient clinic). Outcomes reflect what happened to the patient, in terms of palliation, treatment, cure, or rehabilitation. Obviously, the definitions of structure, process, and outcome are not sufficiently precise to prevent the unreliable labeling of some measures which are used to assess quality. Nevertheless, the conceptual distinction among these three measures is important to maintain, since in essence they measure three different things: the resources necessary to solve a problem, the way the problem was solved, and the results of the problem solving, respectively.

Efficacy and effectiveness are two additional words defined differently within the medical care literature. Efficacy relates to the benefit or lack of benefit a procedure or treatment has when performed under ideal circumstances. Effectiveness relates to the average benefit of a procedure or program when used by the average provider in the average community. A procedure clearly can be both efficacious and effective. It can also be efficacious and ineffective, but the reverse cannot occur. A kidney transplant program at a university hospital may be efficacious but, when done in the average hospital by the average surgeon, may be ineffective in improving the health of patients in renal failure.

QUALITY ASSESSMENT AND ASSURANCE

Definition of Quality: Technical Care and Art-of-Care

The literature is replete with comments about how quality should be defined. From these comments a consensus has emerged that quality of care measurement involves two basic concepts: the quality of the technical care, and the quality of the art-of-care. Technical care refers to the adequacy of the diagnostic and therapeutic processes; and art-of-care relates to the milieu, manner, and behavior of the provider in delivering care to and communicating with the patient. A provider who delivers a higher level of the art-of-care should promote the following behaviors in his patients: willingness to discuss sensitive problems; utilization of medical services in a manner which would maximize the chance of these services benefiting the patient's health; increased compliance with regimens directed at controlling or alleviating chronic diseases (many of which at the time of diagnosis may be only mildly symptomatic or asymptomatic); and adoption of lifestyles and health habits conducive to longevity and decreased morbidity. Virtually all quality assessment studies have evaluated the technical aspects of quality; measurement of the art-of-care is just now beginning.

Examination of these two concepts raises three policy issues. First, the objective of assuring a high level of the technical and art-of-care aspects of quality has improvements in health as its overriding goal. This objective could be accomplished either by raising both the level of the art-of-care and the technical aspects of care simultaneously or by concentrating efforts on improving either aspect alone. Until now, virtually all efforts at raising quality have gone into improving the technical aspects of the delivery of care. Data from community surveys, however, suggest that improvement in the art-of-care may produce greater changes in health than would similar changes in the technical aspects of care. Hypertension, heart disease, obesity, drug abuse, accidents, smoking, and drinking are the major causes of excess morbidity and mortality; their control depends more on improving the art-of-care than on improving the level of technical care provided.

Second, the ethics underlying any attempt to improve the art-of-care must be examined. The most dramatic way to ensure that a patient complies is to lock him up. Although this is done with alcoholics by hospitalizing them in state mental institutions or by confining them to prison—which is considered ethical—most Americans would probably consider the incarceration of smokers, for instance, unethical. In an attempt to improve the art-of-care, other, more subtle techniques, such as biofeedback, personality modification, and motivational manipulation, are being developed. Which of these techniques will be considered ethical when used in the medical care system is an important issue.

Third, at a conceptual level, investigators who have *defined* the term quality of care have always invoked technical and art-of-care concepts, but investigators who have *measured* quality have almost never measured the art-of-care component. Unfortunately, our society emphasizes what is measured;

what is not measured or is unmeasurable is forgotten or ignored. Since improvement in the health of the American people is likely to require greater improvements in the art-of-care than in the technical aspects of care, the development of art-of-care measures must be emphasized. The first set of recommendations, therefore, is as follows:

1. Research priority be given to the development of valid measures of the art-of-care.
2. Simultaneously, efforts should be undertaken to determine the ethics of various procedures used to modify the level of art-of-care.
3. Ethical procedures and techniques focused on improving the art-of-care should be rigorously tested as to efficacy.
4. After better methods of improving the art-of-care are developed, studies should be undertaken to determine the relative costs and benefits of improving the art-of-care versus the technical aspects of care.

Without emphasis now on developing measures of the art-of-care, any quality assurance system of the 1980s is likely to be grossly distorted toward improving the technical aspect of care. This would most certainly not produce the largest increments in health for a given amount of money.

History of Quality Assessment and Assurance

Attempts at improving the quality of care provided are perhaps as old as the concept of healing, but history's message is that interest in quality assurance waxes and wanes. In a few ancient civilizations, if a doctor operated on the eye of a freeman and the man went blind, the surgeon's right hand was amputated. In the 1860s, studies were performed which compared hospital size with the probability of surviving an amputation. The larger the hospital, the greater the case-fatality rate. On the other hand, few studies which measured quality of care were performed from the 1920s to 1950s. The reason for this cyclical interest in quality assurance is unclear. It may reflect questions about the utility of quality assurance activities in improving health in general; it might also reflect concern over the iatrogenic effects such activities might produce on the medical care system. Part of the cyclical disinterest in quality assurance may have been due to the placebo nature of medicine in the pre-antibiotic era. In that era, the choice of technique or procedure made little difference for most diseases, since virtually all therapies were essentially placebos that produced neither harm nor benefit.

Whatever the reasons for this cyclical interest in quality assurance, it seems imperative that one of the objectives in building a quality assurance mechanism in the 1970s should be that of establishing a system which will survive. Survival will be at least partially dependent upon demonstrated effectiveness and efficiency. This will require the testing of various forms of quality assurance systems. The second recommendation, therefore, is as follows:

> Any attempt to develop an *ideal standardized* quality assurance system in the next few years is folly. Instead, rigorous experimentation should be undertaken, with each experiment subjected to careful evaluation.* Quality assurance activities which do not improve the health of people should be ruthlessly eliminated; those that improve health should be expanded. The product of this period of experimentation should be the acquisition of knowledge that will lead to the development of a quality assurance system by 1980 to 1985 which can stand the test of time.

Results of Quality of Care Assessment

In the last 60 years, close to 1,000 studies have been performed to assess the level of quality of care delivered. These studies have used a variety of data collection techniques—from direct physician observation to claims form review. They have also examined either structural, process, or outcome variables. Virtually all of these studies have detected basic problems in the level of quality of care delivered. For example, there is ample information to support the contention that simple, routine tasks are not performed well in the American medical care system. Hypertension is often not recognized; when it is recognized, it is often not treated. Children are not given immunizations. Anemic children are not given iron. Preschool children are not screened for visual problems. Successful completion of such straightforward routine activities is not related to the acquisition of knowledge about the proper use of sophisticated, newly developed interventions, but instead to the development of better practice habits. This implies that a quality assurance system which emphasizes the acquisition of new knowledge may have little effect on health.

---

* The word experiment as opposed to developmental activities is deliberately chosen. One learns little from developmental activities in this field. The results obtained from developmental activities are often biased and are usually interpreted in a misleading manner. On the other hand, experiment is not a synonym for controlled clinical trial; advantage can be taken of the recently developed quasi-experimental designs.

Some investigations have attempted to predict which facility and/or professional characteristics are associated with better care. Variables that have been studied include size and affiliation status of a hospital (such as whether it is a teaching hospital); organization and financing of ambulatory care facilities, including prepayment; and physician characteristics such as age, years in practice, years of postgraduate training, standing in medical school class, medical school of graduation, specialty, and specialty board status. To date, the results from these studies have been disappointing. Little variation in the level of quality of care provided can be predicted accurately by any of these variables (or even by all of them together). In general, care is perhaps slightly better in large teaching hospitals than in either proprietary or community hospitals. Physicians who are younger and board-certified render better care than those who are not. Treating a "modal" patient (a patient who has the condition the physician is trained to treat) is associated with the provision of better quality care. Nevertheless, a patient who is treated by a young board-certified physician is not likely to receive *substantially* better care than one treated by an elderly non-board-certified physician. The difference between the optimal level of quality of care and that given in the average community is far greater than the difference in care between, say, any two types of physicians or ambulatory facilities.

In summary, no matter what method is used to assess it, quality of care is found to be deficient. Many of these deficiencies appear to be related not to physician knowledge but to physician habits and behaviors and, more importantly, to the characteristics of the medical care system. There is wide variation in the quality of care delivered in an average community, but only a small fraction of this variation, unfortunately, can be predicted by a standard set of characteristics of facilities or providers. The third recommendation, then, is:

> Attempts to improve the level of quality of care by requiring mandatory continuing education, recertification, or other efforts to improve solely cognitive skills must be resisted. Furthermore, arguments for or against altering the organization of ambulatory care such as by increasing the number of prepaid group practices or large multispecialty group practices should be made on cost grounds and not on quality grounds, since there is very little evidence that such changes affect the quality of care provided. Finally, since changing physician and/or system-wide behaviors is as important to improving health as is improving physician cognitive knowledge, quality assurance activities should be incorporated only into systems able to assess changes in such behaviors.

The above may appear to be self-evident, but state legislative bodies are moving rapidly toward requiring physician relicensure and mandatory continuing education, etc., in exchange for resolving the malpractice crisis of 1975. These efforts, directed as they are at improving cognitive knowledge and unassociated with attempts to change physician or system behavior, are unlikely to increase health of the citizenry. They are likely to be expensive.

Validity and Reliability of Quality Assessment Methods

Quality of care has been shown to be deficient no matter what method is used to measure it. The *level* of deficiency, however, depends greatly on the method used to assess quality. In assessing quality of care, different data sources and different kinds of data can be used (see Table 1-1). Each combination will produce different assessments of quality, yet very little work has been done to evaluate individual methods of assessment, let alone to compare the results obtained when the same care is assessed by two or more methods. Nevertheless, from the methods work to date, the following conclusions can be drawn.

First, no matter what method is used to assess care, ambulatory care is found to be far more deficient than hospital care. This does not necessarily

Table 1-1

METHOD OF COLLECTING DATA FOR
QUALITY OF CARE ASSESSMENT

Method of Collection	Type of Data			
	Structure	Process	Outcome	Combination
Routinely reported data	X			
Hospital discharge abstract		X	X	X
Claims form		X		
Encounter form		X	X	X
Source-oriented medical record		X	X	X
Problem-oriented medical record		X	X	X
Direct observation of physicians		X		
Simulation techniques	X	X		
Patient interview		X	X	X
Tracer disease strategy		X	X	X
Population survey		X	X	X
Combination of above	X	X	X	X

Source: Institute of Medicine policy statement, see note 4.

mean that, for a fixed amount of dollars, a greater improvement in health would occur from investment in ambulatory care than in hospital care. However, considering the present emphasis in the PSRO and JCAH programs on improving the quality of hospital care while totally ignoring ambulatory care, the above proposition needs testing.

Second, the harshest judgment of quality of care occurs when the process of medical care is judged by a medical record review and *a priori* explicit criteria. If care as judged by this method were to reach "acceptable" levels, the number of procedures given and/or recorded must increase by about 50 percent in the hospital and by 250 percent in the ambulatory care area. This alone would increase the percentage of the GNP devoted to health to between 10 and 14 percent per year.*

Third, very few elements of the process of ambulatory care can be assessed through recorded information, such as in the medical record. Routine activities, such as physical examination, history taking, or patient education, are rarely recorded legibly (or usefully) in the medical record. Perhaps the only reliable, routinely recorded information are the vital signs, medications, and the results of laboratory tests. Thus, only a few aspects (albeit important aspects) of ambulatory care can be assessed by means of the medical record.

If a broader assessment of the quality of ambulatory care is desired, then outcome assessment must be used, the physician-patient relationship must be observed, or the amount of information recorded must be dramatically increased. Outcome assessment would be expensive (contacting the patient is required), but its costs could be contained by sampling patients. Observing the physician-patient encounter would also be expensive and, except for research purposes, not feasible. To acquire a valid assessment of quality of care by observing the provider-patient relationship, an entire episode of illness (multiple visits) must be observed. This could be possible as part of a research study, but otherwise would seem to be totally impossible. Requiring additional recording of information to be used only for quality assessment and not for the subsequent delivery of additional care may be possible, but it would be extremely costly. Physicians in primary care spend, on the average, about 12 minutes with each patient, of which less than one minute is devoted to recording information. If quality assurance activities increased this to

---

* The total medical care bill amounts to approximately 100 billion dollars annually. The hospital care sector consumes about 54 billion dollars of this total, and the ambulatory care sector approximately 17 billion dollars. A 20 percent increase in hospital care would be produced by a 50 percent rise in hospital procedures, and this would amount to 10 billion dollars. A 250 percent increase in ambulatory care services would cost an additional 40 billion dollars. These increases would place the total medical care bill at approximately 150 billion dollars—or about 12 percent of the total GNP.

three to five minutes, this could raise by one-third or more the price of an office visit. On a national level, this would increase the cost of care by about $4 billion ($4/visit × 5 visits/person × 200 million people). Thus outcome assessment, even though it is expensive, is the only practical way of assessing aspects of ambulatory care other than the use of medications, the taking of vital signs, or the performance of laboratory tests.

Fourth, the process of hospital care is recorded far more reliably and completely than is ambulatory care, but recording of physical examinations and history items (especially for patients with acute surgical conditions) may still be incomplete. Studies need to be conducted in the hospital setting to compare the performance and notation of routine medical care activities. In doing such studies, hospitals of different sizes, with and without house staff, and of different ownership should be included. If large discrepancies are found, then either the outcomes of care must be assessed or higher medical record standards mandated. In the hospital setting, the latter seems feasible, since this would increase the cost of care by, at most, 1 to 2 percent. (Physician charges would increase about 10 percent, and physician charges represent 16 percent of total hospital charges.)

Fifth, assessment of either the hospital or ambulatory component of care could be misleading and may result in decisions about improving quality which are not cost-effective. Inhospital care of patients who have acute infectious diseases is approaching an end (except in the elderly and/or immunologically compromised hosts). Most patients who are hospitalized suffer from chronic diseases, and care must be assessed on an episode-of-illness basis, and not on a single-visit basis. For instance, a hospital audit of care given to patients who had suffered a stroke might suggest that the best way of improving the health of the stroke patient is through increasing physical therapy and treating brain edema with steroids. Audit of the entire episode of illness of stroke patients, however, would probably suggest that maximum health could be achieved by earlier detection and better treatment of the hypertensive patient. Thus, two fundamentally different ways of improving care occur as a function of the manner in which the medical care system is assessed.

Sixth, in the last 20 years, criteria used in the assessment of the process of care have changed from implicit to explicit. Implicit assessment was based on professional opinion after the physician had read the medical record, and care was generally graded on a scale from acceptable to unsatisfactory. Judgments generated by this method reflected a gestalt view of medical care. The explicit method, on the other hand, relies on the application of a set of previously agreed-upon criteria to a medical record. Clearly, the reliability of the method is increased through the use of explicit criteria, but changes in the validity are somewhat suspect, due mainly to the nature of the criteria. Explicit criteria, although disease-specific, are not branched, meaning that performance of a criterion is not conditional on the results of a previous criterion. Furthermore, most criteria sets identify only one pathway to achieving a goal as acceptable. Basically, the science of decision analysis has not been applied to the development of criteria, and, in fact, only a handful of clinical investigators even understand the simple principles of decision analysis. Thus, quality of care assessment based on explicit criteria, which in most cases specify a laundry list of items that must be performed on every patient, has replaced the implicit judgment of care which reflected, although somewhat unreliably, the thinking patterns of good physicians.

Seventh, until now, criteria usually have been generated solely by physicians; they tend to reflect physician activities and ignore those aspects of care performed by other providers (e.g., nurses, physical therapists). Yet the care provided by these individuals may be more critical in improving health, especially with respect to care given to patients with chronic diseases. Clearly, a new generation of process criteria which employ simple principles of decision analysis and which cover the whole process of care must be developed. These advances are likely to yield a set of process criteria which are more valid than heretofore; for example, the correlation between the process assessment and the outcome of care will be higher.

The last area of methods research to be addressed is that of outcome assessment. Two major problems exist in this area. The first is that evaluation of the quality of care cannot be based on outcomes which require 10 to 15 years to occur. Long-term outcomes can and should be used to assess the efficacy of different therapies, such as the 20-year survival in patients with breast cancer treated by simple versus radical mastectomy, but they clearly cannot be used to evaluate the quality of that care. Instead, short-term disease-specific outcomes are needed; one to two years following the receipt of care is the longest interval that can be used to assess the quality of care. For some conditions it may be impossible to develop these short-term outcomes, but for most conditions it should be possible. Research to ascertain their validity, however, will be necessary.

The second main problem in using outcomes to assess care relates to the influence of factors outside the medical care system on those outcomes. A poor outcome could be due to external factors, such as housing, and not to poor medical care at all. In order to overcome this methods drawback, patients with a given condition must be grouped into prognostically homogeneous strata. This process would divide patients into approximately five to seven subgroups to account for the variation in outcomes that relates to the initial severity of their disease. Disease taxonomies now in existence, such as

ICDA, generally subdivide patients within a disease category on the basis of anatomical considerations. For instance, a patient with a heart attack is subclassified by the artery whose circulation was disturbed. What is needed is a disease classification system that would predict prognosis (and thus outcome) better. For example, in the heart attack patient, subclassifications should be based on initial systolic blood pressure (e.g., greater than 100) and/or history of previous heart attack. Development of a new type of disease taxonomy based on prognosis will require some effort, but it should be undertaken even if it requires funding of new areas of clinical investigation.

In summary, a large number of potential research studies have been suggested in this section on methods problems in quality of care assessment. Certain generic principles stand out, however, and serve as a basis for the fourth set of recommendations.

First, in the next five years, the only feasible non-research method for quality of care assessment will be process assessment. This is not necessarily a negative statement. Process assessment can be used to detect and correct basic deficiencies in medical care, and the next five years should be spent in this endeavor. Process assessment, however, must be performed with great caution and only valid, easily applied criteria should be used; otherwise the efficiency of the medical care system will decrease.

Along these lines, examples of good criteria would be: (1) using the appropriate antibiotic in children under two years of age with otitis media; (2) performing at least one electrocardiogram or one enzyme determination on patients with symptoms of an acute heart attack; and (3) treating patients with diastolic blood pressure above 110 with any hypotensive agent. These criteria are good because they are based on information usually contained in the medical record and because they have been shown to relate to improved health.

Second, the emphasis on "locally valid" process criteria should be reversed.

Unfortunately, most quality assurance programs permit (if not advocate) the local establishment of criteria. In the long run, this is dangerous (and certainly counterproductive), since it almost guarantees the development and acceptance of invalid (and certainly non-comparable) criteria. Moreover, application of these invalid criteria to current care will dramatically increase the cost of care.

Third, during the next five years, three major research undertakings should be completed: (1) development of criteria which employ decision analysis principles for judging the adequacy of the process of care; (2) generation of new diagnostic taxonomies which are divided into prognostically homogeneous strata; and (3) formulation of diagnosis-specific short-term outcomes. All three activities should be done simultaneously on the same disease category for about 25 disease categories each year. Insofar as possible (or necessary), the process criteria should link ambulatory and hospital care. The process criteria should also be established in a manner which will allow compliance with them to be determined from information available in the new AMA insurance claims form (ambulatory care) or from information in the medical record in the average community hospital (for inpatients).

Completion of this agenda should permit the adoption of a new quality assurance system in the 1980s which is more likely to lead to improved health of the nation.

How Much is Health Worth?

With an operational quality assurance system in place, it will, sooner or later, become painfully obvious to the public what the medical care system is or is not doing and can or cannot do. If the millenium comes five years from now and a reasonably valid quality assessment method is developed, the issue in need of solution will be "how much is health worth?"

Modern medical science has developed a flock of no- or low-risk procedures, many of which are efficacious but also costly. For example, is everyone with a headache to receive a "five-way zap" (i.e., skull X-ray series, a brain scan, an EEG, an ECHO, and an EMI), so that the very rare meningioma can be detected in a curable state? The answer to this question depends partly on the sensitivity and specificity of the tests and partly on the prevalence of disease at issue. Clearly, if the harm caused by the identification of substantial numbers of false-positive cases is greater than the good done by the identification of a small number of true-positives, then the tests will not be performed. But, if the false-positive problem does not arise, and instead the problem is one of the high cost of identifying one true-positive, what then?

The situation described above is not at all facetious. If nothing else, the biomedical revolution has increased the public's expectations concerning the doctor's ability to cure its ills regardless of the amount of self-inflicted damage due to poor health habits. Despite the large expenditures of funds in the antismoking campaign, for example, people continue to smoke. The right to smoke is preserved; cigarettes stay on the market at a cheap price. At the same time, the public expects that persons suffering respiratory failure from chronic obstructive lung disease should be entitled to every means to save them including (at present) a respirator and (in the future) probably an artificial lung or portable membrane oxygenator. Expense is no object. A quality assurance system, if not carefully applied, could accelerate the process by which the public has relinquished its opportunity to control and improve its own health. The public has transferred this responsibility to a medical care system that consumes an ever greater percentage of the GNP.

A workable quality assurance system will make a second major, fact obvious—the maldistribution of effective care (not to mention efficacious care) in the United States. Certain hospitals have better survival rates, fewer postoperative infections, and fewer neonatal deaths, or whatever. What variation in effectiveness then will be or should be tolerated? Will experts construct a normal distribution and declare anything within two (or maybe even three) standard deviations acceptable? This is exactly the procedure followed by the American Board of Internal Medicine in determining who should pass their recertification examination. But the questions are whether the public will accept this level of variation as natural or as a reflection of an external force beyond their control, and whether they will demand greater equalization of quality.

Answers to the above are virtually unknown, and it is imperative that investigation of these areas begin in the next few years. The fifth recommendation, then, is as follows:

> Work should be undertaken to determine, first, the value placed on health by the public and, second, how much inequity in the distribution of the quality of those medical services will be tolerated by the public. Furthermore, work in this area must also vigorously experiment with techniques by which the public can be taught to protect its own health and not shift this responsibility to costly medical technology.

Knowledge About Quality Assurance

If quality assessment is in its infancy, then quality assurance is embryonic. Virtually all previous efforts in the quality field have ended at quality assessment. Little, if anything, has been done about changing the behavior of the medical care system or the provider. Certain basic principles of quality assurance have emerged, however. First, changing physician behavior to improve quality is hard work and a painfully slow process. When changing physician behavior, the physician's cognitive knowledge is not necessarily the critical variable. The quality with which a physician practices may depend more upon his skills in taking a history or performing a physical, or on his habits in providing coverage and follow-up care, than it does on cognitive knowledge. Undoing years of practice habits in these areas will require far more effort than would be required to increase knowledge about the use of the latest medication or procedure. Second, more often than not, critical changes needed are not under the control of the physician at all, but require administrative action or approval.

Recommendation six, then, is as follows:

> The quality assurance system must be designed to include in responsible positions a wide variety of people in the medical care field. Responsibility for the delivery of high quality of care is shared by many professionals; authority for running a quality assurance system must also be shared, since physicians alone cannot be expected to make most of the necessary changes. For reasons stated above, the public must also be intimately involved in such a system.

Changing Physician Behavior and Sampling

When changes in physician behavior are desirable, the best approach to achieve this goal is unclear. A dismayingly large number of questions arise. For example, does local involvement by physicians in setting standards and criteria make it easier to modify their behavior subsequently? How should feedback of information about level of quality be accomplished—in a formal or informal manner, by individual physician, by specialty, by medical society, or by area of the city in which the physician practices? These questions need answers which can only be obtained through well-designed research efforts.

Since virtually all process or outcome criteria are disease or condition-specific, groups of patients with a given condition must be identified. Unfortunately, the average doctor does not usually treat enough patients with one condition in a short enough time period to make statistically meaningful comparisons possible. This is true for both ambulatory and inpatient conditions. For instance, suppose an internist is responsible for about 800 people who will generate about 80 hospitalizations in a year. Even if one diagnosis accounts for 10 percent of these hospitalizations (which is very unlikely), the maximum number of hospitalizations in one year in one diagnostic category would be eight.

Except for common complaints of infectious diseases such as colds, sore throats, and ear infections, sample size problems in the ambulatory area are just as discouraging. Returning to the internist example, one would expect about 10 percent of his patient population—about 80 people—to be hypertensive. In assessing the quality of care in this instance, it would be preferable to review only the care given to newly diagnosed hypertensive patients. Since perhaps 10 percent of this physician's hypertensive population would be newly diagnosed, the sample size is again reduced to eight. The conclusion is obvious: it will be impossible to judge the quality of care given by one physician to one group of patients with a given condition. Data must be aggregated either by doctors or by patient conditions, and this choice is dependent upon two considerations: (1) variation in the quality of care among physician practices compared to the variation within a physician's practice; and (2) the manner in which the data will be used to change physician behavior.

A finite amount of dollars will be spent on quality assessment; this will limit the number of cases selected for study. The variation in quality among physicians treating the same condition is presumed to be greater than the variation within a physician's practice across all conditions, although this has never been demonstrated by any research. Insofar as these presumptions hold, the more efficient sample would involve a large number of physicians and few cases per physician, leading to quality of care statistics for diagnostic categories aggregated across all physicians. Changing individual physician behaviors, however, may be possible only when data concerning his practice are released to him. This would require selecting a large number of cases per physician and aggregating across a variety of different conditions within his practice. Recommendation seven is:

> The need to use aggregated data in quality assurance must be recognized. Exactly how this should be done (either by physician or diagnostic category) and what impact it will have on changing physician behavior is not known at the moment. Since these latter issues are eminently researchable, funds should be provided to study them.

Summary

This first topic has summarized what is known about quality of care, quality assessment and assurance, and physician behavior modification. Seven sets of recommendations, generally relating to increased knowledge about quality assessment and quality assurance, were suggested. The more important parts of this research agenda are: (1) development of a valid art-of-care measure; (2) development of rational sets of condition-specific, explicit process criteria that take advantage of principles of decision analysis;

(3) stratification of disease conditions into prognostically homogeneous groups; (4) development of disease-specific outcome measures; and (5) determination of the value the public places on health. The technology exists to make major advances in each of these areas by 1980, although upgrading the validity of the measures developed may require a longer period.

In the second topic, this paper presumes that the recommendations proposed above have been completed. Were this not to occur, the building blocks necessary to support an operational quality assurance system would be absent, and the following discussion of the future rendered irrelevant.

THE FUTURE OF QUALITY ASSURANCE

1975-1980

The period 1975 to 1980 should be viewed as a transition period. During this transition, the following events will or should occur, each of which will facilitate the development of a quality assurance system for the 1980s and beyond. First, some form of national health insurance will be passed. Second, the Uniform Hospital Discharge Abstract will be instituted in all hospitals nationwide. Third, a problem-oriented ambulatory claims form (which relates procedures to diagnosis or symptom), such as that proposed by the American Medical Association, will be accepted and implemented by the insurance industry. Fourth, mandatory assignment of benefits, such as occurs in the Medicaid program now, will become commonplace. Fifth, better techniques for assessing and assuring quality of care will be developed.

In this environment, the Professional Standards Review Organization (PSRO) and its medical care evaluation studies and the Joint Commission on the Accreditation of Hospitals (JCAH) and its Physician Evaluation Procedures (PEP) will continue to operate. Some modifications in the PSRO program should also take place in this period to permit a smooth transition to the future quality assurance system. First, the public in general and health professionals other than physicians should be given an explicit role in PSRO. Improving the quality of medical care will require both explicit value judgments by the public and changes in components of the medical care system which are not under the direct control of physicians.

Second, some PSRO areas should be redesignated in order to be coextensive with true medical care service areas. This redesignation could consider the relationship between primary, secondary, and tertiary services within an area and should reflect current referral patterns. If necessary, state borders should be crossed when medical care service areas are formulated. Third, national minimum standards which detect basic deficiencies in the process of care should be developed and promulgated. Fourth, review of care should be expanded to include both care financed by nonfederal programs and ambulatory care in general. Fifth, results of quality audits should be made available to the public by PSRO area, by hospital, and, if necessary, by physician or at least by physician characteristics (e.g., age or board-certification status). This latter suggestion assumes that such analysis would be placed in proper context, so that hospitals or physicians caring for sicker patients are not penalized. If these five changes were made in the PSRO program, development of a new quality assurance system will be greatly enhanced.

PSRO can make two other contributions to quality assurance in the period 1975-1980. First, it can identify and correct basic deficiencies in care; indeed, PSRO activities in the quality area should be limited to the correction of these basic deficiencies. (A more aggressive quality assurance system awaits the development of a more valid quality assessment method.) For instance, in two years of operation, the New Mexico Experimental Medical Care Review Organization (a forerunner of PSRO) was able to eliminate 50 percent of the injections given in the ambulatory setting to Medicaid patients by changing physicians' practice patterns. These injections were considered medically unwarranted, and over half of them were potent antibiotics capable of causing severe iatrogenic disease. Thus, misuse of injectables—a fairly basic shortcoming in medical care today—was prevented by a PSRO-type organization; such accomplishments in this and other areas are attainable nationally and should be pursued. Second, if the PSRO program is carefully evaluated, valuable information about quality assurance which is needed to help resolve problems in the 1980s and thereafter will be produced. Such information would include: (1) a national picture of the types of deficiencies existing in quality; (2) knowledge of what needs to be done to improve quality and whether such changes can be produced (i.e., modify the system, increase physician cognitive knowledge, etc.); (3) information about how quality assurance organizations should function at a local level; and (4) knowledge about how much quality assurance activities cost.

1980 and Beyond

Prerequisites

Development of a quality assurance system for the 1980s and beyond has been predicated on the following assumptions: (1) that the fee-for-service system is worth preserving; (2) that any national health insurance plan will contain a provision for setting a national fee schedule for services rendered; (3) that the right to generous health insurance coverage is accompanied by the duty and obligation of professionals and public alike to provide data about the process and outcome of care to a central agency (such as the National Center for Health Statistics [NCHS]); and (4) that most or all of the previous recommendations have been accomplished.

If the fee-for-service system were not worth preserving, a quality assurance system based on mandating the prepaid group practice concept or other organizational changes in the medical care system should be considered and explored. If the national government is to pay for services rendered, it certainly has the right to be an active participant in setting fees for services rendered. A generous health insurance bill will guarantee payment to the physician for virtually all services rendered. In exchange for this, the federal government should retain the right to assess the quality of care given under this insurance system, with the implication that professionals must supply the necessary information. The public, in return for financial coverage of medical care, has an equal responsibility to provide health-related information, similar perhaps to its obligation to participate in the census. The federal government, on its part, would guarantee that health information about individuals must remain strictly confidential. (The experience of the NCHS Health Interview Survey and Health Examination Survey suggests that this confidentiality of patient data can indeed be maintained by the federal government.)

Quality Assurance Institute

The quality assurance system of the 1980s would, like the present one, have federal and local bureaucracies, the latter of which would correspond to perhaps 150 medical care service areas (MCSA) which, in many cases, would be identical to present day PSRO areas. To coordinate nationwide efforts, a quality assurance institute would be implemented at the federal level. Using newly developed tools and techniques, this institute would monitor both the process and outcome of care in each MCSA. One approach to this monitoring would be the identification by this institute of a sample of perhaps 300 patients in each MCSA with one of 100 or so conditions (a total of 30,000 patients per area per year); the sample could be chosen on the basis of information contained on either the ambulatory claims form or the Uniform Hospital Discharge Abstract. Data would be collected from medical record review, patient interview, and, if necessary, a physical examination. At an average cost of $200 per patient, the total cost would be about $1 billion ($200 × 300 patients × 100 conditions × 150 MSCAs), and 4.5 million patients would be contacted per year. Thus, about 2 percent of the population would be interviewed each year; 1 percent of the resources used in the delivery of medical care would be spent in this manner.

The quality assurance institute would have the capability to analyze these data rapidly, and disseminate the following information: (1) relative ranking of quality of care by medical care service area; (2) relative ranking of quality of care by disease condition; (3) relative ranking of quality of care by population demographic features for specific disease conditions and across all conditions; (4) relative ranking of the quality of care delivered by physician characteristics such as board certification, age, or specialty; (5) relative ranking of the quality of care delivered by individual hospitals; and (6) relative changes in the quality of care delivered in each area from year to year.

The first use of these data would be to aid the public in selecting hospitals and physicians that delivered good care. This in itself may have a profound effect on the level of quality rendered. Likewise, it would geometrically increase the amount of available information about physicians and medical care facilities.

The second use of these data would be to regulate the quality of care directly. Before considering how this would be done, it is necessary to examine the relationship between the average observed level of quality of care in a medical care service area as a function of the medical care resources consumed in that area (see Figure 1-1). The curve in Figure 1-1 is not based on real data since none exist, but instead reflects the following: (1) increasing resources will increase quality except in MCSAs in which too many procedures (e.g., unnecessary surgery) are being done; (2) initial increments in resources produce greater changes in quality than do subsequent increments; and (3) too many resources may produce more iatrogenic disease than health improvement.

The curve in Figure 1-1 has four distinct regions (A, B, C, D). MCSAs in Region A do not have enough resources to deliver high quality care; MCSAs in Region B have just a few too little resources; MCSAs in Region C have about the right amount of resources; and MCSAs in Region D have too many resources, are operating inefficiently, and are producing excess iatrogenic disease. If one assumes that the public values the health presumably produced through the delivery of high quality care sufficiently to want all MCSAs to be in the C Region (instead of B or A), the first objective in regulating quality would be to make all areas similar to those in Region C. (Note: It may be necessary to develop a set of curves by type and/or place of care instead of relying on one curve depicting the entire scope of medical care. For instance, an MCSA conceivably could be in one region for ambulatory services and another for hopital services. This is unlikely but should be subject to confirmation by research studies.)

The second objective of regulating quality would be to shift the whole curve up, so that for the same amount of resources larger amounts of quality

Figure 1-1

Hypothetical Relationship Between Quality of
Medical Care and Medical Care Resources Consumed
Per Person for All Medical Care Service Areas

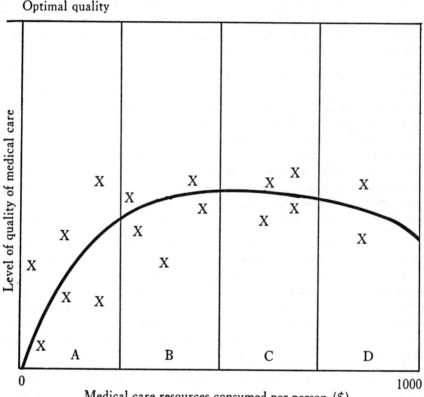

Optimal quality

Level of quality of medical care

A   B   C   D

0   1000

Medical care resources consumed per person ($)

are obtained. The third objective would be to reduce the variation in quality
either produced or received among areas within a region, among provider
groups, and among patient groups such as the black, poor, or elderly.

In order to accomplish the above, some redistribution of medical care
resources must occur. Since physicians generate 80 percent of the medical
care expenditures, this essentially means redistributing physicians. Taking
the extremes (Regions A, C, and D) as cases in point, some sort of "tax"
could be assessed on physicians who practice in Regions C and D and turned
over to physicians in Region A. Physicians in Region D presumably earn
roughly the same amount as those in Region A. Using this tax, the net

income of physicians in Region C and D could be decreased by, say, 30 percent per year until a physician's net salary in Region C was about 10 times the poverty level or some other arbitrary amount. In Region D, the final desirable physician salary could be five times the poverty level. The money obtained from this tax could be given to physicians in Region A as a bonus. Physicians would not be required to leave areas where quality was high and efficacy low (as in Region D), but the maximum amount they could earn would be limited severely; this mechanism could be a strong incentive for redistributing physicians among regions.*

Hospitals might be controlled as follows. From those MCSAs that fall in Region C, an "optimal" number of hospital days per population could be calculated. Using this figure, an optimal number of hospital days for each area in Region D could be calculated. This figure would, of course, consider adjustments for patient demographic variables. The excess number of hospital days which occurred in areas in Region D would not be reimbursed. Instead, this nonreimbursable cost would be shared by all hospitals in proportion to their number of beds. The stimulus, of course, would be to close some beds or possibly even some hospitals, and thus to enhance the efficiency of hospital utilization in Region D.

Other techniques could be proposed to equalize the resources consumed per person in each area. Physician fee schedules for the same services performed in Region A or B could be established 10 to 15 percent higher than those in Region C or D. Since 80 percent of the services performed in the medical care system are physician-generated, this would lead to the consumption of more services by increasing the number of physicians in the area. Finally, grants could be given to MCSAs in Regions A and B to increase the availability of medical care services.

The above proposals, of course, may prove unnecessary. For all practical purposes, all medical care service areas in this country may fall into Region C. Better data will help determine whether the hypothesized differences among medical care service areas really exist, whether those differences can be smoothed out along the horizontal axis of Figure 1-1, and whether the approaches suggested above would serve that goal.

---

* This argument assumes that all MCSAs place equal value on receiving a high level of quality of care, and that this level is typified by the quality of care available in Region C. A more generic argument for the redistribution of resources would recognize that other areas may place greater value on receiving additional money or other types of services than on increased numbers of physicians' services, but that consideration is beyond the scope of this chapter. However, if such a circumstance occurred, in lieu of additional resources to improve quality, services in kind could be provided.

The third major use of these data would be to improve the quality of care in all MCSAs without increasing resources (equivalent to shifting the curve in Figure 1-1 upward). At the end of a two-year period, the quality institute would have data on the care given to patients with one of 100 or so conditions. These 100 conditions would represent over 75 percent of all medical care. Analysis of these data could lead to information about which conditions were being "overtreated" *versus* which were being "undertreated." Models could be built to determine how redistribution of resources among diseases would affect quality of care and thereby health status. Through the reimbursement mechanism, the quality institute could control the proportion of total resources spent on individual conditions and maximize health for a given amount of resources.

Finally, the data collected as proposed above could be put to a fourth use. It would be possible to determine the mean level of quality of care after controlling for differences in patient demographic variables for each area and region (see Table 1-2, which shows hypothetical results for five MCSAs of Region C). Suppose that for Region C, the regional mean for a given disease is 50 and the standard deviation is 5. Compared to those values, Area 1 is providing better quality care which is equitably distributed. Areas 3 and 5 are providing average care, but care is distributed inequitably in Area 3 where the standard deviation is high. Certain segments of the population are receiving much better care than that given to other segments. Areas 2 and 4 are providing poorer care on the average, although the level of care varies widely in Area 4 and little in Area 2.

Table 1-2

HYPOTHETICAL LEVELS AND VARIATIONS IN QUALITY OF
MEDICAL CARE BY AREA AND REGION

Area	Disease	Region	Mean Level of Quality	Variation (Standard Deviation)
1	1	C	70	5
2	1	C	30	5
3	1	C	50	40
4	1	C	30	40
5	1	C	50	5
.				
.				
.				
n				

These two values, the mean value of quality and its standard deviation, could be combined, using a weighting scheme that reflects the public's preference, to give a single figure representative of the quality of care given in an area. This "observed" figure could be compared with the expected value determined by the amount of resources consumed. On the basis of this comparison, the quality assurance institute could implement an incentive system by raising or lowering provider fee schedules. This does not imply that the price of each procedure could or would be determined at the federal level, but rather that the basic worth of a unit would be raised or lowered (as, for instance, with the California Relative Value Scale). This incentive system would be used to reward areas which show substantial improvements in their quality of care from one year to the next, have high levels of quality, and/or distribute quality equitably within their populations.

The incentive system could also be used to address more specific issues. Suppose, for example, that analysis of these data shows that board-certified physicians perform better than their noncertified colleagues across all areas and all diseases. The fee schedule could be adjusted to reward this evidence of professional accomplishment. Likewise, suppose open heart surgery is shown to be much more successful when performed in accredited hospitals attached to university training programs than elsewhere. The quality assurance institute could choose virtually to eliminate surgery performed under any other conditions by refusing to reimburse for it.

The above incentive system is directed at providers, but a quality assurance system need not be oriented entirely in one direction. A number of disease conditions are due in no small measure to patient behavior—e.g., cancer of the lung or cirrhosis of the liver. Perhaps when national health insurance is passed, the quality assurance institute could be given the authority to place excise taxes on toxic substances that contribute to poor health habits, or could raise or lower local and/or out-of-pocket contributions to the health insurance premium (if these occur) as a function of the level of self-destructive health habits in the local medical care area. The former would be a direct incentive to individuals to avoid such toxins, and may increase the patient's responsibility for improving his own health. The latter action would extend that responsibility to the community in general, and may be associated with a greater public awareness of the prevalence of poor health habits throughout the community. Finally, incentives directed at other health professionals could be devised.

The federal function in this hypothetical quality assurance system has been characterized as an objective data gatherer, analyzer, and applier of broad sanctions and incentives. Its purpose is to ensure that quality—both technical and art-of-care—is rising, that quality is equitably distributed across the population, that resources are used more efficiently, and that the public is motivated to take more responsibility for its own health. The system is designed to minimize the amount of regulation. The data-gathering operations will interfere little with the physician-patient relationship. Virtually all of the authority of the quality assurance institute will be exercised through its regulation of fees.

Local Quality Assurance Bureaucracies

The local role in this quality assurance system is vital. A local organization like PSRO must exist in each MCSA. At the end of each year the federal government would give each of these organizations the following: (1) a detailed comparative analysis of the quality of care provided in the area; (2) a decision regarding the level of reimbursement for services rendered in the area; and (3) between 1 to 2 percent of the dollars spent on medical services in the area (for a population of 1 million this is $5 to $10 million or $5 to $10 per person).

The money to be given to these local organizations would have only two stipulations: (1) public access to information except when that violates confidentiality of patient information; and (2) cooperation with evaluators who will use qualitative and quantitative techniques to determine the characteristics of successful quality assurance organizations. This information will be shared with organizations in other areas. No reports would be required. No grants or contracts would be completed. No regulations would be issued. Essentially, the local organizations would be left alone to determine how and by what method the quality of care in their area could be altered. They could organize courses, mandate continuing education, demand relicensure, remove physicians from practice, close down hospitals they know provide poor care, educate their patients regarding proper health habits, or whatever. To accomplish these objectives these local organizations probably should have: (1) elected public members who participate actively; (2) active participation of all health professionals; and (3) the authority and responsibility for disciplining physicians and other professionals.

The success of the local organizations would be determined by the national surveys done by the quality assurance institute. Areas would be compared against empirically derived norms as well as ideal standards. Success or failure would be rewarded promptly, and information describing how to run a successful local quality assurance organization would be freely shared among areas. This system would help ensure the maximum feasible flexibility in allowing a local area to run its own quality assurance program. The local area could not legitimately blame the federal government for overly rigid regulations which minimized its ability to effect true improvements in quality of care.

CONCLUDING REMARKS

The first part of this chapter briefly examined what is known about quality assessment and assurance. Due to limitations in quality assessment methods, institutionalization of a quality assurance program at this time should be limited to the detection and correction of basic deficiencies in care. The major effort in the quality field during the next five years should be in research on measuring quality. In particular, the following should be developed: (1) a valid measure of the art-of-care; (2) disease-specific process criteria that employ principles of decision analysis; (3) disease-specific short-term outcome measures; and (4) disease taxonomies that group patients into prognostically homogeneous strata.

The rudiments of a hypothetical quality assurance system for the 1980s and beyond was presented in the second section. This system is based on a set of assumptions about the adoption of a national health insurance plan and about the value of preserving the fee-for-service system. The federal role in this system consists of determining what regional differences in quality exist and of applying broad incentives to correct deficiencies where appropriate. The incentive system is tied directly to the fee schedule. Local organizations are given almost total flexibility, authority, and responsibility to correct deficiencies in the level of quality provided.

The institution of a quality assurance system will be expensive ($2 to $5 billion per year). Its success or failure must be carefully evaluated. Its success will probably lead to the preservation of the fee-for-service system for a long time, while its failure will most certainly hasten the demise of that system.

NOTES

1. The research reported herein was performed pursuant to a grant from the U.S. Department of Health, Education, and Welfare, Washington, D.C. The opinions and conclusions expressed herein are solely those of the authors, and should not be construed as representing the opinions or policy of any agency of the United States Government.

2. Brook, R. H., Avery, A. D. Quality Assurance Mechanisms in the United States: From There to Where? P-5520, Santa Monica, California: The Rand Corporation, October 1975.

3. Brook, R. H. *Quality of Care Assessment: A Comparison of Five Methods of Peer Review.* DHEW Pub. No HRA-74-3100. Washington, D. C.: U.S. Department of Health, Education, and Welfare, 1973.

4. Advancing the Quality of Health Care: Key Issues and Fundamental Principles. A policy statement by a Committee of the Institute of Medicine, National Academy of Sciences, Washington, D. C., August 1974.

5. Donabedian, A. *A Guide to Medical Care Administration, Vol. II: Medical Care Appraisal—Quality and Utilization.* New York: The American Public Health Association, Inc., 1969.

6. Altman, I., Anderson, A. J., Barker, K. *Methodology in Evaluating the Quality of Medical Care: An Annotated Selected Bibliography, 1955-1968.* Pittsburgh: University of Pittsburgh Press, 1969.

7. Donabedian, A. Promoting quality through evaluating the process of patient care. *Med. Care* 6:181-202, 1968.

8. Klein, B. W. *Evaluating Outcomes of Health Services: An Annotated Bibliography.* Los Angeles: University of California at Los Angeles, School of Public Health, 1970.

9. Mactavish, C. F., Sundeen, J. *Assessment of the Quality of Medical Care: An Annotated Bibliography.* AFR Memorandum No. C-2. Minneapolis: American Rehabilitation Foundation, 1968.

Chapter 2
Problems of Federal Policies and Strategies to Influence the Quality of Health Care

Cynthia Taft
and
Sol Levine

INTRODUCTION

The enactment of PSRO must not be viewed as a unique or unprecedented action to affect the health delivery system but must be examined from the vantage point of past federal policies. An historical view of recent governmental policies provides us with a context and perspective with which to understand the impetus for the PSRO legislation, and to appreciate the kinds of strategies underlying it, as well as some of the problems which may be anticipated as the law is implemented. A brief historical review will not only make explicit past federal approaches to the health delivery system, but may also suggest alternative approaches which should be considered in order to avoid past deficiencies and to make PSRO more effective.

This chapter argues that federal health legislation, for the most part, has served to retain the existing structure and mode of organization of the health delivery system and to augment it by providing additional resources. These efforts have been guided by an assumption that considerable consensus prevails among the major sectors of the health system and that new resources will be utilized rationally and efficiently. Guided by this belief, the federal government has relied mainly on educational strategies to effect change or influence outcomes in the system. Its policymaking efforts have generally focused on the need to deploy resources more efficiently or to improve communication and coordination among providers. Rarely have governmental efforts included strategies which employ economic incentives or the application of coercive methods to influence the system. In recent years, some efforts to apply more leverage on the health system have been evident, but these have still been consonant with the existing structure and power arrangements. For example, the essential prerogatives of the medical profession and the role of the private health sector have not been seriously questioned.

31

The difficulties in achieving centrally planned change in the United States are also pointed out, primarily because (1) divergent interest groups have to be accommodated; and (2) the systems which may be the targets of change tend to resist innovations they find threatening. Accordingly, efforts are often diverted or rendered innocuous by various sub-systems of the health delivery system. And planners in the United States have rarely possessed the necessary authority to implement their plans and to exert leverage on the organizations or health segments in their jurisdiction. It is not unfair to characterize federal planning as little more than a rationalistic exercise.

Will PSRO work? The consensual and rationalistic approaches which have been used in past change efforts are, in the main, still evident in trying to make PSRO successful, but questions should be raised about the need to consider alternative approaches. One strategy which may merit consideration, despite its obvious problems, is the introduction of tight incentives. Specifically, the idea of having an expenditure ceiling or fixed budget in each area for Medicare and Medicaid services should be considered. More information is needed about how individual parts of the health system operate, particularly the ways in which PSROs function, the problems they encounter, and the manner in which they are resolved. Clearly, the PSROs throughout the country offer diverse laboratories for the study of efforts to raise the quality of care and to decrease the costs of health care in the United States.

THE EVOLUTION OF THE FEDERAL ROLE IN HEALTH

The federal government first took action to influence the health care delivery system during the Depression in the 1930s when serious health problems began to emerge in those areas hardest hit by poor economic conditions.[1] The basic problem, as perceived by governmental leaders, was not the health system itself but the fact that people who needed care were not receiving the full benefit the system could provide. What was needed, it was felt, was some mechanism to ensure that more of the population had access to these benefits.

The issue, then, was not the quality of the care delivered, but rather the barriers which prevented the existing service structure from providing for people's health needs. The policies that resulted were thus focused on expanding the system's capabilities through the input of additional resources and information. Specific and restrictive controls on how these inputs would be utilized were not part of the government's strategy because it was generally assumed that the system would use them in a rational way.

What were the major problems which these initial federal policies attempted to correct? The most serious problem was felt to be the shortage and uneven distribution of health facilities and services. In 1935 the first federal action was taken to improve the situation, with the passage of the Social Security Act. Included in this legislation were provisions for federal support of local and state public health programs and for programs specifically targeted to maternal and child health problems.[2] Federal funds were dispersed to support specific categorical programs at both the local and state levels. The provision of these additional resources helped to expand health services in most areas of the country, but because funding was tied to categories based on federal priorities, the program did little to foster local coordination and planning. As a result, these grants did not serve to improve the distribution and relieve the shortage of services and facilities.[3]

The federal program designed to have a direct and substantial impact on this problem was the Hospital Survey and Construction Act (P.L. 79-725), passed by Congress in 1946 and popularly known as the Hill-Burton program. Because of financial restrictions during the Depression and World War II, very little construction and modernization of hospital facilities was possible, resulting in serious bed shortages in many areas of the country. As public concern over the situation gradually increased, support also grew for the government to intervene to help solve the problem. What seemed necessary was a major infusion of funds to encourage both the building of new facilities and the expansion and modernization of existing ones.

The Hill-Burton program was the government's response to the bed shortage problem, and it also represented the first federal attempt at health planning. Under the program, states were required to survey their existing hospital facilities in order to determine their bed needs, and to then use this information in developing a plan for hospital construction. Federal funds were provided for the planning activities, as well as for construction, in an attempt to foster a rational approach to facility development.[4]

Amendments to the original act broadened the scope of the program over the years to include construction and modernization of other types of health facilities. Ultimately, the program helped more than 3,700 communities build hospitals, public health centers, extended care facilities, and rehabilitation centers.[5] However, while there is little question that the infusion of federal resources had a substantial impact on the bed shortage problem, particularly in rural areas, its achievements with respect to rational health planning were minimal. "The federal government failed to require the states to truly plan. Federal regulations failed to stipulate how planning was to be done and in what way performance of the states could be judged."[6]

Planning attempts were bound to fail because there were no explicit criteria to determine facility needs and no real incentives for planning. In most cases, the states did little more than survey their facilities to determine bed-to-population ratios.[7] Thus, although the Hill-Burton legislation included language aimed at utilizing health resources more efficiently, there was little support to achieve such a "rationalization" in the health system.[8]

Federal interest in expanding the resources of the health system focused not only on hospital beds and facilities but also on medical research and training of health personnel. The impetus for major federal support in this area was the transformation which had taken place in medicine following World War I. The practice of medicine had become increasingly complex with the changing patterns of disease in the population. "Diseases such as typhoid fever, dysentery, and diphtheria, which previously had engaged much of the attention of physicians were rapidly disappearing. Other diseases, previously unknown, were taking their place. Such diseases included: allergies, diabetes, arthritis, and diseases of the peripheral blood vessels. And with the new diseases came new specialists."[9]

To study these "new" diseases and to pay for the technology which was revolutionizing medical science, substantial sums of money were needed to support research and to train specialists. The private sector provided some support, but it soon became apparent that the federal government would have to assume responsibility for research and training.

Beginning in 1937, with the founding of the National Cancer Institute, Congress established a series of specialized National Institutes of Health. Each institute was targeted to a specific disease category or set of related conditions (heart disease, neurological diseases and blindness, arthritis, etc.) and was authorized to do intramural research and to make grants to outside institutions and individuals. Federal support for these research activities gradually expanded over the years, as the National Institutes of Health developed into 14 separate institutes and divisions. By 1968, the NIH budget had grown to $1.6 billion, and the staff had grown to over 13,000 full-time members.[10]

The federal government also got involved in health manpower training. Mental health training began as early as 1948, and in 1963 the first broad subsidies were granted for educating health professionals.[11] But, while these programs were intended to address the manpower shortage problem, monies were allocated directly to educational institutions with few specifications as to how they should be used. No leverage mechanisms were included with the authorizations to ensure that funds would be spent where critical manpower problems existed.[12]

As the federal government gradually got involved in building hospitals, in supporting biomedical research and training, and in assisting in the development at the local and state level of programs targeted to specific disease categories, the major objective was always to spread out the benefits of the system. Even though some of the authorizing bills contained reference to planning goals and to coordination of resources, these objectives were clearly secondary to the overriding commitment to expand the system. Even when the main focus of concern shifted in the early 1960s to the inability of consumers to meet the rising costs of medical care, the government's approach to the problem was the same: the provision of additional inputs.

When Medicare and Medicaid were passed in 1965, the federal government took on the enormous responsibility of providing financial coverage for the medical expenses of the elderly and poor. Once again the assumption behind the government's action was that the existing system would respond in a rational fashion to meet the needs and demands of the population if additional financial resources were allocated.[13] The basic problem was not considered to be the structure of the system itself, but instead the economic barriers which prohibited access to that system. With the focus therefore on covering health care costs, no serious attempt was made when Medicare and Medicaid were passed to alter the system by which services were delivered.

Even when the federal government *did* attempt to introduce innovative forms of health care delivery, the effort was not based on a desire to restructure existing patterns of care. · Experiments with new delivery arrangements, such as the neighborhood health centers authorized by the Economic Opportunity Act of 1964, were restricted to specific segments of the population—those whose health care needs were not being met by the system. The objective, therefore, was to *supplement* the existing delivery arrangements and not to reorganize the basic service structure. As one writer comments: "Taken together, these programs left most of the population and health problems untouched."[14]

In describing the basic model behind federal policymaking as essentially a resource input strategy, it is important to note that this represented not only the government's assessment of what was needed but the public's view as well. Although there were individual health planners who spoke out whenever new programs were initiated and predicted their inability to accomplish their objectives, these views were not shared by the general public. The belief that additional resources would solve health problems and assure the availability of needed services seemed to be the prevailing view inside and outside of government.

Beginning in the early 1960s, however, the efficacy of the resource expansion approach began to be questioned. Despite substantial federal allocations little progress was being made in combatting the major health problems: the spiraling rises in costs; shortages and maldistribution of manpower and facilities; and increasing fragmentation of health services. Support for the idea that better planning in the use of health resources was needed began to grow among government policymakers and the general public. This idea also found some support among those in the medical profession who were concerned by how long it took for the fruits of medical research to reach the public. As these concerns began to surface, support was generated for programs that would not only infuse more resources into the health system, but which would also ensure better planning in the way these resources were to be used.

The first federal program which attempted to tie health spending to more active planning was initiated in 1965 with passage of the Heart Disease, Cancer, and Stroke Amendments (P.L. 89-239), commonly known as Regional Medical Programs (RMP). The primary mission of RMPs was to promote, through "regional cooperative arrangements," the extension of new medical knowledge about disease treatment from the medical centers into the offices of general practitioners and community hospitals. The need to reduce the "health technology-application gap"[15] had been one of the major conclusions of the DeBakey Commission, appointed by President Johnson in 1964, to study the problems associated with treatment of heart disease, cancer, and stroke. The original RMP legislation which resulted from the DeBakey Commission's work was thus designed to work toward closing this gap, with the hope that by making available to more patients the latest advances in the diagnosis and treatment of these target diseases, the health system as a whole would be upgraded.

Despite agreement on such long-term goals there was considerable confusion as to what the specific mission of the RMP should be. Much of the confusion resulted from political maneuverings surrounding the final enactment of the bill, when language was added ensuring that activities would be carried out "without interference with the patterns, or the methods of financing, of patient care or professional practice, or with the administration of hospitals."[16] This was interpreted by many to mean that the new program, like its predecessors, would not attempt to restructure or "regionalize" the health service system.

Confusion about the program can be attributed not only to its statutory language but also to the direction provided by Washington in implementing the program. As one writer points out: ". . . unusual emphasis [was placed] on voluntary local initiative, rather than mandatory federal direction."[17] The ideas for the projects which received federal funding came from each individual RMP grant applicant, and regional boundaries were defined locally as well. No overall national strategy guided allocations toward specific goals of service delivery improvement or coordination. And, although some RMPs did attempt projects specifically focused on service arrangements,[18] most of the projects were aimed at expanding research activities related to the three targeted diseases.

This emphasis on research, however, should not be viewed as a departure from the original intention of the law. For although much attention was placed on removing the "science-service gap," as recommended by the DeBakey Commission, another major conclusion of the Commission was that basic and clinical research was receiving insufficient federal support.[19] This concern was reflected in RMP funding stipulations, which provided that 60 percent of the funds would be allocated to basic and clinical research and 40 percent to "service." But, as Komaroff points out, a substantial portion of the 40 percent flowed into research facilities to support their "service" efforts in disseminating research results.[20]

Thus, the RMP effort represented an attempt to merge two goals: the promotion of scientific research, which was a traditional focus of federal health policymaking; and the development of improved service arrangements in the application of knowledge. The fact that achievements in the service area were generally uneven can probably be attributed to two factors: (1) little direction from Washington as to how service improvements could be accomplished; and (2) little public understanding of the role health planning and coordination could play in solving the major problems of high costs and limited accessibility. These factors, together with the medical profession's overriding interest in research activities, did little to encourage a strong movement toward health planning.

Second Attempt by Government

The federal government's second attempt to tie spending to better planning, the Comprehensive Health Planning and Public Health Service Amendments (or Partnership for Health Act, P.L. 89-749), was enacted in 1966, one year after RMP, and shared many of the same problems. Under the act, state and areawide comprehensive health planning (CHP) agencies were set up to assess health needs and service capabilities, and to establish priorities for future federal and state funding for health programs. Like the RMP experience, one of the major problems with the program was its limited authority to enforce better coordination of services.

Although the preamble of the new law called for the "marshaling of all health resources to assure comprehensive health services of high quality for every person,"[21] it is difficult to see how the CHP agencies, in fact, could "marshal resources" over which they had no formal authority. They could hold meetings and foster communication between the parallel groups which control resources in the health sector, and even reach decisions about what should be done.[22] However, they were not given control over the funding that could achieve action on these decisions. Part of the reason for the agencies' limited authority over parallel agencies stemmed from the fact that administrative control over health activities was also diffused at the federal level.   The agency administering CHP was placed on a parallel level, organizationally, with agencies administering health facility and health manpower programs, thus making it very difficult to improve coordination between them.[23]

As with RMP, the actions authorized by the law were to be carried out "without interference with existing patterns of private professional practice of medicine, dentistry, and related healing arts."[24] This restriction severely limited the number and kinds of corrective actions a CHP agency could take in attempting to correct inadequacies in the present pattern of services, since almost any action at all that deviated from traditional practice could be called "interference."

As a result of these restrictions on CHP operations, it is understandable that CHP agencies have had only very limited impact on existing patterns of care.   Part of this is due to the fact that there has been very little commitment, either at the federal or local level, to the idea of effecting changes in the system.   The government's major interest in establishing these agencies appears to have been to encourage discussion among the various parties, but not to hold anyone accountable for the performance of specific health planning tasks.   The evidence confirms the lack of enforcement.   A 1972 study showed that only 20 percent of 128 health planning agencies surveyed could project facility needs in their area, and less than 50 percent knew the bed needs in their area for the current year.[25]

Much more could be said in evaluating the strengths and weaknesses of this program.   But most relevant to this analysis is the fact that although CHP was meant to represent a new departure in federal policymaking, moving toward better coordination and control over federal spending for health problems, it actually was not very different from earlier policies.   CHP neither provided sufficient funds nor firm incentives for effective planning.   It is not surprising that it failed to achieve some of its main purported objectives.

Given these difficulties with policies attempting to solve problems through mandated health planning, the federal government also became involved in activities aimed more directly at solving specific health problems.   The containment of rising health costs has been a major concern of the government, particularly as its share of these costs has increased, and several attempts have been made to institute some measure of control.

The first federal attempt was a requirement included in the Medicare legislation (Social Security Amendments of 1965, P.L. 89-97, Title XVIII) that hospitals and extended care facilities institute "utilization review" (UR) procedures as a condition of participation in the program. A physician-run UR committee had to be set up in each facility to consider (a) whether the medical services covered under the program were necessary; and (b) whether the services were provided in the appropriate facility.[26]

The government's objective in requiring such review was to ensure some way of controlling costs. To do this, it was felt that the peer review activities which already existed in some facilities had to be expanded from "a process of technical self-evaluation and education among physicians to one concerned with wider elements of patient care, including service costs and administrative mechanisms."[27] The cost-containment goal of UR procedures was made even more explicit when they became mandatory for the Medicaid program as well, under the 1967 Social Security Amendments (P.L. 90-248). It was stated then that the regulations would "safeguard against unnecessary utilization" and ensure that payments would be "not in excess of reasonable . charges consistent with efficiency, economy, and quality of care."[28]

However, although the institution of these procedures was required by law, for the most part they have been ineffective in influencing the cost escalation which has occurred under these programs. During the initial stage following enactment of Medicare and Medicaid, the federal government was preoccupied with enlisting the support of health providers in order to get the overall programs launched. Consequently, the importance of UR procedures was downplayed to avoid antagonizing those in the medical profession who saw them as potential greater governmental intervention and policing of professional practice. The de-emphasis of the government's role in UR also rested on the expectation that the intermediaries and carriers would achieve effective controls.[29]

Whatever the rationale for weak enforcement of the peer review process, it became quite clear that the government's plan for cost control under Medicare and Medicaid was not working. A Social Security survey of hospitals in 1968, for instance, found that almost half the hospitals were not reviewing any admissions, even though this was a statutory requirement.[30] Gradually, increasing evidence of serious cost escalations in Medicare and Medicaid expenditures[31] stimulated the government's interest in devising more effective cost-containment procedures. The major concern was over-utilization, for in hearings held by the Senate Finance Committee testimony was given that a "significant proportion of the health services provided under Medicare and Medicaid are probably not medically necessary."[32] Obviously, such over-utilization would have a significant economic impact on the costs of the programs.

In response to the growing concern, Senator Wallace Bennett of Utah, the ranking minority member of the Senate Finance Committee, introduced a proposal for peer review in 1970 which was modeled after the review systems already being used by doctor-sponsored foundations for medical care. Although his amendment was unsuccessful in 1970, it was re-introduced in

1972 and passed as part of the mammoth Social Security Amendments of 1972 (P.L. 92-603).

The Professional Standards Review Organization (PSRO) Amendment was designed to overcome the deficiencies in the UR system by changing the organizational structure of the program, broadening the scope of review, and ensuring that better use would be made of review determinations.[33] The law removes primary responsibility for review from the hospitals and assigns it instead to local organizations of physicians (and osteopaths). These organizations, known as PSROs, are now in various stages of development throughout the 203 designated areas of the country, and will have the responsibility of ensuring that health care paid for under the Medicare, Medicaid, and the Maternal and Child Health programs is: (1) medically necessary; (2) consistent with professionally recognized standards of care; and (3) provided in the least costly setting possible.[34]

To make these determinations, each PSRO must develop criteria and standards for the diagnosis and treatment of the cases it reviews. Thus, the mechanism the government is relying on to control utilization and unnecessary costs under its financing programs is the procedure of self-regulation by physicians, with assessments as to the medical necessity, quality, and appropriateness of care made on the basis of physician-determined criteria.

With physicians in each area developing the standards for the reviews to be carried out in that area, it seems likely that the standards will be based on what is customary practice. But, as one writer has pointed out, the "custom" may or may not be "the standard of the reasonable physician critically evaluating the need for a service."[35] A review program that essentially promotes the adoption of customary practice, therefore, will probably not induce physicians to evaluate critically the necessity of services which have been provided. Potential cost-savings under the program will thus be limited to those services *now* considered to be unnecessary under customary standards. It is not likely to lead to the more substantial cost-savings which would probably result if critical review of the customary standards themselves were required.

One problem that has contributed to the skepticism about the program's potential effectiveness stems from the confusion which surrounded it from the beginning. Although the program was clearly designed on Capitol Hill as a way of ensuring more effective cost controls in federally financed health programs, this objective was obscured somewhat initially by the government's attempt to implement PSRO without antagonizing the medical profession.[36] The key phrase relied on to rally support and get the program moving was "quality assurance." Even though most physicians were aware of the government's interest in cutting unnecessary costs, they were also told that "quality" would be a major objective of the program.

Cost-containment and quality assurance are, of course, not necessarily incompatible objectives. The problem in the PSRO program, however, is that very little attempt has been made to clarify how they are to be related. If the two goals continue to be pursued independently, as they are now, it seems unlikely that the program will be able to have a significant impact on either one. For, at present, there is no effective mechanism to tie the concurrent review process, which is focused on controlling unnecessary utilization of hospital services, to the procedure of retrospective medical audit, which is viewed essentially as a quality assurance device.

Some method must be devised to join these two efforts, so that quality-related audit decisions are able to guide (and also lend "respect" to) cost-cutting through utilization review. Otherwise, the force of the "quality imperative" for more and better care[37] will tend to cancel out any hope for achieving the cost-containment objectives of the program. If this happens, PSRO will fall into the same category as earlier federal programs, which attempted to solve health problems through "inputs," with little effort made to integrate them into the system in a rational way. In this case the input would be mechanisms to ensure quality in the delivery of care. Although some improvement in care might result, depending on how audit procedures are carried out in each area, there would be no improvement in the government's ability to assess rationally what it should and should not be paying for in health care.

The discussion thus far has attempted to enumerate some of the weaknesses in federal strategies to achieve certain health-related goals. Simply describing how particular strategies have been employed with different degrees of success and failure, however, does little to further understanding of the steps needed to achieve a more appropriate interface between government and the health system. As the government continues to expand its role in guiding health delivery, either by fostering such alternative forms of delivery as health maintenance organizations[38] or by attempting to foster more effective planning and regulation of services,[39] more attention is needed to the question of how policies are influenced both in their development and implementation by numerous forces which are outside the sphere of formal policymaking. These forces, or constraints, must be understood if the federal government's involvement in health care is to become more productive.

CONSTRAINTS IMPEDING EFFECTIVE POLICYMAKING

There is no blueprint of how a health service system should be constructed. Given the pluralistic nature of American health care institutions, the continually shifting body of technological knowledge, the existence of regional and local differences in health care resources (and perhaps also in the relative financial and social value put on health services by members of the population), one ideal system may never be attainable, and is probably undesirable.[40]

Probably the most pervasive force affecting the formulation of health policy is captured in a key phrase from the quotation above: "Given the pluralistic nature of American health care . . ." It is a fundamental axiom of health policymaking that the matrix of services which collectively are called the American health "system" is actually the sum of numerous and quite diverse interests operating independently. According to this view, policymaking involves devising ways of coordinating these competing interests, but only at certain points and times when such intervention in what is essentially a private sector operation is felt to be both necessary and beneficial for society as a whole. The general operating principle is that power in the health system is not held by any one group but shared by a wide range of private and governmental bodies, where each has some influence over how the system functions.[41]

The interests which thus collectively "control" the system include everything from institutions like hospitals and medical schools, to organizations representing health professionals, insurance companies, pharmaceutical firms, the individual providers and consumers, and the various levels of federal, state, and local government. Even though the final policies are issued by government officials, all of these groups have a part in the determination of exactly what form these policies have and how they are subsequently implemented. The American Medical Association is well-known for its influence on policy, particularly for its ability to mobilize a majority of practicing physicians to support or reject specific proposals which affect the practice of medicine.

In the face of these wide-ranging and independent forces, the process of policymaking takes on special characteristics. Rather than viewing policy formulation as the result of conscious decision making, it is instead seen as a bargaining process where competing groups work out the agreements and adjustments on which policies are based. The government's role is thus not one of creating policy but of ratifying these agreements and ensuring that all interested parties are able to participate freely in the bargaining process.[42] Such a process is more likely to lead to incremental rather than large-scale changes, since each of the major parties' tries to preserve its power in the interchange.[43] Any attempt by the government to force large-scale change on the system is not considered to be legitimate since the government is viewed as an external force. What *is* legitimate is the free competition among the various interest groups, for the outcome is then felt to be the product of a "fair game" type of interaction.[44]

To allow this to happen, therefore, the government essentially delegates to private parties or abnegates its own power to make public policy. In the case of the Regional Medical Programs, for instance, the federal government for the most part gave individual applicants the power to decide how cooperative arrangements should be fostered in their regions. Even though the government decided whether or not to fund certain projects, it has been the customary policy to rely on private groups to determine the kinds of programs which should be established. The strategy of delegating power in this way is based on the assumption that there is much consensus within and among different segments of the health system and that health providers, guided by their professional norms, will work in the public interest.

Unfortunately, this assumption fails to take into account that each interest group also has internal objectives which are not always consistent with the overall goal of maximizing the public good. As David Mechanic points out, "medical care involves a variety of interest groups that tend to view priorities from their own particular perspectives and interests, and it is enormously difficult to achieve a consensus."[45]

The separation between "public" and "private" goals occurs in two ways. First, the service orientation of physicians represents essentially a micro-level perspective, for their primary concern is the welfare of their individual patients and their own individual self-interest. In some cases this orientation may conflict with the "public good." For instance, physicians may expend an inordinate amount of resources to prolong the life of a hopelessly dying patient and divert resources which might be employed in ways which are more beneficial to society as a whole.[46] The micro-macro problem is evident at the organizational level as well, where internal decisions aimed at helping an organization survive may conflict with larger societal goals.[47] An example of this is the administrator who struggles to keep his hospital open even though the state has decided that the facility is no longer needed.

Policymakers thus must face the challenge of competing goals in designing and implementing policy. Yet, in studying the development of the federal role in health, it is clear that although the diversity has generally been acknowledged, very little strategical planning has been directed at how these private interests actually influence policy implementation or even how they might possibly be utilized to make policies more effective. Instead, the usual strategy has involved first identifying the overall goals of a program and then attempting to promote their achievement through the allocation of additional resources. The expectation has thus been that "the combination of need, knowledge, and resources will generate, at some point, a rational reorganization."[48]

The difficulty with this type of approach is that its effectiveness depends to a large extent on whether, and to what degree, the target groups will take the necessary actions. In the area of health care, it is expected that they will comply because of the normative orientation providers have—an orientation which is assumed to take precedence over any individual considerations. Additional incentives or sanctions are felt to be both unnecessary and a violation of the autonomy traditionally granted to those involved in professional work.

Thus, the strategy derives both from the belief in a professionally based normative consensus and from the pluralist notion that a system built primarily on bargaining interest groups will be perfectly self-corrective. Theodore Lowi describes this philosophy as the "myth of the automatic society granted us by an all-encompassing, ideally self-correcting, providentially automatic political process."[49]

Lowi is not alone in his belief. Critics of the pluralist perspective, called "bureaucratic reformers" by one author,[50] point to the unresponsiveness of providers to health needs of the public, generally blame market competition for the defects of the system, and call for increased administrative regulation and central planning. The ultimate goal, according to this view, is the creation of "a rational, efficient, cost-conscious, coordinated health delivery system."[51]

Although definitions of central planning and bureaucratic management are many and varied, the terms have generally been used most often to refer to one or all of the following:

1. the reorganization of structure and activities into comprehensive systems to improve coordination and achieve economies of scale;
2. the use of quantitative analysis and computerized information systems to improve decision making; and
3. the reliance on experts and technique, rather than politics, in decision making and in dealing with conflict.[52]

When applied to health care the focus has generally been on the undesirable overlap and duplication of services and facilities, and the potential for improving the overall quality of care through better coordination.

Although most critics of the bureaucratic approach acknowledge the need for more rationality in the administration of health programs, they question whether it is either possible or desirable to substitute efficiency for politics. In one writer's view, management science is a "seductive ideology" which tends to underestimate the strength of market mechanisms and pluralism, and which can lead to misguided assumptions about the ability of planning strategies to control all of the factors in health production.[53] Attempting to remove politics from health policy decision making fails to take into account the fact that politics is the result, not the cause, of conflicting aspirations.[54]

Yet, the central management attitude toward these conflicts is that they will be absorbed as mechanisms are created to unify and integrate the entire system.

This is the philosophy behind the certificate-of-need programs and other regulatory schemes which are based on the assumption that there is a "best" solution which can be obtained through the application of technical knowledge to specific health problems. What this perspective obscures, however, is the fact that "management by objective" is no less dependent on goal consensus than is the pluralist strategy. The difference is that in this case it is the bureaucratic managers who set the goals instead of relying on the political process to define objectives and determine priorities. The assumption "that it is possible for a competent and disinterested decision-maker to find in any situation a value premise that uniquely determines the content of the public interest" is seriously questioned by Banfield, who feels that there is likely to be a systematic bias in the decision maker's choice of value premises, away from those which are controversial or problematic and toward those that can be measured and controlled.[55]

The problem of limited knowledge is a common criticism leveled against the bureaucratic management approach. Without acceptable measures of quality and knowledge about the relationship between good health and medical care, it is said, there is great potential that regulatory requirements will produce unanticipated and, in some cases, harmful results. The major difficulty, the critics say, derives from the administrators' assumption that they can both establish overall goals and employ a predetermined set of bureaucratic procedures to achieve them. What this overlooks, however, is the manner in which these directives are received by the target groups and the interplay which results. It ignores the fact that programs create social interactions, which "may create new needs, or produce shifts in priority on the basis on newly-realized feasibilities, out of which a new set of goals should emerge."[56]

Thus, in analyzing both the pluralist and central management strategies, a key factor is the degree of flexibility involved. The pluralist approach might be viewed as too flexible in the sense that goals and resources are put forth without the administrative mechanisms needed to produce the desired results. The administrative strategy, on the other hand, ties goal setting to specific implementation procedures, but in relying on a predetermined plan tends to be unresponsive to the influence of external forces on the intended results. Both strategies, therefore, are essentially based on a simple input/output model, where goals and goal achievement are the central concerns. But, as the former director of the Social Security Administration, Robert Ball, points out:

> Given the observable fact of the great ingenuity of man in getting
> around law and regulation, supervision, and attempted education, it
> is a matter of some amazement how little attention tends to be paid
> to the intervening steps—the difficult steps grouped under the
> heading of administration—that must be taken between the ex-
> pression of a goal and the achievement of that goal.[57]

In the input/output approach to health policymaking these intervening steps
are de-emphasized, leaving the success of the strategy totally dependent on
whether there is sufficient consensus regarding both the value of the goal and
the proper method of achieving it.

The existence of such a consensus in the health system is highly questionable. For although most health providers might agree in principle that
certain goals are worth pursuing, they very often differ considerably when it
comes to determining how they should be pursued. For instance, the question
of how to reduce fragmentation in health care delivery is approached very
differently by providers, depending on what relationship they have to the
organizational structure of the delivery system. A physician in private
practice might believe that the solution lies in changing insurance reimbursement policies so that a broader range of services now covered only on an
inpatient basis could be provided in his own office, thus enabling him to offer
patients a unified package of services. The hospitals, however, might view
such an action as producing greater duplication and fragmentation of
services, and would probably recommend instead a closer coordination and
centralization of services within and between existing facilities. Blame for
the fragmentation might in this case be placed on the growth of free-standing
ambulatory clinics like surgicenters and family planning clinics, which focus
on specific health needs but make no attempt to provide total patient care.

In many cases such as this there is general consensus that something must
be done about a particular problem, but the specific methods favored to solve
it are quite different and often contradictory. Given this, it seems highly
unlikely that policies which depend on goal consensus and rely essentially on
an input/output strategy to achieve goals, will be effective. Whatever change
strategy may be adopted, we need more precise and systematic information on
the process of policy implementation and how different segments of the health
system respond to policy thrusts. Too often policymakers base their
prescriptions for action on an implicit and incomplete judgment of how the
system operates. While an attempt may be made in setting policy goals to
accommodate the specific concerns of one or two of the dominant factions in
the target population—organized medicine, for instance—this is generally
not done for other groups to be affected. Whatever attention is given to
projected policy impacts on specific groups is usually confined to estimates of

the probable reactions of these groups to policy goals. What is customarily ignored is how individual target groups will receive and respond to the specific mechanisms through which policy goals are to be reached.

Morris and Binstock identify four key questions which policymakers should be able to answer before judgment is made on the feasibility of certain goals:

> 1. How does the overall goal fit with the primary interests of the dominant groups involved?
> 2. What kinds of influence are these groups responsive to?
> 3. What kinds of changes are needed in each of these groups in order to achieve the overall goal? Which of these changes is most and least likely to be resisted?
> 4. For each of the given changes sought, what types of resources are likely to prove effective in influencing the groups to change in these ways?[58]

A key distinction must be made between this type of assessment and that embodied in the bureaucratic management strategy discussed earlier. The managerial approach begins with the setting of a goal and then continues by attempting to devise techniques that will foster its achievement. The type of strategy being proposed here, however, focuses not on a particular goal but on developing a working model of how the system operates. The basic premise is that policy development must be preceded, and accompanied, by a realistic assessment of what is actually happening in each sector of the delivery system.

Amitai Etzioni believes this "systems model" approach is an improvement over the goal-consensus framework for policymaking and evaluation. In following a systems approach one does not "confront a social unit with an ideal and then grade it according to its degree of conformity to the ideal," but instead an attempt is made to determine "the external and internal conditions that enable it to function."[59] The first question, then, is: what are the actual organizational goals of each unit in the system, and what conditions foster their achievement? If we know the mechanisms which operate in a particular organization and how they respond to external events, it is then possible to design policies which utilize these same mechanisms to maximize fulfillment of a new goal. This assumes, of course, what has customarily not been the case—that policymakers possess authority to implement their policy objectives.

The value of this approach is that it recognizes that those responsible for a particular subsystem tend to identify with the interests and values of their individual unit.[60] In Etzioni's view,

> ...the system model is a prerequisite for understanding and bringing about social change. The goal model leads to unrealistic,

Utopian expectations, and hence to disappointments ... The system model, on the other hand, depicts more realistically the difficulty encountered in introducing change into established systems, which function in a given environment.[61]

It is this "given environment" which has been too often either ignored or given too little attention in health policymaking. For in most cases federal policymaking efforts have relied almost entirely on goal-oriented strategies and have not had the benefit of a realistic understanding of how individual units in the target population function. Again, policymakers have had little authority to implement their plans. This has produced isolated policy directives aimed at single sectors of the health system, and has resulted in frustration when the expected outcomes did not occur. One prerequisite to a more coordinated approach to policymaking is to understand the inter-relationships among individual sectors of the system. It is this kind of knowledge that is needed to make the federal role in health more productive.

The next section addresses the specific question of how the systems model approach could be utilized in health policymaking, and specifically to improve the knowledge base on which policy decisions rest.

RECOMMENDED:
A NEW MODEL FOR HEALTH POLICYMAKING

Given the traditional role which the federal government has played in health, where resource expansion has been the dominant pattern for over 40 years, the suggestion that significant changes in that role are possible may seem highly speculative. Major shifts in government policies are not the norm. But the suggestion that significant role changes are needed is hardly a novel one, and has in fact become quite commonplace. Probably the most significant point about the growing interest in a new federal role is the fact that the suggestion comes not only from a wide range of private groups and individuals but is also gaining support inside the government itself.

First, the Congressional committees and now most federal health agencies have expressed deep concern over the apparent inability of existing programs to control the inflationary costs in the health delivery system. As the burden of the federal budget increases every year, and as the costs of government health programs like Medicare and Medicaid continue to escalate, more and more attention is being directed at the dual problems of controlling hospital charges and physician fees. In addition, there is growing consumer concern over exorbitant medical expenses. In short, there is now more pressure to change the role which the federal government has played.

One factor working against any change in federal policy is the lack of consensus among those who profess to favor changes in the federal role. For, as discussed earlier, the varying perspectives of individual units in the health sector do not represent a unified view, either as to what is wrong with the system or what should be done to improve it. Competing concerns are manifest in the manner in which the government has attempted to deal with the cost-containment challenge. Although it is clear that the impetus for passage of the PSRO amendment derived chiefly from concern over cost escalations, the program has been "sold" or presented to the medical profession primarily as a quality assurance effort, with cost control a secondary factor.[62]

Given these constraints, both inside and outside of government, to achieving anything resembling consensus on how to rationalize the health system, it should be clear that the traditional goal-consensus model for federal policymaking is inappropriate. Recognition and acceptance of this fact is strongly resisted, however, both by those who view policymaking as the "natural" result of open negotiation among competing interests, and by those who see it as a mechanism for synthesizing these competing elements to enable the system to function rationally. In each case goal consensus is viewed as the basis for policymaking, either consensus through bargaining or through planning. But, despite the appealing characteristics of each of these approaches—the first because it allows the "natural order" to function freely and the second because it proposes to make the system more rational—neither has been very effective in resolving the major problems confronting the health system.[63] The difficulty lies in the fact that their effectiveness is dependent on a consensus which simply does not exist. For such a consensus does not evolve naturally, and it cannot be imposed mechanically on the system by a master plan, especially when no leverage exists.

Once this fact is recognized, progress can begin to be made toward developing a strategy which can be effective. The crucial first step is to develop a working model of how individual components function in the system, specifically what their operative goals are and what interrelationships exist between them. Then, rather than devising policies which represent simply an add-on to the existing structure, it may be possible to tie policymaking directly to each unit's operational goals. What this represents, then, is a dual but simultaneous process whereby knowledge about the functioning of the system serves as the basis for policymaking, which in turn generates additional knowledge and leads to further policy development.

The PSRO program will be used to illustrate how the process could work. As discussed earlier, the key issue underlying the government's interest in the program is cost-containment, and the need for improved decision making in government spending for health care. Rather than assuming direct responsibility for instituting cost-cutting measures, however, the government decided to delegate this responsibility to physicians. The major problem here is that physicians are unlikely to be responsive to the fundamental policy objective of cost-containment. Since physicians are to develop the criteria and standards by which they and their peers will be held accountable, it is unrealistic to expect that new information about evaluating medical care will be forthcoming. Much more likely is that the process will produce criteria based on what is "usual and customary practice." There are simply no incentives in the present law which stimulate the kind of critical evaluation of existing practices which might lead to cost-containment.

A different type of approach is needed to ensure that this kind of critical assessment does take place, so that the new knowledge produced can be utilized as the basis for policymaking aimed at reducing unnecessary costs. It is unreasonable to expect physicians to get involved in this difficult task voluntarily, not only because the immediate benefits are few, but because such an expectation assumes a level of cost-consciousness which most physicians do not have. As Havighurst and Blumstein point out:

> ... the physician's 'micro' view makes it hard for him to recognize 'macro' problems of limited access to care and ever-rising costs outpacing benefits, or at least to accept the proposed remedies which threaten his ability to do for his patient whatever he may think they need. Medical tradition and the values inculcated from the very beginning of medical education make the physician unreceptive to 'macro' conceptions of the health care system and resistant to benefit/cost calculations.[64]

To overcome this resistance and ensure that serious attention is given to developing the information needed to make decisions involving trade-offs between costs and quality, physicians must be given stronger incentives. The present approach in federal policymaking does not provide sufficient inducement for physicians to spend the time required to develop this information, particularly since it is time away from more remunerative activities. The strength of these material motives must be acknowledged by building into federal policies the kinds of financial incentives which will ensure the critical evaluation of medical practice which is needed.

Until now every proposal made for building financial incentives into federal health policies has been successfully blocked by the numerous arguments mounted against them. Despite the strength of this opposition, however, it may soon be overruled by another perspective which is rapidly gaining support—the realization that a much more serious attempt must be made to allocate our limited resources more rationally.

Acceptance of the fact that our resources are finite is the key to developing an effective mechanism for containing costs and maintaining quality in our health delivery system. A recognition of this fact would require that limits be set on health care expenditures and that physicians either make the appropriate decisions or assume a financial responsibility for not doing so. The motivation for such a strategy is that, while medical training and peer influence encourage physicians to be quality-conscious, there have been no comparable mechanisms to ensure equal attention to the cost implications of their actions. The only effective way to stimulate cost-consciousness is by making physicians face a personal cost, by placing them in a position where their decisions are associated with tangible risks or benefits.

This approach is similar in concept to the health maintenance organization (HMO) strategy, where prepayment acts as a ceiling giving providers a strong incentive to provide effective care in the most economical way possible. But while HMOs offer great potential for stimulating cost savings, both internally and in other delivery systems through market pressure, sufficient opposition to some of their special features (for instance, salary *vs.* fee-for-service payment to physicians) has hampered their development and makes it difficult to predict what their ultimate impact will be. The approach suggested here is similar in many respects, but its implementation is not dependent on adoption of a strict HMO-type organization.

The fixed-budget concept can be implemented in several ways. One method would be to utilize the PSRO organizational structure, where physicians are responsible for all care in a given area. But instead of merely requesting that providers review services, the government would establish a fixed budget in each area for reimbursement under Medicare and Medicaid, to hold federal spending to the total amount spent in that area in the previous year. The purpose of such a ceiling would be to induce physicians to critically evaluate services to ensure that they are both medically necessary and provided in the most economical way possible. Any expenditures above the ceiling would be borne by the physicians themselves, but the PSRO would be given a percentage return on any cost savings which resulted, to be reallocated as the PSRO saw fit.

These remunerative incentives would have to be balanced, however, by strong normative controls to guard against possible underservicing or other quality-related abuses. The peer review process should be effective in preventing such abuses. For relying on peer review as a check on overzealous cost-cutting is far more realistic than the expectation embodied in the present PSRO strategy that peer review and existing controls will initiate serious cost-cutting efforts. The traditional bias of physicians to provide more and better care for their patients regardless of cost is not conducive to generating the kind of "macro-level" decisions which are required. But this quality bias can serve as an effective check on abuses which financial incentives might produce.

The strategy proposed here gives hospitals a more active role in the review process. Instead of simply carrying out reviews as delegated by the PSRO, the hospitals would be an integral part of each PSRO's operation. Based on reimbursement costs from the previous year, each hospital would be given a fixed amount from the PSRO's overall budget to cover its Medicare and Medicaid services. Thus, hospital administrators and medical staffs would have a strong incentive to devise ways of making their hospitals more cost-effective. And because the PSRO would have ultimate responsibility for any cost-overruns, for the first time physicians would have a real stake in helping the hospital to operate economically. This "shared-fate" incentive may lead to much more cooperation between physicians and hospitals than is likely under the current PSRO strategy.

To ensure that the cost-cutting decisions made by PSROs are based on a comprehensive assessment of the full range of service options, the government should include in the budget ceiling the full amount of Medicare and Medicaid reimbursements for ambulatory services provided in each area. Providers would thus be given a real incentive to consider the potential cost/benefit trade-offs between inpatient and outpatient care, an incentive which until now has not existed.

Ideally, the proposed strategy should cover the full range of services and not be limited to services covered by federal reimbursement programs. This restriction, combined with the fact that no attempt is made to reduce existing federal costs, since budget ceilings represent prevailing costs, could inhibit the program's overall cost-cutting potential. But one of the practices this proposal is designed to put an end to is policymaking based on insufficient knowledge. Rather than attempting full-blown reform of the system as a whole, the first concern must be to develop a working model of how the system actually functions. For while it may have once been possible to pour money into our health system without the benefit of this knowledge, it should be clear that this time has passed.

The fixed-budget strategy proposed here is one example of the kind of fundamental change which is needed in federal health planning and policy-making. For to be successful, federal policies must utilize incentives and sanctions which have a direct and inescapable impact on those areas in the health system where change is needed. If the objective is to reduce unnecessary and costly hospitalization, for instance, it is not enough for the government to simply ask physicians to review services with this goal in mind. To stimulate the kind of critical decision making that this entails necessitates giving physicians and other health providers a vested interest in the choices to be made. Only in this way will their full attention and expertise be directed at generating the knowledge which is needed about cost and quality trade-offs in the delivery of health services. Without this information, the federal government cannot move ahead on its own and devise ways of reducing hospital services and cutting costs. For, in order to utilize its authority to take this kind of corrective action, federal planning and policymaking must be guided by solid evidence of how the system functions and what the components of quality health care actually are. It is only through the use of direct and unavoidable incentives that this kind of information will be produced.

CONCLUSION

The federal government has encountered numerous problems in its attempt to respond to deficiencies in our health care system. Despite vast sums of money expended, the basic problems confronting the system have remained—the uneven distribution of services and facilities, the fragmentation in care delivery, and the many problems associated with seemingly uncontrollable health costs. The various federal strategies employed to improve these conditions, including, among others, the categorical grants, hospital construction funds, manpower training assistance, comprehensive health planning, and utilization review, either seem to have exacerbated the problems or left them basically unchanged.

Numerous studies have been done to determine the weaknesses in each strategy, and often these assessments have formed the basis for subsequent policies. What has generally been overlooked, however, is the fact that all these federal programs have embodied essentially the *same* strategy. For even though there was a gradual shift away from resource expansion programs as the need for better planning became apparent, the basic pattern has been the same: each program represented an attempt by the government to supplement the existing system in some way—not to change the system.

In some cases, funds were allocated to meet a specific health need, while other times providers were asked to participate in planning activities. But in each case, no attempt was made to interfere with the basic operation of the system. Given the basic assumption about the rationality of the system and the dedication of physicians to provide the best possible care, it was assumed that solutions could be achieved by additional resources and better planning.

The fact that this has not happened can be attributed to a fundamental and persistent misconception about our health care system: the assumption that there is sufficient consensus among the individual actors and organizations to ensure compliance with stated health goals. In fact, such an orientation to promote the "public good" is only one of many different goals which may be pursued by individual units in the health system. Self-fulfillment and institutional survival are also key operative goals, and in some cases conflict with the more "macro" needs of the system as a whole. The needs and interests of individual groups have not been taken into account.

What is proposed here is a new model for health policymaking. It essentially involves a two-part strategy, although the two steps are inter-related and must be undertaken jointly: (1) priority must be given in policymaking to mechanisms which will generate explicit knowledge about how the system functions and what the actual components of quality health care are; and (2) policies designed to both generate this knowledge and act on it must consider the operative goals of the individual units which make up the system. Although there have been individual researchers who have addressed these questions, policymakers have generally avoided them and have concentrated instead on goal formulation. The assumption in government has been that its task is to articulate the public's needs and develop specific plans of action for meeting them. Too often, however, these plans have been conceived with little understanding of how the system actually operates. They have been based instead on broad conceptions of how a system which is guided by professionals and dedicated to serving the public is expected to behave. Thus, when policies have not turned out as planned, the failure has been attributed to inappropriate goals rather than to misjudgment about the system itself. Finally, planners have not possessed the authority to exert leverage on the system.

The new model proposed for health policymaking will change this pattern. For if the mechanisms designed to meet specific health needs are based on solid evidence of how target groups function and what incentives they respond to, policymaking is much more likely to have positive results. To generate the information which is needed to bridge this gap between knowledge and public policy, the initial target must be physicians and other direct providers of care, since they have the expertise needed to identify the technical components of quality care. The method suggested here to induce them to produce this information focuses on the question of how these quality factors in health care are to be balanced with crucial questions of cost. To stimulate the difficult decision making this requires, specific recommendations are made for utilizing both normative and remunerative incentives.

As these actions begin to expand the knowledge base, policies can be aimed at additional targets in the health system. For instance, the information gained about alternative utilization patterns under Medicare and Medicaid can be the basis for policies directed at changing insurance company benefit packages, thereby broadening the scope of cost-containment and quality assurance to include privately insured patients; or cost/benefit studies on the utilization of allied health personnel could lead to changes in insurance company reimbursement policies. In addition, the states could use the knowledge gained about facility utilization trade-offs and potential cost-savings to strengthen certificate-of-need and rate-setting policies.

But it is the public in general which will benefit the most from this new knowledge. For, if explicit information were available on health cost and quality trade-offs, educational programs could be developed which would benefit consumers not only in the form of personal savings on medical expenses but also in terms of their share of publicly-supported services. Even more importantly, it is clear that if this information were both known and communicated to them, consumers' expectations about high quality care at the lowest possible cost would be far better served.

NOTES

1. William L. Kissick, "Health Policy Directions for the 1970's," *New England Journal of Medicine* (June 11, 1970), p. 1345.

2. *Ibid.*

3. David F. Bergwall, Philip N. Reeves, and Nina B. Woodside, *Introduction to Health Planning* (Washington, D. C.: Information Resources Press, 1974), p. 17.

4. Judith R. Lave and Lester B. Lave, *The Hospital Construction Act: An Evaluation of the Hill-Burton Program, 1948-1973* (Washington, D. C.: American Enterprise Institute for Public Policy Research, 1974), p. 25.

5. Kissick, *op. cit.*, p. 1346.

6. A. L. Levin, "Health Planning and the U. S. Federal Government," *International Journal of Health Services* (August, 1972), p. 368.

7. *Ibid.*

8. Bergwall, Reeves, Woodside, *op. cit.*, p. 21.

9. Rosemary Stevens, *American Medicine and the Public Interest* (New Haven: Yale University Press, 1971), pp. 179-180.

10. *Ibid.*, p. 358.

11. Kissick, *op. cit.*, p. 1346.

12. Levin, *op. cit.*, p. 368.

13. Kissick, *op. cit.*, p. 1346.

14. Kissick, *op. cit.*, p. 1348.

15. Roger M. Battistella, "The Course of Regional Health Planning," *Medical Care* (May-June, 1967), p. 149.

16. P.L. 89-239, Title IX, Section 900 (c).

17. Anthony L. Komaroff, "Regional Medical Programs in Search of a Mission," *New England Journal of Medicine* (April 8, 1971), p. 759.

18. This was more common after the new RMP law, passed October 30, 1970, placed new emphasis on primary care, preventive care, and care of the poor. Komaroff, *op. cit.*, p. 762.

19. Komaroff, *op. cit.*, p. 758.

20. *Ibid.*, p. 759.

21. P.L. 89-749, Section 2 (a).

22. However, the notion that this occurred frequently is best dispelled by a scenario suggested by Krause, who likened CHP to "a group of people closely gathered around a table, holding their breath and watching one of their number delicately building a castle out of playing cards. Suddenly someone sneezes, and the house of cards collapses." Elliott Krause, "Health Planning as a Managerial Ideology," *International Journal of Health Services* (Summer, 1973), p. 457.

23. Levin, *op. cit.*, p. 369.

24. P.L. 89-749, Section 2 (a).

25. Clark C. Havighurst, "Regulation of Health Facilities and Services By 'Certificate of Need,'" *Virginia Law Review,* 59 (October, 1973), p. 1198; although the CHP law declared planning to be an "imperative," Kissick raises the point that at the time of its enactment there were not enough professionally trained health planners to staff the new agencies: "Considering the existing state of the art, an authorization to support and foster comprehensive health planning is somewhat premature. Ideally, training (314c) should have preceded efforts toward comprehensive planning (including 314a and 314b) by several years." Kissick, *op. cit.*, p. 1349.

26. P.L. 89-97, Title XVIII, Section 1861 (k).

27. Stevens, *op. cit.*, p. 460.

28. P.L. 90-248, Section 1902 (a)(30).

29. Stevens, *op. cit.*, p. 460.

30. Stevens, *op. cit.*, p. 461.

31. "A 1970 report of the Senate Finance Committee noted with concern that 1965 estimates of the cost of Medicare for 1970 was $3.1 billion, but by 1969 it was apparent that the cost would be approximately $5.8 billion. Similarly, the federal share of Part B had increased from $623 million in 1967 to $1245 million in 1971." Michael Rapp, "Federally Imposed Self-Regulation of Medical Practice: A Critique of the Professional Standards Review Organization," *George Washington Law Review,* 42 (May, 1974), p. 823 (footnote #4).

32. Senate Report No. 1230, 92nd Congress, 2nd Session, 254 (1972).

33. Rapp, *op. cit.*, p. 825.

34. P.L. 92-603, Title XI, Part B, Section 1151.

35. Rapp, *op. cit.*, p. 843.

36. A strategy which was very similar to that used in implementing the Medicare program, where utilization review was de-emphasized to encourage physician cooperation.

37. Havighurst and Blumstein define the "quality imperative" as a "societal bias toward more and better care." See Clark C. Havighurst and James F. Blumstein, "Coping With Quality/Cost Trade-offs in Medical Care: The Role of PSROs," *Northwestern University Law Review* (March-April, 1975), pp. 20-30.

38. Federal support for the development of health maintenance organizations was authorized by the "Health Maintenance Organization Act of 1973" (P.L. 92-222). Its impact on the overall delivery system thus far has been limited by legislative restrictions impeding widespread development. Congress is currently debating provisions to modify the restrictions in the original legislation.

39. The The federal government has mandated a more active role in planning and regulation at the local and state levels with the signing into law on January 4, 1975 of the "National Health Planning and Resources Development Act of 1974" (P.L. 93-641). The eventual impact of this legislation is difficult to assess at the present time because much depends on how the law is

interpreted in federal regulations still in various stages of development.

40. Stevens, *op. cit.*, p. 523.

41. Theodore J. Lowi, *The End of Liberalism: Ideology, Policy, and the Crisis of Public Authority* (New York: W.W. Norton & Co., 1969), p. 42.

42. *Ibid.*, p. 71.

43. Eli Ginzberg *et al.*, *Urban Health Services: The Case of New York* (New York: Columbia University Press, 1971), p. 226.

44. Edward C. Banfield, *Political Influence* (New York: The Free Press, 1961), p. 331.

45. David Mechanic, *Public Expectations and Health Care: Essays on the Changing Organization of Health Services* (New York: John Wiley & Sons, 1972), p. 6.

46. Havighurst and Blumstein, *op. cit.*, p. 28.

47. Robert M. Sigmond, "Health Planning," *Milbank Memorial Fund Quarterly* (January, 1968); reprinted in John B. McKinlay, ed., *Politics and Law in Health Care Policy* (New York: PRODIST, 1973), p. 119.

48. Robert R. Alford, *Health Care Politics: Ideological and Interest Group Barriers to Reform* (Chicago: University of Chicago Press, 1975), p. 186.

49. Lowi, *op. cit.*, p. 54.

50. Alford, *op. cit.*, p. 1.

51. *Ibid.*, p. 204.

52. Roger M. Battistella, "Role of Management in Health Services in Britain and the United States," *The Lancet* (March 18, 1972), p. 628.

53. Alford, *op. cit.*, p. 205.

54. Battistella, *op. cit.* (1972), p. 629.

55. Banfield, *op. cit.*, p. 330.

56. Richard Sasuly and Paul D. Ward, "Two Approaches to Health Planning: The Ideal *vs.* the Pragmatic," *Medical Care* (May-June, 1969), p. 239.

57. Robert M. Ball, "Background of Regulation in Health Care," *Controls on Health Care,* Papers of the Conference on Regulation in the Health Industry, January 7-9, 1974 (Washington, D. C.: National Academy of Sciences, 1975), p. 22.

58. Robert Morris and Robert H. Binstock, *Feasible Planning for Social Change* (New York: Columbia University Press, 1966), p. 140.

59. Amitai Etzioni, "Two Approaches to Organizational Analysis: A Critique and a Suggestion," *Administrative Science Quarterly* (Sept., 1960), p. 26.

60. Etzioni, *op. cit.*, p. 276.

61. *Ibid.*

62. See Havighurst and Blumstein on this point, *op. cit.*, esp. pp. 41-45.

63. A third and more radical assessment of the health care system, which Alford calls the "institutional or class perspective," rejects the piecemeal view of reform espoused by both pluralists and bureaucratic rationalizers, and challenges the assumption that health care problems can be dealt with in isolation from the broader social ills existing in society as a whole. Alford, *op. cit.*, pp. 265-266.

64. Havighurst and Blumstein, *op. cit.*, p. 28.

Part II

Inpatient Quality Assurance Activities:
Coordination of Federal, State,
and Private Roles

Chapter 3

Regulating the Quality of Hospital Care— An Analysis Of the Issues Pertinent to National Health Insurance

Michael J. Goran, James S. Roberts, and John Rodak, Jr.

INTRODUCTION

The last decade has seen a tremendous increase in efforts to implement hospital quality assurance mechanisms. The Professional Standards Review Organization (PSRO) program—the latest in a series of efforts to require the review of hospital services—is implementing a well-defined review mechanism throughout much of the country. The Joint Commission on Accreditation of Hospitals (JCAH) has established extensive hospital audit requirements, and Medicare and Medicaid continue to require utilization review (UR) in those areas where PSRO review is not in effect. The next major step appears to be national health insurance and its attendant review requirements. It is certainly timely, therefore, that, in anticipation of the enactment of national health insurance, there be a conference which identifies and examines the major public policy issues related to quality assurance in hospitals. We hope that such discussion will result in a set of review requirements for national health insurance which is both realistic and effective.

To assist in this discussion, important public and private quality assurance requirements are used to help identify major public issues related to hospital quality assurance. Specifically, the two major mechanisms designed to help assure that care provided in hospitals is both necessary and of high quality are examined. These mechanisms are: (1) the accreditation/certification process and (2) medical care review. We will outline the genesis and objectives of these requirements, the manner in which they have been enforced, and then identify the major public policy issues which should be addressed for each prior to their extension to national health insurance.

BACKGROUND

The hospital is a unique and highly important institution in our nation. In recent years inflation, rising personnel costs, increasingly complex medical technology, and expanding third party coverage which encourages hospitalization have combined to result in alarming increases in expenditures for hospital care. There is evidence that unnecessary care is being provided in hospitals. The courts have rested responsibility for hospital quality assurance with the hospital's governing board. The federal government has focused more and more attention on the quality and appropriateness of hospital care. The JCAH has expanded its emphasis on inpatient quality assurance. Unlike any other health care institution, the hospital represents a relatively closed system in which the professional staff is organized, continuing education is an ongoing process, patient health problems are relatively circumscribed, and data on the care provided are readily retrievable.

All of these factors have resulted in the high visibility given to inpatient quality assurance, and given rise to expectations which may go beyond the state of the art of quality assurance. More importantly, this attention has resulted in the establishment of a wide variety of objectives for hospital quality assurance—many of which cannot be realized.

Quality assurance has simultaneously been looked to both as the means by which hospital and health care costs can be controlled and as a mechanism to maintain and improve the health status of the population at large. Neither of these expectations is, of course, realistic, but unless they are tempered, inpatient quality assurance is certain to be judged a failure. While the potential of inpatient quality assurance to improve the quality of health care services is substantial, this in no way should be confused with broader issues of health care cost control and the health status of the general population.

The economic problems related to the financing of health services in this country are not going to be solved by inpatient quality assurance. At best they will be effected only at the margin. All that inpatient quality assurance can offer in this regard is a mechanism that ensures better use of whatever is spent on health care services. Similarly, quality assurance mechanisms are not going to markedly affect health status. Health care services per se do not appear to have as much of an effect on health status as do other factors such as environmental, genetic, psychosocial, economic, and cultural. Both of these major health care public policy issues exceed the scope of quality assurance activities, yet influence expectations about them dramatically. The amount of the nation's gross national product which is to be devoted to health care, the means by which health care financing is to be regulated and controlled, and the relative emphasis that this country will place on the provision of health care services vs. efforts to improve health status through other means, such as improving general environment, are all critical issues.

During the interval before national health insurance becomes a reality the need to discuss these public policy issues has reached crisis stages. None can be substantially effected by either the success or failure of quality assurance programs. Unless positive steps are taken to come to grips with these issues, however, it appears inevitable that quality assurance mechanisms will in part be judged a failure because they have not helped to cope with these broader issues.

Within these constraints, the promise of quality assurance is exciting. While the focus here is on inpatient programs, ultimately quality assurance must be viewed as a mechanism for the entire health care delivery system on a community level. It is here that its real potential will be realized as a major tool to regulate practice patterns and assure, in conjunction with regulatory activities that effect resource allocation and financing, that the public has access to high quality care.

Realistically, the goal of inpatient assurance programs is to assure the quality of the health services provided in hospitals throughout the country. This goal is achieved through the implementation of a review system consisting of three components: (1) the ongoing performance of medical care evaluation studies to identify problems of quality or the administration of health care services through application of the scientific method utilizing objective criteria, study, and the correction of problems through education and appropriate remedial action; (2) the conduct of ongoing programs to assure the appropriate use of hospital services; and (3) periodic analysis of the performance of the health care delivery system, including review, comparative and trend analysis of the aggregate patterns of experience of patients, practitioners, and institutions. Responsibility for this hospital review system rests with the PSRO, but it is also impacted by a variety of programs, including state-administered review efforts and utilization review required under Medicare. For example, hospitals seeking voluntary accreditation by the JCAH are required to maintain an effective ongoing quality assurance program.

While there is a consensus that these mechanisms, particularly PSRO, are intended to meet the goals described above, this consensus is an informal one and is to some extent contradictory. Though there are a variety of federal laws which address facets of quality assurance, there is no comprehensive statement on the subject, and there has been little public discussion of the overall purposes, intents, objectives, and methods that are currently in use. That analysis has yet to occur and, in fact, supports the need for a conference such as this. Yet today there seems to be a consensus emerging in this country that the quality of health care is legitimate regulatory issue. There continues to be controversy regarding how such regulation should be performed or who should perform it, but there is not much dispute that quality assurance is an issue of public accountability that should be subject to regulation.

The basis in law for federal hospital quality assurance requirements is derived from the financing programs. Historically, the passage of Medicare marked the beginning of full-scale federal intervention into inpatient quality assurance. It is through requirements relating to eligibility to participate in financing programs that federal quality assurance requirements have their effect. Even today, 10 years since the passage of Medicare, there is no statutory base that authorizes the direct federal regulation of quality. The Medicare Act itself requires that nothing in it be construed to interfere with the practice of medicine. Section 1801 of Title XVIII of the Social Security Act which authorized the establishment of Medicare states:

> Nothing in this title shall be construed to authorize any Federal officer or employee to exercise any supervision or control over the practice of medicine or the manner in which medical services are provided, or over the selection, tenure, or compensation of any officer or employee of any institution, agency, or person providing health services; or to exercise any supervision or control over the administration or operation of any such institution, agency, or person.

Yet, elsewhere, the Act requires that hospitals participating in the Medicare program must, as a matter of obligation, conduct ongoing utilization review to assure the necessity and quality of services provided and paid for by the program. Further, there are extensive additional requirements imposed on hospitals as conditions of participation that relate to organization and administration.

Thus, contained within the Medicare Act itself, are the very contradictions that today have yet to be resolved. In the following sections of this chapter, the impact of these contradictions on the efforts to conduct hospital quality assurance are examined. Over the past 10 years, considerable progress has been made in upgrading the quality of hospital care, yet there is reason to believe with resolution of some of these fundamental issues substantial additional improvement can still be expected.

ANALYSIS OF CURRENT REQUIREMENTS

Hospital Accreditation and Certification

The Accreditation and Certification Functions

Hardly any aspect of hospital operations, from the organization and responsibilities of its professional staffs to the methods for disposal of wastes, remains free from external controls imposed by public (official) and voluntary (professional) "approval" agencies whose purposes, ostensibly, are to maintain an acceptable level or improve the quality of patient care provided in the hospital. The discussion in this section focuses on the processes of accreditation, notably that of the JCAH, and on certification, as applied under the Federal Health Insurance for the Aged, or Medicare program.

Joint Commission on Accreditation of Hospitals (JCAH). Upon the establishment of the American College of Surgeons in 1913, the improvement of patient care in hospitals was advanced as an explicit goal.[1] The concept of hospital accreditation as a formal means of assuring quality hospital care dates back to 1918, when the American College of Surgeons inaugurated its Hospital Standardization Program.[2] This organization established a set of standards which put emphasis on records, medical staff organization, conferences for review and analysis of professional services, and clinical laboratory and X-ray facilities. The result of the first survey of hospitals in 1918 under this program pointed out the severe problem facing the nation at the time in the status of hospital care. Of the 692 hospitals surveyed, only 90 (or 12.9 percent) were approved. This small number so shocked the medical profession, hospital administrators and trustees, as well as the general public, that the College's program began to receive considerable support.

By 1950, of the 2,429 hospitals surveyed, 94.6 percent (2,297) qualified for approval. However, with the growth of the nonsurgical specialties after World War II, and with the general recognition of the success of the College's program of accreditation, it became clear that standards should be developed for the nonsurgical aspects of hospital activities, and that the approval program should be supported by the whole medical and hospital field. Accordingly, in 1952, the JCAH was established to take over from the American College of Surgeons the responsibility of the approval program. The sole purpose of this new organization was to encourage the voluntary attainment of uniformly high standards of institutional medical care. The founding sponsors of the JCAH were the American College of Surgeons, the American College of Physicians, the American Hospital Association, the American Medical Association, and the Canadian Medical Association. The Canadian Medical Association continued its participation in the JCAH until 1959, when the Canadian Council on Hospital Accreditation established its own program. Although the standards established by JCAH were directed to minimal achievement, in terms of the essential supportive elements of the hospital, accreditation served as a yardstick to those institutions that wished to achieve a level of care set by a professional and nationally recognized voluntary organization.

The objectives of the JCAH, which have served as its fundamental guidelines since its creation in 1952, are: (1) to establish standards for the operation of hospitals and other health care facilities and services; and (2) to conduct surveys and accreditation programs that will encourage members of the health professions, hospitals, and other health care facilities and services voluntarily to: (a) promote high quality of care in all aspects in order to give patients the optimal benefits that medical science has to offer; (b) apply certain basic principles of physical plant safety and maintenance, and of organization and administration of function for efficient care of the patient; and (c) maintain the essential services in the facilities through coordinated effort of the organized staffs and the governing bodies of the facilities.[3]

The standards which the JCAH has established for hospital accreditation cover virtually all facets of hospital operation. For example, standards have been prescribed for the physical plant and environment, including its safety, functional efficiency, and salubrity; its organizational form and administration; the organizational form and responsibilities of the professional staffs, including policies and procedures for the rendition of services; personnel qualifications; equipment; etc.[4] The assumptions underlying these structural-process criteria are that they can serve to measure and indicate the capacity of the institution to provide good quality care and that if prescribed form and procedure are complied with, then the professional judgments and actions made in this environment will have the best chance of being optimum. The revised JCAH hospital accreditation standards, published in 1971, updated in 1973, and currently again being modified, reflect new and intensified attention to form and procedure, and more explicit concern about the assessment, through medical peer review processes, of the quality of medical services rendered in the institution.

Although the JCAH standards are comprehensive in scope, and despite the demonstrated efforts to strengthen them, the requirements continue to be minimum. Significantly, however, at least one state (New York) requires JCAH accreditation for licensure purposes, and in some states, third party payors, such as Blue Cross, also require accreditation as a condition for reimbursement.

On-site inspections of hospitals seeking to be accredited or re-accredited by the JCAH are performed by staff employed by the organization. Prior to 1961, when the JCAH began to develop its own field staff, the accreditation surveys were conducted by representatives of three of the member organizations, concurrently with their performance of other functions on behalf of their organizations. Currently, the Commission employs a full-time field staff of approximately 49 full-time and 28 part-time[5] surveyors who visit approximately 2,600 hospitals annually. A survey fee was established in 1964 to make the field program self-supporting. The survey fee is based on the number of hospital beds; the average cost per surveyor-day is approximately $450. Depending on the size of the institution, an accreditation survey may take between one to three days. For teaching hospitals of 500 or more beds, the surveys are conducted by a team comprised of a physician, nurse, and hospital administrator. Other hospitals are visited by a two-person team comprised of a physician and a professional nurse, or a hospital administrator. In January 1976, JCAH proposes to have, on a trial basis, a three-person team visit each hospital.

The findings made by the survey team are recorded on a survey report form keyed to the accreditation manual (standards) and are discussed with appropriate key hospital staff. The approach used is a consultative, educational one. The documents in which survey findings are recorded are not released to the institution involved, although findings and recommendations are subsequently communicated in writing to the hospital. Depending on the results of the accreditation survey, the hospital may be granted accreditation for either one or two years, or not be accredited. Because of insufficient manpower, JCAH is, generally, unable to make periodic followup visits to the hospitals once they have been accredited. Followup visits are made when the institution appeals the JCAH decision, or to investigate substantial, documented complaints about accredited facilities.

The JCAH consistently has safeguarded the confidentiality of the information obtained through the accreditation process, and this was one area in which the commission recently undertook legal proceedings against the Department of Health, Education, and Welfare (DHEW), in connection with that agency's program to validate JCAH surveys.

It should be pointed out that the accreditation requirements of the JCAH are applicable to all hospitals seeking accreditation, regardless of their size. The principles underlying the application of the standards are that the methods used to meet the requirements may vary with the type and size of the hospital, and that professional judgment must of necessity be used in dealing with individual cases. Where locally applicable governmental requirements are higher than those prescribed by the JCAH, these higher requirements prevail for accreditation purposes.

Certification of Hospitals Under Medicare. On the federal level, the Sheppard-Towner Act of 1921, the Social Security Act of 1936, the Emergency Maternity and Infant Care Appropriations Act of 1943, and significantly, the Hospital Survey and Construction Act of 1946, which fostered the development of state licensing programs, all served as stimuli to increase control and regulation of hospitals. The passage of Public Law 89-97, the Social Security Amendments of 1965, which established the Medicare and Medicaid programs, however, marked the beginning of augmented direct involvement of the federal government in the control of hospitals and other providers and suppliers whose services were covered under the programs.[6]

With the enactment of the Medicare law, specific statutory authority was provided, for the first time, to define and apply uniform national standards in order to ensure the Congressional intent that only those medical services that met professionally acceptable standards of quality would be paid for under the program. Significantly, in Section 1861(e) of the law, which sets forth the definition of a hospital, Congress prescribed some 10 fundamental, statutory requirements (e.g., that the care of every patient must be under the supervision of a physician, that professional nursing care be available 24 hours a day, seven days a week, that a medical record be established and maintained for every patient, etc.) which were mandatory for all hospitals seeking to participate in the Medicare program. Also importantly, the law authorized the Secretary of Health, Education, and Welfare to develop and apply other standards ("Conditions of Participation") that were deemed essential to ensure the health and safety of program beneficiaries and the quality of care rendered to them.

In addition to authorizing uniform national standards as a minimum for participation in the Medicare program, Congress also required the Secretary to use "willing and able" state agencies to "certify" that providers meet and continue to meet the conditions of participation.

Under Medicare, the term *certification process* is generically interpreted to include the standard-setting activities in the program; the application of standards to individual providers and suppliers of services by designated state agencies; the recommendation (certification) by the state agency to the Secretary that the provider/supplier is eligible for participation (i.e., reimbursement for covered services rendered) in the program, on the basis of having demonstrated compliance with the standards; and the approval of the provider/supplier for participation by the Secretary.

As suggested earlier, the general objectives of the certification program are to ensure that services reimbursed under Medicare meet professionally accepted standards of quality, and to safeguard the health and safety of program beneficiaries. The specific operational objectives of the program might include: (1) to establish and apply uniform national (minimum) standards as a means for determining the capability of providers and suppliers of services to deliver quality care; (2) through onsite inspection and survey processes, to identify the degree of compliance with the established criteria and the areas in which deficiencies exist; (3) through consultation, technical assistance, and other remedial efforts, to assist providers and suppliers of services to meet and continue to meet the prescribed standards; (4) to encourage providers and suppliers of services to exceed, whenever possible, the minimum levels of quality that have been specified for approval; and (5) to encourage states to adopt, where possible, standards which are higher than the minimum requirements prescribed by the Medicare program.

For independent clinical laboratories, extended care facilities (skilled nursing facilities), and home health agencies, the Medicare program provided an opportunity to break new ground in the definition of national standards for these categories of providers and suppliers of services. The law set no accreditation floor or ceiling in regard to the development of standards for these groups, and little was available in terms of licensing and accreditation criteria that could serve as guidelines for such development.[7]

For hospitals, however, the Congress made crucial decisions on the standards which determined the level at which these standards could be set. For example, Public Law 89-97 specifically recognized the accreditation program of the JCAH and required the Secretary of DHEW to accept JCAH-accredited hospitals as meeting all the conditions of participation, except those requirements pertaining to utilization review. (Hospitals accredited by the American Osteopathic Association also were deemed to meet all Medicare requirements.) Further, the Congress prohibited the Secretary from establishing for hospitals standards that exceeded those of the JCAH.

Upon an assessment of the JCAH accreditation requirements, it was determined that the accreditation standards were minimal and could be adapted for national application under the Medicare program. Accordingly, the Medicare conditions of participation for hospitals were drafted to be equivalent to those of the JCAH.[8] Like the comparable standards of the JCAH, the Medicare standards for hospital care require, to ascertain the institution's capacity to meet at least the minimum standards deemed essential to ensure an acceptable level of quality, and because of the subjective language in which the standards are written, considerable professional judgment and discretion in their application.

Like the hospital accreditation standards of the JCAH, the Medicare regulations for general hospitals cover virtually all aspects of hospital operations. There are some 16 separate conditions of participation (e.g., covering governing body and management, medical and nursing staffs and their responsibilities, physical plant and environment, dietary services, pharmacy, clinical laboratory and pathology services, etc.) which incorporate some 100 separate standards and several hundred factor items. Theoretically, it is assumed that conformance with each and every criterion will be assessed in determining the institution's compliance with the overall set of requirements.

As indicated earlier, the Medicare law prescribed that willing and able state agencies be delegated responsibility for applying the conditions of participation to individual providers of service participating or seeking to participate in the program. For the most part, these state agencies have been those units of state health departments which have had responsibility for conducting facility licensure programs. Indeed, in most states now, in order to reduce duplication of effort, maximize the use of personnel, and cut costs, one on-site inspection is generally conducted for purposes of both state licensure and Medicare certification. In order to be certified for participation in the Medicare program, individual nonaccredited hospitals, as well as other providers and suppliers of services, must undergo an on-site survey, or inspection, conducted by personnel employed by the designated state Medicare agency. A number of the state agencies delegate certain of the survey functions to other units of state government, and to units of local government. For example, fire safety considerations may be delegated to the state fire marshal, or to local official fire safety experts. Nationally, a wide variety of health personnel, including, for example, professional nurses, physicians, pharmacists, medical care and hospital administrators, medical records administrators, sanitarians, engineers, social workers, etc., are involved in the survey/certification process.

For the most part, state Medicare agencies employ the team approach in conducting the on-site surveys of facilities. The composition of the team is not standardized nationally, and these teams represent a heterogeneous mix of health disciplines. Predominantly, however, where the team approach is employed, the team is comprised of a professional nurse, sanitarian, and a hospital administrator. The team may also be comprised of "generalist" surveyors who have been trained (largely under DHEW auspices) to survey across the various areas of an institution; in most instances, these generalist personnel draw upon available consultant assistance in specialty areas. Nationwide, there are approximately 2,000 survey personnel who perform the onsite inspections for Medicare certification purposes. Of this group, approximately 50 percent are directly involved in surveying hospitals.

Equipped with the conditions of participation, related interpretive guidelines, and survey report forms, these state agency survey personnel spend an average of 12.5 hours (per surveyor) per hospital survey in assessing the degree of the facility's compliance with the prescribed requirements.[9] On the basis of assessing conformance with the various standards and factors which comprise a given condition of participation, the surveyor is expected to make a judgment as to whether that condition is or is not being met. In addition to checking a series of "yes" and "no," and "met" and "not met" boxes on the survey report form, the surveyor is expected to document, in an "explanatory statements" column, the rationale for the decision made.

A finding of noncompliance with any of the statutory requirements automatically results in the denial of the facility's eligibility for participation in the program. Further, eligibility can be denied (exclusive of noncompliance with statutory requirements) if the documented findings reflect that deficiencies constitute a serious hazard to the health and safety of patients. A hospital can be found eligible for participation, even when deficiencies may be significant (but not a threat to the health and well-being of patients), provided that an acceptable plan of correction is submitted and the facility demonstrates progress, over a prescribed time period, toward rectifying the problem situation. Hospitals, as well as other providers and suppliers of services under Medicare, are surveyed on an annual basis. Unlike the case for skilled nursing facilities, which may be certified for participation for periods under one year (through the mechanism of time-limited agreements), hospitals deemed to be in compliance with the standards are certified for a period of one year.

After the certification survey has been completed, the state agency forwards its findings and recommendations to the Regional Office of the Bureau of Health Insurance, Social Security Administration, for review. Professional staff of the Public Health Service, in an advisory capacity to the Bureau of Health Insurance, may also participate in the review process. The findings reported by the state agency, and as accepted by the Bureau of Health Insurance, are then reported in writing to the provider institution with recommendations regarding plans of correction, if indicated. State agencies are expected to monitor progress toward the correction of deficiencies, through periodic followup visits and contact, and to provide needed consultation and technical assistance in order to help the provider remove deficiencies and thereby advance toward compliance with the standards. Hearings and appeals procedures have been established for all categories of providers and suppliers of services to provide an opportunity for clarification or resolution of problems related to survey findings and certification decisions.

Assessment

JCAH Hospital Accreditation Program. The JCAH appears to have had a salutory influence on the improvement of hospital care in this country. Particularly in recent years, however, the JCAH hospital accreditation program has come under strong criticism, and charges of ineffectiveness and less than satisfactory progress have surfaced in both the public and private sectors. Many of the constraints which have served to limit the effectiveness of the JCAH program are not singular to this organization, but are shared with other voluntary and public standard-setting and approval programs, including the certification program under Medicare.

When Title XVIII legislation linked the Medicare hospital standards to the JCAH standards, accreditation became officially established as the norm for nationally acceptable quality. In effect, there no longer was an indicator of the "high quality" facility, since the minimum requirements prescribed under Medicare were equivalent to those set for accreditation by the JCAH. Further, because JCAH accredited hospitals were deemed to meet the Medicare requirements, and they were not subject to federal review except for matters related to utilization review, this linkage raised the issue of how much authority and responsibility can appropriately be delegated to organizations that cannot be held accountable to the public.

Public Law 92-603, the Social Security Amendments of 1972, removed the limitation that had been initially placed on the Secretary's standard-setting authority, in regard to his not being able to prescribe standards exceeding those established by the JCAH. Further, these amendments authorized the Secretary to arrange for state agencies to conduct on-site inspections, on a selected sample basis, of JCAH accredited facilities in order to validate their "deemed" status under the Medicare program. This validation activity has precipitated a number of volatile issues, which in essence represent a test of roles, responsibilities, and authorities between the private and public sectors. It has resulted in litigation and the interim suspension of such surveys by DHEW. Some of these issues include: (1) the validity with which the results of the survey process reflect the quality of care provided by an institution; (2) the rapidity with which survey measures are modified to reflect changing technology and practice; (3) the limitations in numbers and qualifications of those conducting the surveys; (4) the nature of the relationship which should exist between the Medicare and JCAH survey processes; and (5) under what circumstances and to what degree survey results should be considered privileged information.

Medicare Certification Program.   Although some would argue for hard data to substantiate the claim, it is our firm conviction that the Medicare certification program has had a salutary effect on the quality of hospital services delivered to all patients.   The significance of the federal/state presence in health facilities, both in terms of surveillance and consultative, supportive assistance, together with the incentive of federal dollars, cannot be disregarded.   Further, the program has contributed significantly to the upgrading of performance of state agency survey personnel through formal university-based and other programs of training and professional development.   The Medicare certification process is far from optimal, however, and we are acutely cognizant of the need for improvement of current operations as well as the need for defining, testing, and applying innovative approaches in our standard-setting and enforcement activities.

A continuing challenge in our standard-setting activity is to develop criteria that are appropriate, cogent, objective, and conducive to measurement of performance, and easily administerable. Although we have made some progress along these lines, the language of the regulations is still too highly subjective and conducive to misinterpretation. The validity of the assumptions underlying the rationale for applying a uniform set of criteria to a heterogeneous mix of facilities, such as hospitals, has not been rigorously tested. Our experience suggests that this approach has some merit, however. For example, well over two-thirds of the small hospitals, predominantly in rural areas, which initially were certified in a special limited access category because of their distinctive characteristics and deficiencies, have been assisted and upgraded to near full compliance with the regulations.

As indicated earlier, state agencies are delegated responsibility for applying the conditions of participation to the several categories of participating providers of service. Clearly, such delegation is in conformity with traditional intergovernmental relationships and has some advantages in terms of effectiveness for both federal programs and state government. For the states, the delegation of responsibility for selected aspects of the Medicare program has served to considerably strengthen their standard-setting activities. Of advantage to the federal programs is the state agency's cognizance of local needs and realities, and its ability to observe effectiveness first-hand. However, despite our efforts to improve the survey/inspection capabilities of the state agencies, through strengthened training programs for example, there remains a high degree of variability among the states in the application of program standards. Further, questions can be raised as to whether the state agency survey personnel truly strike a reasonable balance between matters of substance—e.g., the significant aspects of patient care rendered and environmental safety—and those items of lesser significance which are more process oriented—e.g., minutes of committee meetings, written procedures for staff, etc. In deciding whether to call something a deficiency, we wonder if surveyors generally apply the professional judgment needed to determine whether a particular situation bears a significant relationship to patient health and safety. We wonder, also, if surveyors by their "findings" and actions impress providers and stimulate them to achieve meaningful improvements in patient care, or whether the process results in a cynical or irritable response to standards enforcement, where the provider performs superficial motions and may not commit itself to achieving a meaningful or continuing improvement in things that really count.

Although considerable progress has been made in coordinating standards development and regulatory programs, the need for further improvement along these lines still remains. The lack of coordination among federal programs in regard to quality assurance dilutes the impact of the various programs on the health system and reduces the leverage of these programs for accomplishing federal health objectives. This lack of coordination and duplication of effort among standard-setting agencies in the public and private sectors is inefficient and wasteful of limited resources. In the area of fire safety, for example, many of the problems are directly related to conflicting requirements of various federal programs. Because of differing interpretations of requirements, a facility constructed under the auspices of one federal program (e.g., Hill-Burton) may be denied approval/certification by another federal program (e.g., Medicare/Medicaid) unless excessive costs are incurred to comply with the requirements of the latter agency.

Policy Issues

Looking ahead to national health insurance, the challenges at this juncture are to determine: the fundamental essentials of an effective standard-setting and enforcement system; the extent to which the federal government should coordinate or direct such a system; and the alternative approaches that might be pursued. Some specific policy issues are given below.

The Nature of the Standards. Accreditation and certification have used the approach of minimum-level structural-process standards, on the assumption that, at the time of the approval survey, capability to perform at a level considered the minimum acceptable provides a high probability of continuing acceptable performance. Capability does not necessarily guarantee satisfactory performance, however. The relationship between structural-process standards and quality outcomes has not been adequately determined, and while performance and outcome measurements may be more promising, more research and evaluation in these areas are needed.

Another basic policy issue is whether standards for providers and suppliers of services should be uniform nationally in terms of the level of quality required, or whether the standards (and hence the quality) should vary geographically in accordance with local and regional capabilities. Clearly, the ability of providers/suppliers of services to meet standards ensuring capacity to deliver an acceptable quality of care varies greatly. If even minimum standards are set too high, and if providers/suppliers are unable to meet these requirements, citizens will not have access to the care to which they are entitled under the federal program. If standards are set at the level of the lowest common denominator, providers/suppliers will lack motivation to exceed these requirements and to provide care of high quality.

If one of the standard-setting objectives of federal programs is to set minimum requirements to ensure against outright poor quality, the question can be raised as to the appropriateness of the federal government's setting requirements which exceed the accepted minimum. Theoretically, this should be the role of the professions and their representative voluntary professional organizations. If the latter default, however, can the public sector appropriately remain complacent when it is responsible and accountable to the citizenry whose interest it is supposed to safeguard? In lieu of exploring and testing potentially feasible alternatives, the federal approach has been to maximize the authority for standard-setting, and the result has been the proliferation of higher requirements which are developed within and appended to the frame of the underlying standards system. The issue then becomes whether this is rational and whether it serves any real purpose in terms of quality where there are serious questions about the foundation upon which these additional requirements have been built.

Clearly, the quality standards must be appropriate and reasonable, and reflect a sense of practical reality. In the area of manpower, for example, where shortages are reported in virtually every category, the requirements should not constrain these limited resources, and career mobility should not be blocked. Without sacrificing quality, personnel requirements must be sufficiently flexible to allow for maximum utilization of available health manpower. In accordance with authority provided under Public Law 92-603, the Social Security Amendments of 1972, the department is currently administering proficiency examinations as a means of qualifying under the Medicare/Medicaid regulations certain categories of health personnel who do not meet the formal education and training requirements prescribed in these regulations. While the methods used to design these examinations have been tested as part of the examination development process, no external validation has been performed to confirm the validity of the examinations and to ensure that only those who are truly qualified are identified.

Limitations of the Survey/Standards Enforcement Process. The Medicare program has established uniform national minimal standards, but the application and enforcement of these standards vary widely, given that over 50 separate jurisdictions (state Medicare agencies) are involved in the certification process. The issues are related to the classic problems of decentralization *vs.* centralization. States continue to have difficulties in attracting the number and quality of personnel essential for the conduct of effective survey programs. Misinterpretation of the regulations/standards and deficiencies in survey techniques continue despite significantly strengthened efforts to train state agency surveyor and supervisory personnel. The findings obtained through federal monitoring and surveillance of state agency performance (e.g., through biennial administrative program reviews) reflect that states continue to have many of the same administrative and programmatic problems year after year, despite federal remedial assistance efforts.

The Medicare standards establish minimum requirements for a heterogeneous mix of facilities within the specified provider/supplier category. All providers and suppliers meeting these requirements, and thereby certified for participation, are reimbursed for all covered services rendered, regardless of the degree to which they meet the prescribed standards. Facilities that are judged to be demonstrating a higher level of performance than others are not rewarded for this achievement; in effect, there is no financial incentive for improved performance and the correction of deficiencies. Legislative authority for varying conditions of participation for providers rendering different types and levels of services is provided in the Medicare law. It is not clear, however, whether there is current legislative authority to limit the reimbursable services under Medicare in accordance with the specific set of conditions of participation met by the provider. If such authority does not exist, the question is whether it should be sought or whether the federal role should be confined to the establishment and enforcement of minimal standards, with more optimal standards being developed by private organizations.

Public vs. Private Roles. As has been noted, with the exception of the assessment of compliance with utilization review requirements, JCAH accreditation has allowed a hospital to be certified for participation in Medicare. Further, the standards established for both programs are virtually identical. Thus, hospital accreditation/certification represents a situation where there has been an active attempt to merge an important public and private regulatory process.

The findings of validation surveys conducted as a result of requirements of the 1972 Social Security Amendments have substantiated the congressional concerns about this relationship. Are the interests of the public and private sectors different enough to warrant a separation of the surveys processes? Does the fact that the JCAH process is primarily educational and the Medicare process dependent upon the ultimate sanction of nonparticipation make the two processes different enough to warrant their separation? Therefore, is it necessary to explore the feasibility and cost/effectiveness of establishing not only a minimum set of standards but also an additional, graded, set of more optimal standards which are designed to help guarantee the delivery of quality medical care? If this approach seems to have merit, is it appropriate to view the federal responsibility as the establishment and enforcement of compliance with the minimal standards, and that of the private sector as being to define the optimal standards and conduct for the education and training necessary to move toward their achievement?

Medical Care Review

History

The health professions have traditionally concerned themselves with assuring that their individual practitioners deliver necessary care which is of high quality. This has been accomplished in a variety of ways including licensure, control of privileges, specialty certification, and review by peers of actual performance. Medical societies and hospitals have created committees which have the responsibility for performance of these functions.

With the advent of widespread third party involvement in the financing and reimbursement for health care, mechanisms began to develop which were designed to assure that care provided to individual patients was medically necessary—the intent being that the use of limited resources be constrained by the parameters of medical necessity. The need to construct such mechanisms has been increasingly apparent as the costs for health care have continued their remarkable rise.

Parallel to and often overlapping with this recent effort to rationalize the utilization of services has been a significant increase in attempts to create formal mechanisms within the hospital to assure that high quality care is being provided. This has been spurred, in large measure, by a growing log of case law which has concluded that the hospital, as a public institution, has a public responsibility to assure the delivery of high quality care. The board of directors of the hospital is identified as the group responsible for assuring the existence of quality assurance mechanisms. This, coupled with the widely accepted notion that the results of performance analysis should be used when making determinations of hospital staff privileges and when designing the topics for the wide variety of hospital continuing education activities, has resulted in quality assurance being considered, at least conceptually, as a major focal point of activity of a hospital.

Thus, the last decade has seen rapid evolution of the traditional concept that the medical professions are responsible for assuring the adequate performance of their peers. Government at the federal and state level, the courts and voluntary agencies such as the JCAH have generated significant external pressure on the profession in this regard. This has been reflected in development of a wide variety of guidelines, rules, and regulations and with them a plethora of enforcement mechanisms.

Predictably, this has resulted in resentment, confusion, tacit and active noncompliance, and lack of uniform success. By way of illustration, the current requirements for a hospital with regard to medical care review are outlined below. Also discussed are the enforcement procedures used. These discussions will be used to highlight the major public policy issues related to the regulation of the quality of health care.

Medicare

Since the inception of Medicare, a hospital has been required, as a condition of program participation, to conduct utilization review. The objectives of such review are to assure that hospital level care is medically necessary and that the quality of care meets the expectations of the medical staff. To accomplish this, a committee must be formed (either external or internal), and a plan for the conduct of review developed. In this plan the committee defines how it will accomplish a review of admissions and conduct medical care evaluation studies (medical audits).

By the early 1970s it had become apparent that utilization review (UR), as required in Medicare, had not successfully met its objectives. The review was often conducted in a pro forma manner, and there were few, if any, examples of true success. Recognizing this, Congress developed major changes in the review requirements which were enacted as part of the 1972 Social Security Amendments. The major substance of these amendments as they related to UR was that UR, as it had traditionally been performed, was abandoned to be replaced by review conducted by local PSROs.

Recognizing that widespread implementation of the PSRO program would take time, Congress also enacted changes designed to upgrade the UR conducted prior to PSRO. Uniformity in methods between Medicare and Medicaid became a requirement. Medicare mechanisms were to be used in both programs unless a State Medicaid Agency could demonstrate that it had a superior system in operation. Further, for Medicaid, DHEW was required to reduce its payments to states found out of compliance with utilization control requirements.

These general statutory requirements were given more detail in DHEW regulations which required concurrent review of all admissions and periodic review (on a concurrent basis) of the appropriateness of continued hospital stay. While these regulations are currently being rewritten, the basic requirements for admission and continued stay review and medical care evaluation (MCE) studies will not change. Only the required methods by which these reviews are to be accomplished will undergo alteration.

In addition to these UR requirements, Medicare, Medicaid, and PSRO require physicians to periodically certify the need for a patient's continued stay in a hospital. These certifications were designed to provide additional assurance that care provided in the hospital was medically necessary by periodically focusing the attention of the attending physician on the need for continued hospitalization.

As discussed above, hospitals and physicians must comply with a number of federally developed requirements if they are to participate in the Medicare program. These include the requirements for UR and physician certification. The principle method used to assess compliance with these requirements is an annual survey made by agencies of each state government. These are broad-ranging surveys in which the hospital's organization, operation, and physical plant are inspected. The survey covers such diverse topics as compliance with fire codes, architectural requirements, quality control of clinical laboratory operation, and compliance with the UR and physician certification requirements. The surveyors spend only one or two days in each facility. For UR they examine the hospital's review plan, the frequency of UR committee meetings, the attendance at the meetings, and whether the committee conducted admission review and MCEs.

To assess compliance with physician certification requirements, the surveyors check to see if certifications were conducted on the required days of hospitalization. As noted above, the survey teams do not have the training and expertise necessary to determine if UR had been conducted in an effective manner or if problems identified by review had been acted upon. For physician certification, the surveyors are not trained to determine if certification was appropriate in individual cases. Thus, compliance with the only mechanisms which require physicians to directly review the medical necessity and quality of their care is determined by personnel trained and qualified only to assess whether the processes occurred and not whether they were performed in the right instance or conducted effectively. Further, despite the fact that most compliance with requirements for UR and physician certification is *pro forma,* a hospital has never been barred from participation in the Medicare program because of lack of compliance. This may be appropriate because in these requirements we may have a classic case of an attempt to shoot a fly with a shotgun. The treatment is too potent for the disease. As will be discussed later, we must move toward the point where compliance with requirements for health care assessment is enforced by methods which follow the maxim—"First, do no harm."

Medicaid

UR became a requirement in Medicaid in 1967. State agencies are required to develop a UR plan for each type of service provided by the state program (e.g., hospital care, drugs, etc.). Because the states were given great latitude to design their review mechanisms, there is a wide variety of plans in existence. The 1972 Social Security Act Amendments recognized need for Medicare and Medicaid to be compatible and mandated the use by Medicaid of the Medicare UR structure and methods. There was provision, however, for the use of a Medicaid review system for both Medicare and Medicaid if the Medicaid system was found to be superior in effectiveness.

For a variety of reasons, this required compatibility between Medicare UR and Medicaid UR has not yet been achieved. Thus, in several states, hospitals continue to either conduct separate internal (medical staff) UR for Medicare and Medicaid or conduct internal review for Medicare and external state agency review for Medicaid.

Mechanisms to assess compliance with Medicaid UR requirements vary from state to state. In some states the mechanisms link with the results of the Medicare survey, while in others an independent survey is conducted. In many states there is no attempt to assure compliance.

For some hospitals, additional survey burdens were added by Section 207 of PL 92-603 which required a substantial decrease in federal payments to those states found out of compliance with Medicaid UR requirements. To implement this requirement, DHEW surveys are conducted by DHEW Regional Office staff. These surveys concentrate on: (1) the degree to which the state's written UR plan conformed to statutory requirements; and (2) the degree to which selected hospital's review complied with statutory requirements. As with the Medicare survey process, the intent was to determine compliance with structure and process measures. No attempt was made to assess the impact of compliance on patient care.

Professional Standards Review Organization (PSRO)

As noted above, the 1972 Social Security Act Amendments contained provisions to upgrade utilization review and created PSROs. It was envisioned that, in most areas, the new UR requirements would be implemented prior to PSRO. Further, the law required that PSRO review replace UR when a PSRO was found capable of conducting effective review. The UR regulations were designed, therefore, in close conjunction with PSRO guidelines to help assure a smooth transition from one to the other. It was further envisioned that this transition would be enhanced by the requirement that PSROs utilize the services of those hospitals with the capability to conduct effective review.

Because of this close link between PSRO and UR, the review required in each program is similar. Despite this, however, when viewed from the hospital's perspective, the transition from UR to PSRO will be a confusing one. Some of the reasons for this will be outlined below.

The PSRO program represents a major shift in the locus of reponsibility for review of Titles XVIII and XIX patients. Whereas the vast majority of hospitals under both Medicare and Medicaid retained this responsibility as part of the activities of their medical staff, in PSRO the responsibility shifts to an external organization.

Even this shift, however, will be an involved one because of the requirement that PSROs "utilize the services of and accept the findings of" hospital committees which the PSRO feels are capable of conducting review effectively [Section 1155(e)(i)]. This requires the PSRO to enter a formal process in which it solicits from each hospital in its area an expression of interest in conducting review under delegation. For all interested hospitals, the PSRO must assess the past performance and current capability of the hospital and judge whether or not it appears capable of conducting PSRO review. As part of this process, the hospital must submit a review plan to the PSRO. The PSRO will then use predetermined criteria, known to each hospital, to help it make its determination. A hospital may conduct either concurrent review, MCEs, or both. When delegation does occur, the PSRO will continually monitor the performance of the hospital and may modify its delegation decision as appropriate.

Whether review is delegated or not, the PSRO will require the collection of a common set of data on all patients. New mechanisms will be required to assure that the decisions of PSRO review are meshed with the claims submission process. The PSRO will focus much more attention on the need for hospitals to conduct effective discharge planning. Site visits will be made by the PSRO to examine individual medical records and to observe and evaluate the review process. The PSROs will generate profiles of the care provided in individual hospitals and will expect the hospital—through its organized medical staff—to examine and correct any deficiencies which may be found. While MCEs will be required of each hospital, the PSRO will often coordinate the performance of an MCE across several hospitals—a process which has rarely been attempted in the past.

Responsibility for enforcement of PSRO program requirements will also shift. Medicare intermediaries and Medicaid state agencies will monitor PSRO review but only in an advisory capacity to the DHEW central and regional offices. Staff in these offices will focus their attention on PSROs rather than hospitals. The manner in which this will be accomplished and the consequences of poor performance have yet to be detailed.

Despite the fact that PSRO unifies the review required for Medicare and Medicaid, it does not cover the large number of patients whose care is financed by other means. While this will occur in some areas, it will take new legislation—most likely as a part of national health insurance—to mandate total patient coverage by PSROs. Thus, a hospital may be subject not only to PSRO review requirements but to the requirements made by other financing programs. While such requirements are not currently prevalent, the rising cost of care is likely to result in their development in the near future.

Joint Commission on Accreditation of Hospitals (JCAH)

Over the last decade, the JCAH has given much more emphasis to the manner in which the hospital conducts medical care review and the way in which review results are used to determine staff privileges and orient continuing education efforts. As previously noted, this has been prompted by two forces: (1) the court decisions which rest responsibility and legal accountability for the performance of quality assessment with the hospital; and (2) provisions of the PSRO law which require the PSRO to delegate review to hospitals proven capable of conducting such review.

The new effort by the JCAH has resulted in policies requiring that a minimum number of MCEs be conducted by each hospital. Not only has the JCAH changed the number required, but their requirements have never been the same as those required by either Medicare under UR or by PSRO. Further, it is not clear that MCEs done for PSRO purposes would count on a JCAH tally. Finally MCEs for JCAH purposes must cover all patient groups, but PSRO requires MCEs only for Medicare, Medicaid, and Title V patient groups.

Much of this confusion results from apparent differences between DHEW and the JCAH on the most appropriate manner in which to conduct MCEs. DHEW accepts a wide variety of approaches. The JCAH had conducted a large educational campaign designed to instruct hospitals on one particular way to conduct MCEs. While there are conflicting statements from the JCAH on whether other methods of review will "count," there has never been a firm statement discussing the relationship between PSRO, MCEs, and the JCAH requirements.

Hospitals, then, are in the position of trying to deal with varying MCE study requirements—both in terms of number and methods—and this has significantly slowed the momentum previously generated for the performance of MCEs.

Except for UR results, the survey process of the JCAH has been accepted for Medicare certification purposes. Survey for compliance with UR requirements has always been a function retained by the state survey agencies. Thus, a JCAH accredited hospital would be certified for Medicare only if it was found by the state survey process to be in compliance with UR requirements. Of the approximately 7,000 hospitals, over 5,000 are JCAH accredited. Thus, each of these hospitals is surveyed by the commission for accreditation purposes a minimum of once every two years and surveyed at least annually by the Medicare State Agency for UR. As indicated earlier, no hospital has ever been denied Medicare certification on the basis of noncompliance with UR requirements. Though JCAH accreditation is voluntary, it is required by any hospital which wishes to be approved as a teaching institution. Finally, in some states, hospitals must receive either JCAH accreditation or submit to a state inspection if it is to be licensed.

Public Policy Issues

While there are a number of public policy issues which could be discussed in the context of a discussion of utilization control and quality assurance, the focus will be on four issues which directly impact hospital review efforts. These are:

1. Variation in Review Requirements, Compliance Measures, and Enforcement Mechanisms;
2. The PSRO-Hospital Relationship;
3. Limitations of Health Care Review Methods;
4. Cost Containment *vs.* Quality Assurance.

Variation in Requirements, Compliance Measures, and Enforcement Mechanisms

Currently hospitals are obliged to comply with medical care review requirements imposed by Medicare, Medicaid, and possibly by other third party financing agencies if they are to be reimbursed for the care provided to their patients. In addition, the JCAH requires performance of medical review as a condition of accreditation. The lack of uniformity in these requirements may only, in part, be solved as a PSRO assumes responsibility for Medicare and Medicaid review.

Also, the survey process which is used to judge compliance with these requirements is fragmented such that, to a large extent, each program conducts its own independent assessment. The replacement by PSRO of UR will relieve a hospital of only a small part of the Medicare survey process. In fact, the relationship established between a PSRO and a hospital will be much more complex and involved than that which currently exists between a hospital and the state survey agency. Further, PSROs will not replace the vast majority of the JCAH survey process.

Finally, the sanctions for noncompliance with UR requirements will continue to differ somewhat, despite the fact that the PSRO legislation provides for uniform Medicare and Medicaid sanctions. It also appears that, because the ultimate sanction for noncompliance will continue to be decertification or nonaccreditation, sanctions will continue to be an ineffective tool to encourage compliance. Ongoing operation of a patient care facility will, and always should, receive priority over enforcing review requirements. Thus, as it relates to the assessment of health care, a hospital is compelled by outside agencies to comply with a wide variety of requirements, submit to a number of surveys, and face a variety of sanctions all designed to help reach common goals shared by both the hospital and the agencies—the provision of medically necessary, high quality care.

That confusion and resentment result from this fragmentation is certain. The extent to which it detracts from the effective performance of medical care review is unknown as is the means by which a more rational system of requirements and enforcement techniques could be developed and accepted.

The PSRO-Hospital Relationship

As was discussed above, court cases have established the fact that the board of directors of a hospital has overall responsibility for assuring the quality of care which is provided in their hospital. Major efforts have been mounted in the private sector to help assure the fulfillment of this responsibility. While the UR regulations by and large are consonant with the view that the internal organization of a hospital is responsible for the review of care provided in that hospital, the PSRO law potentially confuses this relationship.

Section 1155(e)(1) of the PSRO legislation requires that review be delegated to those hospitals found capable by the PSRO of effectively conducting review. It is clear, however, that, while delegation will occur, the overall responsibility for the continuing effectiveness of review rests with the PSRO. Because this is true, the PSRO, both in instances of delegation and nondelegation, is responsible for assuring that when ineffective or inefficient review does occur, necessary changes are instituted.

Thus, with the implementation of PSRO review in an area, two focuses of responsibility exist for each hospital as it relates to medical care review—the PSRO and the board of directors of the hospital. Each has legitimate responsibility to assure that medically necessary care of high quality is delivered to the patients in that hospital. What has not been explored is the manner in which both can effectively assume their responsiblity. Some have suggested that at least in those instances where PSRO review is not delegated, the hospital continues to be responsible for creating its own internal review system. This approach would create duplication of effort and potential conflict between the hospital and the PSRO.

What precisely are the objectives of PSRO review and the review required of a hospital to meet its public responsibility? Do they differ to the extent that each must establish its own review, or are there potential areas of common purpose which will allow an integrated PSRO-hospital review program?

Limitations of Health Care Review Methods

As has been mentioned, the tremendous pressure to implement hospital quality assurance is a phenomenon of the last decade. It has been spurred by a variety of forces: the rapid rise in hospital costs; the belief that there is a significant amount of unnecessary care being provided in hospitals; evidence that the quality and efficiency of hospital care needs improvement; and the desire to fulfill a public responsibility to assure the quality of care. Therefore, the objectives established for hospital quality assurance vary widely. These diverse objectives will not and cannot be met in total by any current methods of review.

Even if the objectives can be brought within reasonable bounds—to assure that hospital care is medically necessary and of a quality which is locally acceptable—the ability of current review methods to meet them is unproven. It has not been proven, for example, that: (1) concurrent review consistently results in the provision of only medically necessary hospital level of care; (2) medical care evaluation studies can result in enduring change in physician or institutional behavior; and (3) profile analysis can consistently identify problems of high priority which can be addressed by more detailed review.

In addition to these limitations in review methods, much more work must address the question of incentives. What are the incentives or disincentives necessary to ensure that quality assurance is viewed as an important, ongoing responsibility of health professions and health institutions? How can these pressures be best applied—by the hospital, health professionals, the public, or all three?

Finally, more appropriate methods to assess compliance with review requirements need to be designed. The currently fragmented survey process must be changed, and one which can focus on the key measure of review system effectiveness must be produced.

Cost Control vs. Quality Assurance

There has been a great deal of debate concerning the principal objectives of UR and PSRO. Some say they are oriented to cost control, while others view them as mechanisms to assure quality. The existence of such debate again highlights the need to more clearly articulate program objectives. Outlined below is our perception of PSRO and UR objectives. This chapter later discusses the steps necessary to obtain broad consensus on these objectives and move toward their realization

PSROs are given circumscribed authority. They are empowered to review the care provided to Medicare, Medicaid, and Title V patients, as well as to determine: (1) if the care provided is medically necessary; (2) if the quality of care meets locally accepted standards; and (3) if the care is to be or was provided in the most economical setting consistent with the health care needs of the patient. Experience from similar past efforts indicates that, at least for the first year or two, PSROs will decrease the number and possibly the length of hospital admissions. This should result in cost savings which may or may not be recognizable, as they are mixed with the multitude of other factors which influence the level of health expenditures.

Further down the road the net impact of PSRO review on expenditures is less predictable. This is particularly true when it is realized that the emphasis of PSRO review will probably change with time.   Currently, PSROs focus considerable attention on the necessity for hospitalization.   As the maximum impact of such review is reached, PSROs will address problems with less impact on health expenditures, such as case finding and under-utilization of hospital services.   If they find unmet health care needs which are then addressed, the result will be an increase in expenditures.   What effect medical care evaluation studies, especially when they include review of ambulatory and extended care, will have on the long-term health of the population and the resultant change in levels of disability is unpredictable and possibly unmeasurable.

In summary then, PSROs and all other health care review mechanisms that have been established, have limited, albeit important, authority.   In ex-ercising this authority health professionals will broadly assess the quality of care provided by their peers.   They will specifically assess the medical necessity of care, the degree to which the health care process and its outcomes comply with local expectations and the appropriateness of the setting.   Thus, PSRO review directly addresses the quality of patient care.   The impact such review will have on health care expenditures is unpredictable and is likely to change with time.

If quality improvement rather than cost control is the fundamental objective of PSRO review, what then is necessary to reach broad-based acceptance of this objective with the commitment necessary to have a fair chance for its realization?

CONCLUSION

It has been the intent of this chapter to examine the public policy issues having to do with current inpatient quality assurance programs and their potential for national health insurance.   The goals and objectives of voluntary and government quality assurance programs have been described. The extent to which these goals are being achieved has been examined.   The barriers that prevent the promise of quality assurance programs from being achieved have been analyzed.   The overlapping, inconsistent, and fragmented nature of the current requirements with their heavy emphasis on procedural and paper compliance has been described.   By examining their impact on hospitals, several major public policy issues have been identified.   If the potential of quality assurance programs is to be realized, these issues and others like them must be addressed and consensus reached on their resolution.

Analysis of these issues reveals that there continues to be debate over the fundamental issues of the role of government in quality assurance.   There is not agreement as to the extent and appropriateness of that role.   Each of the major public policy issues requires debate and discussion alone and in relation to the others. In order to make this debate productive, the public mandate for quality assurance requires re-examination. The prohibition against interfering in the practice of medicine contained in the original Medicare Act should be reviewed in the public forum of the legislative process so that a consensus can be achieved regarding the extent to which government is to regulate the quality of care.

Once the public, profession, and government achieve a workable consensus, the Medicare prohibition can be revised and replaced with a mandate that does not contain the contradictions inherent in today's program. Then, against this framework, each of the quality assurance public policy issues can be researched and evaluated. As a result, quality assurance requirements and programs can be revised and tested in time to be relied upon as a major regulatory mechanism in national health insurance.

NOTES

1. John D. Porterfield, "The External Evaluation of Institutions for Accreditation," in *Quality Assurance of Medical Care,* Regional Medical Programs Service, Health Services and Mental Health Administration, U.S. Department of Health, Education, and Welfare, Washington, D.C., February 1973, p. 111.

2. The discussion on the evolution of the Joint Commission on Accreditation of Hospitals has been extracted from: Pearl Bierman; Beverlee A. Myers; Douglas G. Weir; John Rodak; and Jay S. Reibel; "Standards and Methods: Development and Effects," an unpublished position paper prepared for the Secretary's Advisory Committee on Hospital Effectiveness, Standards and Methods Branch, Division of Medical Care Administration, U. S. Department of Health, Education, and Welfare, November 1, 1967, Appendix, pp. 3-4.

3. Joint Commission on Accreditation of Hospitals, *Accreditation Manual for Hospitals,* (Chicago: Joint Commission on Accreditation of Hospitals, 1973), p. 1.

4. Porterfield, *op. cit.,* pp. 113-114.

5. The JCAH field staff complement (as of November 1975) is distributed as follows: physicians—19 full-time and 19 part-time; hospital administrators—21 full-time and 4 part-time; and professional nurses—9 full-time and 5 part-time.

6. Bierman *et al., op. cit.,* Appendix, pp. 1-2.

7. John W. Cashman and Beverlee A. Myers, "Medicare: Standards of Service in a New Program—Licensure, Certification, Accreditation," *American Journal of Public Health,* Vol. 57, No. 7, July 1967, pp. 1109-1100.

8. *Ibid.,* p. 1108.

9. Division of Provider Standards and Certification, Bureau of Quality Assurance, Health Services Administration, U.S. Department of Health, Education, and Welfare, *Inventory of Health Care Facility Surveyors, United States—1974,* DHEW Publication No. (HSA) 75-6503, 1975, p. 56.

Chapter 4
Inpatient Quality Assurance from the Viewpoint
of the Private Physician

Kenneth A. Platt

This chapter is designed to present inpatient quality assurance from the perspective of the private physician. It is not meant to present a consensus viewpoint since, at the present time, a consensus is hardly feasible in the turmoil and controversy which swirls around a formalized peer review and utilization review mechanism. It will, however, present a broad stroke overview of inpatient quality assurance as viewed from the private sector and contain an attitude and an approach which represents the views of a significant majority of the private physicians working in the sector of utilization review and quality assurance. The chapter is in large part a personal perspective gleaned from several years of working in this field and of discussing the problems with many people throughout the country who are interested in a form of public accountability such as that formalized in Public Law 92-603, signed in October of 1972. This law presented the health professions with a "new game in town." It was "new" in the sense that it formalized utilization review (UR) and quality assurance, and held the profession publicly accountable for quality assurance and utilization of health care facilities paid for by the public sector.

Before we can really discuss the rules and regulations of the "newest game in town," we must ask why, indeed, this occurred. Is it a unique situation in which the health profession has been singled out by the public and held publicly accountable for the funds expended in that sector? Or, is it merely part of a broader trend throughout the country and, indeed, throughout the world in which social conscience, public awareness, and public accountablility are being increasingly demanded, not only of the service sector but of the manufacturing sector of the world's economies?

Thomas Mann rhetorically said, "One looks at revolution and calls it progress; one looks at progress and calls it tomorrow." Certainly we are living in a time of social revolution, world-wide in scope, and with as yet undetermined consequences. A basic tenet of many oriental religions is that change is the only constant. Change that evolves slowly and with rational planning is acceptable to most of us. However, change which is rapid and often accompanied by violence or inflammatory rhetoric is frequently met with resistance and fear. The pace of change in the world-wide community has now reached a dangerous velocity and has been accompanied by war, political assassination, and military coups with repressive measures as a frequent outcome.

Some feel that the United States remains the only country with the political institutions capable of adjusting to the increased pace of social change without suffering the agony of violent revolution. Certainly, our Constitution and political systems have been put to the test over the past two decades and have served us well, thus far. We have already gone through two centuries of dramatic change. Our country was born in a revolution concerned mainly with change in the conduct of government. That revolution, as history shows, was successful, and representative democracy replaced a less responsible parliamentary monarchy.

In the succeeding 100 years, this country was largely preoccupied with establishing territory through westward expansion and in settling its internal conflicts of Federalism vs. States Rights through debate, political maneuvering, and finally in the white-hot crucible of civil war.

Following the Civil War, a second century began which was largely devoted to advanced technology, the industrialization of society, the exploitation of vast resources, and the creation of an affluence unparalleled in the human experience. It seemed as if there was no end to the golden dream of collective and private wealth, and materialism became the goal rather than the reward of much human endeavor.

Walter Reuther is said to have remarked, "The beauty of America is that the pie is constantly enlarging and each one's share enlarges with it." No one can say for sure when this phase of our revolutionary society ended, but I would suggest that this end occurred in the 1950s and the early 1960s when we entered the current phase of our continuing revolution. It is a phase marked by a vast set of social changes as we try to adjust to a plethora of domestic problems.

The affluence we enjoy has created the demand that it be more equitably shared. As a result, the number of transfer payments by local, state and federal agencies has multiplied like rabbits over the past two decades. Racial and sexual discrimination has been attacked on many fronts but has largely been handled by the courts through such mechanisms as busing, fair housing laws, and job guarantees. Consumerism is the rage of the moment, as the public demands a more active role in guiding its destiny and protecting its future.

A natural outcome of such rapid social change with its attendant conflicts has been a skepticism toward our most venerable institutions and a cynicism as to their capabilities to adjust to the pressures of our times. The family has been declared passé; religion has been removed from the classroom; politicians have suffered from an eroded image climaxed by presidential disgrace; and the military has lost its hero status by failing to win its last two wars. We are a nation faced at the present time with a recession, diminishing resources, inadequate energy supplies, and a blurred vision of our "manifest destiny." Confronted with problems of this magnitude, is it any wonder that sincere, dedicated citizens are questioning the capability of our institutions to survive?

Viewed from this perspective, we can arrive at a more rational understanding of the problems confronting the health industry. Certainly we too have been enamored in the past with our expanding technology. In the space of some three or four decades, medicine has literally conquered most infectious diseases, largely eradicating the scourges of smallpox, infantile diseases, and other significant problems such as tuberculosis, pneumonia, etc. The physician has advanced from the horse and buggy, circuit rider type of practitioner to a superb, technologically trained individual capable of transplanting or replacing worn-out organs or vessels. We are making steady progress in researching the problems of aging and of cancer, and may be on the threshold of breakthroughs in these areas potentially of equal significance. Should this occur, the likelihood of prolonging useful life would be greatly enhanced, and the quality of life, which is indeed related to good health, would be improved.

The general public through the media of television, the popular magazines, and the daily newspapers, has become better informed on the capabilities of medical technology to prevent or to adequately treat many of their medical problems. They also have become painfully aware of increasing costs of this applied technology and are concerned about their ability to purchase it, either individually or collectively. Exposed to the political debates raging in many quarters as to medical care as a "right" instead of a "privilege," the public is understandably unwilling to be denied the benefits of sophisticated care merely because of a personal inability to purchase it.

Such concerns have not escaped the attention of many powerful political figures who have added their voices and legislative clout to the current debate. Thus, medical care has entered the center stage on the domestic scene and promises to remain so for the next five to 10 years. This country, during that time, will be developing its own unique medical care delivery system, designed to take care of the problems as perceived by the public and the public's representatives, but leaning somewhat upon the experiences of other countries of both the western and eastern hemispheres, and upon the problems already confronting our health care delivery system and its federally funded programs.

RESPONSE OF MEDICAL PROFESSION

Faced with an expanding technology, inflationary costs, a sometimes hostile political environment, and rising consumer expectations, the medical profession has responded in diverse ways. One would like to say that it has been uniformly positive with a coordinated, constructive, and cooperative approach to commonly perceived problems. Such a response has, of course, not been forthcoming, and it would be naive to expect it. The health professionals are, after all, merely a highly trained segment of our general society and, as such, as diverse in their opinions as any other segment.

Such diversity of opinion carries over not only into the solution of the problems confronting the medical care delivery system in this country, but even to the perceptions of the problems themselves. Some maintain that a crisis exists in one area or another of the system. They cite manpower figures, maldistribution of specialties, lack of primary physicians, over-bedding in hospitals, etc., as flash points in the smoldering fires of public controversy. Others maintain that no true crisis exists, either in total or in part, and that the solutions to our problems lie in less governmental tinkering and larger doses of the status quo. Happily, the truth, as usual, lies somewhere in between these extremes, and more and more dedicated, concerned professionals are striving for the middle ground.

It has become apparent to many in the medical profession that their traditional medical society structure is somewhat inadequate to address these largely social and economic problems. Medical societies are traditionally organized to further the exchange of scientific knowledge and to promote the social amenities peculiar to a highly technical profession. They were never meant to be active in the truly socioeconomic arena or to serve in an advocate role in a rapidly changing social scene. Perceiving this, a new mechanism was sought by the professions through which they could respond to the concerns of the day.

In the 1950s, the Foundations for Medical Care were formed as the profession's answer to this dilemma. Largely a California phenomenon, the foundations recently have spread rapidly across the country under the increasing pressure for public accountability. It would be less than candid not to admit that it was largely the advent of consumerism with its attendant demands for public accountability that spurred the rapid spread of the foundation movement.

In 1972, Public Law 92-603 formalized congressional concerns about public accountability by the medical profession for the federal dollars spent in such programs as Medicare, Medicaid, and Maternal and Child Health. The Professional Standards Review Organization (PSRO) program was created as part of this law and opened to mixed reviews. Viewed by many as a graphic illustration of further governmental encroachment on the physician-patient relationship, it has been actively opposed by some concerned professionals since its inception. Others have viewed it as a mechanism by which they can participate actively in the evolving national health care delivery system, and as merely a more formal mechanism of peer review with which they were already familiar. Again, the truth lies somewhere in between, with the perils of governmental interference in UR and quality assurance plainly visible and potentially dangerous. Despite these potential dangers, the program affords the profession the unique opportunity to participate in designing and implementing proper utilization and quality assurance mechanisms against which their practices will be judged.

The implementation of the PSRO program has been slow and halting. Many of its problems have resulted from lack of experience with such a formal mechanism of peer review and from such common political realities as under-funding and the usual territorial disputes. Implementation is proceeding at an increasing tempo as the profession and the federal agencies develop a better understanding of their respective roles. Although we will ultimately address the problems of skilled nursing facilities and ambulatory review, the initial and current emphasis has been on inpatient utilization and quality assurance mechanisms in the acute care institutions across the land. It is this arena, and the role of Foundations for Medical Care and the private physician in designing and implementing the review processes in such institutions, that concern us here.

Concern with the quality of care, like most things, is not new. Alexander the Great is quoted as saying, "I die by the help of too many physicians." Although most of us are concerned with the quality of medical care delivered to the public, there is no unanimity of opinion as to how to measure it. Much of the initial effort in the PSRO field has been concerned with utilization review, which has, at best, only a modest quality assurance aspect to it.

One of the chief indictments of the PSRO program by the physician community is that its main thrust is in the cost containment area, and certainly UR has a cost control flavor to it. To the general public and to their elected representatives concerned with the spiraling costs of medical care, the emphasis on outpatient *vs.* inpatient care has a natural appeal and explains their fascination with UR to begin with. It is relatively easy to measure and to regulate, when compared to the more difficult task of quality measurement.

Admission certification, length of stay review, and discharge planning are familiar guideposts in assessing provider and institutional performance. This familiarity is comforting in these uncertain times. To the practicing community, however, UR is synonymous with cost containment and not related to quality. They feel that so far, the PSRO program has paid only lip service to quality assessment and thus are beginning to demand a more valid indication of concern about quality of care.

Accepting for the time being the emphasis on UR, what about the future? When and how will quality of care be measured, and who will do the measuring? What role will the practicing physician play in setting quality standards by which his practice is judged, and to whom is he accountable? Where does the consumer fit into the evaluation of the quality of care he receives for his specific problem, and what measurements are available to him in making his judgments? How confidential are the results of quality evaluation, and what role will these results play pro and con in the current malpractice problems? Will quality standards lead to "cookbook medicine," in which a physician uses the guidelines as a defensive maneuver? These are all current and vital considerations in the quality of care discussions and are addressed briefly before the specifics of a quality assurance mechanism in the acute care institution are discussed.

The emphasis at the present time under the PSRO is on UR in the acute care institutions. The emphasis is a natural one—firstly, because UR is more readily measured; secondly, because there is a cost containment mechanism in UR and control; and thirdly, because the question of quality assessment or measurement of quality of care is as yet a controversial one with the actual measures needed to assess quality of care under intense study.

Most physicians are familiar with the audit method of assessing the quality of care rendered within their institutions. This is mainly a retrospective assessment of the care rendered to an individual patient and is frequently process oriented. Tissue Committees, Departmental Audit Committees, and Executive Audit Committees are familiar turf to most of us and pose little or no threat.

The newer methods of evaluation of the quality of care rendered by using comparative criteria and standards are somewhat experimental and, therefore, highly controversial. Although the criteria used are broad screens and designed largely to raise questions rather than to provide answers, many physicians view them with concern, afraid that they may result in stereotyping care and contributing to a median area of mediocrity known as the "safe zone." Safety in this case means that if one conforms, one is not hassled by the reviewing authority and, indeed, can point to his dutiful adherence to previously determined criteria as proof of his competency.

Although there may be some validity to these fears, they are greatly exaggerated and arise from unfamiliarity with criteria and their intended usage, rather than with the results of current quality assessment programs. It is mandatory, however, that the criteria be developed locally and by competent professionals well-respected by their communities, and that they be used as screens rather than definitive measurements of quality. To do less is to fortify the critics of the current quality assessment programs and will result in increasing resistance by the profession.

In the future, the emphasis on utilization review will diminish, and it is likely that UR will become oriented to spot review, such as a certain percentage of all incoming cases; to problem review both as to problem providers and problem diagnoses; and to institutional review on a more local basis, based upon deviations of the institution's profile when compared to its peers. Program emphasis will shift from UR to more direct measurement of the quality of care rendered to the patient population. The practicing physician, as has been previously mentioned, must be actively involved in setting the quality standards by which his practice is judged, and basically this extends not only to setting the screening criteria for utilization review, but to the more definitive criteria for quality assessment. He will be held accountable ultimately not only to his peers, but to the public through the local PSRO, or more directly from the Bureau of Health Insurance, Social Security Administration, or even the Secretary of Health, Education, and Welfare, should PSRO fail.

CONFIDENTIALITY PROBLEMS

Another concern in the current program implementation is the confidentiality problem, both through the individual provider, institution or patient profiling, and through the action taken by the reviewing program on any individual case. This concern revolves around several sensitive areas such as:

1. The release of sensitive data about a patient's illness or his emotional status.

2. The misinterpretation of deviation from the published criteria implying either incompetency or malpractice.

3. An interpretation by the patient when notified of an adverse decision by the reviewing authority that this denotes either incompetency or malpractice by his attending physician. This will be an especially sensitive issue if the patient is given the specific criteria and standards upon which an adverse decision was based.

4. The possible use by a plaintiff's attorney of the deviation from published criteria and standards as evidence of malpractice, despite the disclaimer that they are intended only for screening and not as definitive measurements.

5. The problems that arise from the fact that more and more details about a patient's private life are being stored on computers and even with unique

identifiers and scrambled codes. The details are potentially open to disclosure by unauthorized individuals.

6. The very definite possibility that some or all the information stored in an individual provider's profile may be subject to subpoena and admissible as evidence in court.

Having stated the concerns, how about the remedies? It is obvious to those who work daily with the problem that information gleaned from data must be strictly confidential. Despite obvious political pressure for public disclosure of at least the institution's comparative profile, this must be resisted. This is not a matter of whitewashing the guilty or protecting the incompetent, but an essential part of obtaining factual data upon which accurate profiling can take place and upon which objective decisions can be made.

If we then keep the data gathered under the various quality assurance programs confidential, how does a patient evaluate the quality of care he receives? Unable to judge the care rendered by process, he is most likely to judge it by end result. Since this is subjective to a large degree and dependent upon many factors such as the mood of the patient, his rapport with the provider and the institution, experience in previous medical care situations, the time of assessment, etc., it will differ from the objective criteria method of quality assessment and, thus, may not correlate with the program evaluation.

What may appear to be good care by the process measurement and with an adequate or even spectacular outcome may appear to be a dismal failure when evaluated by the patient. Those who have tried to measure quality from the patient's perception have found that the overall level of the patient's satisfaction with the care rendered was related to the amount of information he received. Changes in the patient's response because he knows he is being evaluated may cause these responses to inaccurately reflect the patient's real opinions and distort the assessment outcomes. Certainly, this is an area where more study is needed to accurately evaluate quality of care from the perception of the patient who receives that care.

When one considers all the problems associated with the quality assessment of health care, such as confidentiality, data collection, profiling, criteria development, process vs. outcomes measurements, concurrent assessment vs. retrospective audit, medical care evaluation studies, and provider education, one wonders whether it is possible to adequately carry out this program.

Having detailed some of the problems of profiling, criteria, confidentiality, and patient evaluation, let us now turn specifically to quality assessment in our acute care institutions from the viewpoint of the practicing physician and the organizations he has formed to represent him, such as Foundations for Medical Care. What is their current role and what may it be in the future? How do the Foundations for Medical Care movement and the private physician relate to the federal and state agencies under the current program, and how do they relate in turn to acute care institutions in doing inpatient evaluation? There are many public policy issues implicit in the formation of quality assurance mechanisms for the inpatient population. Some of the more important ones may be stated as follows:

1. Should the care rendered in any single institution be the sole responsibility of that institution's medical staff, or should it be done by outside reviewers or be subjected directly to outside evaluation?

2. Who pays for such review?

    a. The programs for which review is done as a recognized reimbursable expense, billed for and collected by the institution?

    b. The agency responsible for such review activities such as the PSRO?

3. Should we separate utilization review, which is essentially a cost containment mechanism, and assign this responsibility to an organization such as the PSRO and leave quality assessment to the individual institutions, as in the quality assurance program of the American Hospital Association?

4. What is the best method for dealing with the problems that are discovered in the assessment process in order to improve the care rendered?

5. If the medical care evaluation (MCE) studies' approach, as currently envisioned by the Joint Commission on Accreditation of Hospitals (JCAH) and the PSRO is to be effective as a quality assessment tool, who should initiate the studies? Also, who should develop the criteria for carrying out the studies, and who should assess their impact on inpatient care?

The Foundations for Medical Care vary in their approach to inpatient review in the acute care setting. Many of the early entrants into the PSRO program established outside review authority with complete assumption of the review mechanism. They, with few exceptions, hired and trained the nurse coordinators, educated the physician advisors, and gathered and stored the data obtained from the patients' charts through the abstracting process. Screening criteria were developed independently, although a certain amount of cross-pollination obviously took place. Convinced that the loyalties of the nurse coordinators to the PSRO were strengthened if they were employed by the organization itself, PSRO tended to look upon delegated review as potentially "incestuous" and subject to divided loyalties.

More recently, Foundations for Medical Care have been developed entirely as a response to the PSRO law and have initially delegated all or almost all of the review process to the acute care institutions in their areas of responsibility. This has been partly a philosophical decision but, more importantly, is based on the hard economic facts of life under chronic, under-funding of PSRO. Whether or not the results of total delegation will compare favorably with nondelegation or partial-delegation is as yet conjectural but fascinating.

REVIEW PROCESS

Initially, the controversy in the review process arises at the moment a patient is admitted or considered for admission to an acute care institution. The first decision is whether a pre-admission certification process should be instituted or whether post-admission screening will suffice. If a pre-admission screen is set up, should it be only on elective admissions, or should it concern itself with the urgent or emergent admissions? From the private physician's viewpoint, any pre-admission screen is viewed as an unwarranted interference with the physician's right to decide what is best for his patient. Tested recently in the utilization review (UR) regulations suit brought by the American Medical Association against the Department of Health, Education, and Welfare (DHEW), the rulings currently handed down make this process, at this time, a moot subject with few, if any, pre-admission screens under the federal programs.

However, there is a great deal of interest in screening out such things as unnecessary surgery prior to the admission to the hospital. Certain studies done under union programs have suggested that as many as 25 to 30 percent of elective surgical procedures may not be done if mandatory consultation takes place prior to admission. Although this is not as yet widespread, it may become so if only as a cost savings mechanism by the carrier. Certainly, there is a quality element to this type of pre-admission review, since prevention of unnecessary surgery would also prevent inevitable complications.

If pre-admission screening is moot at this point, what about post-admission certification within the first 24 hours or the first working day thereafter? This is done now largely by the nurse coordinators using previously approved professional guidelines. When necessary, advice is sought from the physician advisor regarding doubtful cases prior to rendering an appropriate decision, with whatever dialogue is necessary taking place between the physician advisor and the attending physician.

Here again, there is a tenuous, but definite quality aspect to the review process. Anyone in an institution for tests or therapy that could be done as easily and appropriately in an outpatient setting should be discharged from the institution. This would prevent the occasional mishaps to this patient group such as acquired infections, errors in medication, the disorientation of the elderly, falls from bed/chair, etc. Once again, physicians view this as an unwarranted intrusion into the physician-patient relationship and feel indignant when informed that the program will not assume fiscal responsibility for further care. In actual practice, however, the percentage of patients affected by the 24 hour screen is quite small, but the profession's concern about its necessity persists. This aspect of review is a clouded issue because of the recent AMA-DHEW litigation.

The most significant part of the review process from the utilization aspect is the length of stay assignment and concurrent stay monitoring. This is a time when utilization and quality become entwined, and when the likelihood of quality impact could conceivably be the greatest. Given a well-trained, well-intentioned nurse coordinator and an astute and sensitive physician advisor, working with well-documented, essential criteria, a reasonably objective evaluation of the care being rendered could be obtained. Since this is a concurrent evaluation, change could be implemented at a time when it would have its greatest impact—i.e., during the actual care of the patient rather than by retrospective analysis following discharge.

This is an extremely sensitive area in which to work and could be a source of real concern by the attending physician as far as direct interference in the physician-patient relationship is concerned. Retrospective audit of the patient's care is the most widely used method of quality evaluation in most acute care institutions today. Audit studies are not new and have been a source of information gathering for educational as well as disciplinary acts for years. Under Medical Care Evaluation Studies mandated by the PSRO and the JCAH, a new impetus has been given and some promise for improving care in the future has been shown.

They may be generated by the staff of the institution concerned about a specific problem identified by their own audit, or identified for them by the PSRO. Using criteria developed internally, the data necessary to carry out the study can be generated and the results analyzed. The presentation of the final outcome to the general staff or specific staff department is an educational process for all concerned, and followup studies to evaluate impact on future performance are mandatory. Most private physicians will accept this type of evaluation and actively participate in the program. Genuinely concerned about the care their patients receive, private physicians have real concern about their performance as compared to their peers. How much of an impact the results of these MCEs will have on their long-term performance is still open to question, with some studies suggesting that the impact is of short duration with old habit patterns soon returning unless continuous monitoring takes place.

MCEs may also be generated by the PSRO as single or multiple institutional projects or even regional or state-wide in scope. These may be generated by apparent problems discovered in the monitoring process or may be motivated by scientific interest in specific areas of medical care or medical epidemiology.

For the first time, a specific organizational entity, the PSRO, has been charged with the responsibility of monitoring MCEs in its area of concern and for keeping its member institutions aware of reduplication of effort and/or of significant outcomes of the studies completed. Although the PSRO does not serve any direct role as an educator, it can coordinate and direct the existing educational mechanisms in order to address the problems elucidated by the studies.

DATA GATHERING

The final step in the current approach to UR and quality assurance mechanisms in our acute care institutions is post-discharge abstracting and data gathering. In the institutions whose admission rate for the Medicare/Medicaid programs is of sufficient volume to justify a full- or part-time coordinator, the abstracting process falls naturally in their job description. For the smaller urban and rural hospitals, a member of the hospital staff usually associated with the medical records unit must be trained to do the job. Both groups do an excellent job, and the data collected appear to be reasonably accurate.

One of the chief obstacles to timely accumulation of data is the delay in obtaining a final diagnosis from the attending physician. In our experience, it takes approximately six months to obtain a 95 percent sample for truly valid data. Since the required Professional Management Information System (PMIS) does not allow such a time lag, it may be necessary for the review coordinators to insert a final diagnosis for those abstracts over 30 days old. With proper training, these should be reasonably accurate, although not ideal. The data collected from these abstracts will form the basis for decisions regarding utilization patterns and MCEs. Quality elements are conspicuous by their paucity in these early abstracts and report forms. The initial emphasis is, again, on admission and utilization rates and patterns, length of stay data, percentage of denials, etc. Once again, the private sector of medicine views this as further proof of an undue emphasis on cost containment rather than quality assurance.

As these programs mature, it will become increasingly important to shift the emphasis to data elements having to do with quality such as the use of ancillary facilities in a sequential time frame; the treatment patterns and time instituted; drug action and interaction; outcomes measurement both by professional and patient standards, etc.

Having briefly touched on the present approach to utilization review and quality assurance under the governmental programs such as the PSRO program, what about the private sector? Are we creating a two-class inpatient population—those formally reviewed because they are governmentally subsidized, and those not reviewed because they are covered by private, third-party payors or are self-insured? The Health Insurance

Association of America has been concerned about this possibility for some time. They have both an altruistic and a pecuniary concern about the problem.

There is the potential, of course, for reducing both the number of inpatients admitted under Title V, XVIII, and XIX, and shortening their average length of stay. Although no hard and fast data as yet are available, early analysis in our state suggests that this is, indeed, happening. It would appear from the very early and as yet inconclusive analysis of the utilization patterns in the Colorado Medicaid Program, that both the admission rates per 1,000 eligibles and their average length of stay has diminished approximately 11 percent. If this is factual, then the hospitals are facing diminished revenues from the public sector in a highly inflationary time. Since they have fixed costs not directly proportional to bed utilization, there is a fear that the private sector will have to carry a heavier burden in the form of increased charges. There is also the obvious altruistic concern with the two-class inpatient population—is it fair to spend tax payers' money on a very formal, highly sophisticated monitoring of the tax subsidized patient, and at the same time not expand the same programs to cover the tax payer who funds them?

Most private physicians are concerned with this problem and feel the entire inpatient population should receive equal attention. The Health Insurance Association of America supports this view, and is encouraging its members to work with the Foundations for Medical Care and the PSRO to broaden the review to include the private sector.

The responses to this suggestion have varied from carrier to carrier and from area to area. Some carriers have embraced the Foundations for Medical Care concept and promoted peer review and UR as an accepted item of expense in their insurance contracts. Industry is beginning to accept the need for quality assurance and utilization screening as testified to by such programs as those of Inland Steel, Samsonite Luggage and Motorola, etc. Gradually, the concept of utilization review and quality assurance as a part of the total health care package of insurance benefits is being accepted.

This is not to suggest that all the critics have been stilled nor the skeptics convinced. There is still a great deal of wait-and-see on the part of industry, and the insurance companies, and no one can fault them for this. Those of us who have been working in this field for some time now can quote cost figures for ambulatory and inpatient review based on current procedures. We can describe in glowing terms the potential in both control of over-utilization and the assurance of quality. However, much of what we honestly believe is as yet hard to document and must be taken with a measure of faith.

The extension of this review process to the entire inpatient population, however, is inevitable, and time is the only criterion. Certainly, if national health insurance becomes a reality, the population covered by the federal programs will expand enormously. The private carriers, faced with increasing pressure at the state and local levels to institute UR procedures and quality assurance methods, will have to accept the concept in some form or another. Whether they elect to contract with Foundations for Medical Care, the PSRO, or go their own way is not as yet fully determined. Given a climate of mutual concern and cooperation, however, it would seem natural to use existing mechanisms.

We have taken a look at the philosophy of UR and quality assurance, and at the pros and cons of the existing programs. It is obvious that these are elaborate programs, complete with bureaucratic, data processing, and educational costs. It is impossible to do an adequate job "on the cheap." The question then arises, how will these be funded?

The choices under the PSRO program lie between total line item funding as a part of the annual federal budget, with all costs flowing through the PSRO; a continuation of line item fundings, and in addition, direct reimbursement for a portion of the UR costs by the Bureau of Health Insurance and the State Departments of Social Services directly to the acute care institutions; and finally, reimbursement for the cost of UR and quality assurance by the governmental funds and private carriers as a reimbursable expense with the funds flowing through the PSRO to pay for the program in both delegated and nondelegated hospitals. Although this decision is still pending, some problems with each are readily apparent. If all costs flow through the PSRO as a line item in the annual budget, the program stands a good chance of slow starvation. Any line item is obvious to both supporters and opponents of the program and subject to all the political pressures and tradeoffs of any other item.

Given the current economic and political climate, it is unlikely that adequate direct funding will be readily obtainable. If this is true, then what about the combination of direct funding for certain common costs such as central administration, data processing and reporting, elements of common training and education and technical assistance, and indirect funding to the acute care institutions for the cost of the nurse coordinators, physician advisors, appeal mechanisms, and MCEs from the federal health trust. Certainly, it is an established fact that UR is a reimbursable item under current governmental programs, and tapping the trust funds would ensure a more stable level of reimbursement from a less obvious source.

There are certain drawbacks to that approach, however, which have created a great deal of concern amongst some Foundations for Medical Care and their PSRO counterparts. Although part of the concern is undoubtedly due to the matter of "territorial imperatives," much of it is genuine concern about the question of adequate and timely reimbursement to the institutions by the trust funds and the Medicaid State Agencies and of the difficulties potentially created for the PSRO in maintaining a uniform and responsive program without direct fiscal responsibility for the entire program.

It would seem from the viewpoint of the private sector, charged with the responsibility of the success or failure of these utilization review and quality assurance programs, that compromise is a necessity. Let the funds from all sources—i.e., direct budgetary funds, trust monies from the Bureau of Health Insurance, and cost reimbursement by the private carriers—be funneled through the PSRO which would then be fiscally responsible for the program in both delegated and nondelegated hospitals. This would guarantee reimbursement to the institutions on a timely and equal basis, while allowing the PSRO to maintain a uniform program with common training of nurse coordinators, physician advisors, appeals committees, etc., as well as to ensure the program against the problems of divided loyalties amongst the program participants.

The final outcome of this public debate on the funding mechanism for the PSRO will have a great impact on how well the program functions and how responsible it is and to whom.

Finally, no discussion of quality assurance in our acute care institutions would be complete without a brief look at the politics involved. On the local level, there is a fear by the private physician and the individual medical staffs that this mechanism will become too federally dominated. The charge is frequently leveled at those involved in program implementation that the private sector is merely setting up the control mechanism by which the federal government will ultimately dominate both utilization and therapy with an emphasis generally on cost containment. Undue emphasis on cost, it is felt, results inevitably in poor medicine, practiced in inferior institutions by indifferent physicians. These are genuine concerns not generated as a self-protecting mechanism but out of fear of what medicine may be like under total federal domination.

A common criticism is directed at the use of criteria and standards as accepted indices of quality care or utilization patterns. The fear is deeply rooted in a mistrust of governmental motives with the specter being raised of using these criteria and standards as a cost control device if the federal government takes over the program and develops national criteria. Although some reassurance is possible by pointing out the dominant position given the practicing community under the current Professional Standards Review Organization Law, critics are quick to emphasize that the final arbitrator is the Secretary of Health, Education and Welfare, and that laws can be both amended and appealed given certain political pressures.

In addition to local concerns, the problems of dealing with the carriers, state departments of social services, state health departments, hospital associations and other providers, the medical schools, and others further complicate the implementation of these review entities. Various aspects of these problems are given detailed analysis in other chapters. It will suffice to say that early dialogue and direct participation by elected representatives of these groups are essential to a successful program.

Chapter 5
Inpatient Quality Assurance Activities: Coordination of Federal, State, and Private Roles—The Hospital's Views

David M. Kinzer

MY OWN BIASES

Starting with the positive, and also the personal, I will state my own views about the Professional Standards Review Organization (PSRO) program—views that I held when the law passed and views which I still believe. I think it has a potential for improving the quality of medical practice in our hospitals, a potential greater than what has been accomplished under such "voluntary" accreditation programs as Joint Commission on Accreditation of Hospitals (JCAH), or from the multiple voluntary reporting services using data that permits institutional comparisons, or even from numerous continuing education programs of the specialty societies, our medical schools, and others. Having the force of law and the power of economic sanctions, no matter how much they are used, does give us a totally new frame of reference for validating medical (and hospital) performance. A lot of people don't like this, but it is still difficult to argue convincingly that something like PSRO wasn't needed.

More specifically, I am interested as a hospital person in the positive things that can happen through the exercise of PSRO's power to give delegated status to hospitals. Assuming the criteria for delegation will be sufficiently challenging and exacting, we can make the job of the hospital administrator a good deal less frustrating and maybe have better hospitals, too. The core problem in hospital administration over the years has been trying to persuade medical staff to do certain things because the hospital is at risk if they don't. These things might include keeping medical records current, getting voluntary staff to take their rotational assignments in the emergency room, and more recently, seeing that the recertifications for Medicare patients are done on time. The recent history of hospitals in this country is replete with examples where the hospital becomes the loser when an individual medical staff member fails to deliver on a responsibility—a failure that does not put the physician at risk. The difficulties of having medical staff discipline are often compounded by an attitude that is still widespread in the medical profession—i.e., that the hospital through its board has no "right" of discipline, and that this "right," if it belongs anywhere, is an exclusive province of the medical staff. The administrator's problem is compounded further in situations, widespread in this country, where the same specialist is on three or four different hospital staffs. Too threatening an approach, or even too much jawboning, poses the risk that the physician in question will depart the scene and take all his future admissions to the other hospitals.

With this problem in mind, delegated status looks like it might have helpful results. My assumption is that there will be, under PSRO, strong incentives for medical staffs to do the things needed to achieve delegated status. The incentive is to escape the unknowns, and potential dangers, of peer review by anonymous and possibly unqualified external sources. Peer review within the hospital is a known and therefore more comfortable quantity. It also seems more workable and effective, or at least it can be. Peer relationships have their most productive results in practice settings, such as in a good hospital or a well-organized medical group practice.

In short, delegated status under PSRO will give the board and the hospital administrator a "handle" to achieve a level of medical staff accountability that heretofore did not really exist. The potential positive impact of PSRO on quality of care is much more significant than its potential for saving government significant amounts of money. But more about that later.

THE MAIN PLAYERS IN PSRO
AND WHO THEY PLAY FOR

Since the passage of P.L. 92-603 with its Bennett Amendment, the scenario of implementation has been fascinating to behold. My position as a representative of the agencies most vitally affected (or economically punished) by the law has obliged me to watch these developments closely and at least try to understand them, if not influence them. As an individual who is totally unqualified to sit on a review panel and knows it, I still feel a heavy responsibility to do what I can to make PSRO a credible and effective process. My frustration, which is shared by all the administrators of hospitals I represent, is that under the law hospitals are granted a voice in PSRO only if the medical leadership of the PSRO decides to give them one. It is not a secure position, but it is the law.

What has been most fascinating about the implementation scenario is that it has surfaced all of the competing vested interests affected by the program in ways which have sharply identified their diverse and contrasting perceptions of PSRO. For anyone familiar with the medical care scene, all of these interests or concerns were easily identifiable in advance of the passage of the law. The three-plus years of effort to make PSRO operational only serve to emphasize the problems that confront implementation of this kind of law.

Federal Government

For government, the hope is to save money and lots of it, under Medicare, Medicaid, and Title V. Improving quality of care would be a welcome dividend, too, but nobody on the hospital side is deceived about the primary motivation that produced the votes that passed this law. It was the pure fright about mounting hospital care expenditures and the sense, still growing in legislative circles, that any idea with any potential for diminishing the outflow of government health dollars is worth a try. A corollary of this, which seems just as indisputable, is that, if the program doesn't prove to be as a big saver, legislative and executive support (and appropriations) will soon diminish.

There are also distinctions in government motivation, depending on the level of government and between affected and involved government agencies. At the federal government level there has been continuing and predictable hassling between BQA, OPSR, BHI, and SRS* to get and stay on top or at least maintain their identity and autonomy. We also have the predictable drive from involved bureaucrats at the federal level to maintain maximum control over what happens locally. After all, the "feds" are putting up all of the dollars for the program.

State Government

At the state government level, there is a significantly different perception. The drive for states' rights is already evident in Medicaid where program administrators are showing notable reluctance to sign the memoranda of understanding that will give Medicaid review responsibilities to the PSROs. Their problem is that big chunks of state money are involved, and they fear the consequences of turning over to essentially independent physicians' organizations total power to decide on how this benefit money is to be spent.

Consumer

On the consumer side, the voice of Ralph Nader has already been heard and will be heard again and again. The question that arises here, of course, is how to give the consumer a voice in decisions that vitally affect his welfare

---

* Bureau of Quality Assurance, Office of Professional Standards Review, Bureau of Health Insurance, and Social and Rehabilitation Service.

but which involve professional judgments that are beyond his capacity to second guess. At the root of this is a longstanding and deeply held suspicion that all medical organizations are essentially mutual protection societies. Consumers are already raising the issues of how the PSRO will affect their rights to privacy, their right of access to now privileged information about specific physicians and hospitals, their right to know what's in their own medical records, and how to make a PSRO publicly accountable for its performance, which must somehow be accomplished since tax dollars are involved.

Health Planners

The health planners have interests that resemble those of the consumers. The Comprehensive Health Planning (CHP) agency types, soon to move over and become the Health Systems Agency (HSA) types, view the PSROs with suspicion. They see the PSROs as groupings of doctors "doing their own thing" and not subject (and glad of it) to consumer control. In health planning, of course, consumer control is an established reality. Looking ahead just a little bit, battles for turf between the HSAs and the PSROs are totally predictable. Because the enabling acts for the two programs specifically establish their independence without defining their interdependency, confusion seems certain to reign. Because utilization control is so relevant to planning decisions, the HSAs will be dependent upon the PSROs for vital input. It seems safe to predict that the HSAs, with their consumer-dominated boards, will be insistent that PSROs be responsive to their interests and needs. Trouble looms just around the corner here, in view of the heavy bias in medicine against health planners.

Blue Cross and Blue Shield

For Blue Cross and Blue Shield there are specialized concerns. As the predominant Medicare intermediaries and with increasing involvement in Medicaid and with their own millions of subscribers, Blue Cross and Blue Shield feel that they have to be a major player in the PSRO game, if someone would just let them be. One of their points is that they helped pioneer UR in hospitals. They know a lot about its strengths and weaknesses and have in their data banks a wealth of baseline information that PSRO badly needs as a point of reference. Like state government, they also have some fears about turning over to independent organizations, whether they be PSROs or medical care foundations, any real control over how their subscriber dollars are spent. They at least don't see their claims review rights and responsibilities being abrogated very soon. In fact, in the context of national health insurance (NHI), their push has been to expand their intermediary roles so that they can be something more in the NHI world than a passer or processer of government dollars and claims. Though PSRO does not apply to private health insurance or prepayment, Blue Cross and Blue Shield view it as the handwriting on the wall for control programs that ultimately impact all patients. In other words, Blue Cross and Blue Shield have a huge stake in what happens with PSRO. It is, of course, interested in the most effective possible utilization controls, but there are few plan administrators who as yet feel really comfortable with PSRO as the appropriate vehicle for accomplishing this.

Commercial Health Insurance

For commercial health insurance, as represented by the Health Insur.nce Association of America, the main interest is to get a "seat at the table" whenever a seat is offered. They, of course, are officially enthusiastic about PSRO for whatever its spillout effect might be on their own claims costs, but they feel as protective of their own claims review prerogatives as does Blue Cross. As a competitor of Blue Cross, they have another concern that is relevant to PSRO—they don't want Blue Cross to have a favored position with PSROs as a data processor or informational or technical resource because this can give Blue Cross additional competitive advantages.

Medicine

For medicine it is a considerable understatement to say that the perceptions of PSRO are mixed. We must start with the individual medical practitioner. His entire training and professional conditioning has as its central theme the predominance of his individual judgments on what is best for his patient. If he is a good physician, he knows these judgments are usually better than any that can come from a committee of peers, if only because he knows his patient's problem in more depth, which of course is his professional obligation. If he is a good physician, his concern for the welfare of his patient also overrides external economic considerations. It shouldn't surprise anyone that this individual is suspicious of PSRO and of the UR regulations from the Social Security Administration (SSA). He has deep misgivings, both instinctively and scientifically based, about the "norms, standards, and criteria" now being generated by these programs. He is suspicious, too, of the motives of the physicians and the bureaucrats now waving the PSRO banner. It all smacks of an effort to control his life and his livelihood. If he is heavily immersed in his practice, the whole business of PSRO seems peripheral and unreal.

For political medicine, as represented by the American Medical Association (AMA), the individual characterized above is the predominant force. The split in AMA is not between those who are for or against PSRO; it is between those who are against PSRO and want to fight it openly on principle and those who are also against PSRO but want to accommodate it as a matter of political prudence. The schizophrenic resolutions passed by AMA are adequate testimonials to the depth of medical feeling on this issue. I really don't think you could assemble a group of physicians in any part of the country, including the groupings that have signed up with PSRO, and find a majority on a closed ballot referendum who really believed in the program.

There are some finer and more specialized divisions of medical attitudes towards PSRO. The Medical Care Foundation movement unquestionably had as its primary recruitment appeal the fears ascribed above to individual medical practitioners. They are, to a large degree, a herding for mutual self-protection, not only against government control but against individual hospital control and against the potential competitive threat of Health Maintenance Organizations (HMOs). Some of the campaigns to build membership in statewide foundations, such as the one in Illinois, openly declared that their goal was to "put doctors in the drivers seat" *vis a vis* hospitals. In other areas, the foundations came into being as a counterforce to HMOs. Because so many of the foundations are indistinguishable in their leadership from the PSROs and, in effect, control them, they will be a highly significant force in the future development of PSROs. They and their national parent, the American Association of Foundations for Medical Care, seem to have, because they are positively in the peer review business, much more political leverage on PSRO than does AMA and its state and county medical societies.

Another clearly separate attitude grouping is in academic medicine. The PSRO law clearly gives the "town" segment of medicine dominance over the "gown." The doctors on medical faculties who hold the key clinical chief positions in teaching hospitals are watching the PSRO scenario with quiet apprehension. The prospect of being reviewed by a peer who is on fee-for-service in a suburban community hospital fills these physicians with distaste, if not alarm. They are deeply skeptical about the credibility of PSRO in its present design. In Boston and in other metropolitan centers, the failure of the town leaders of PSRO to tap the impressive fact-finding and investigative resources on the medical faculties is regarded as a danger signal. The fears of academic medicine in Boston are being aroused also by open declarations by Medical Care Foundation leaders (who also control the PSRO movement) that they intend to channel more routine surgery to community hospitals instead of teaching hospitals, where it always costs so much more. So, just below the surface, PSRO is beginning to pose a threat to established referral patterns vital to the economic salvation of the big Boston teaching hospitals.

The medical specialty groups have their own distinctive perception of PSRO. Over the years, their thrust (and their substantial contribution) has been the upgrading of the capabilities and performance of members of their individual specialties. This thrust never pertained to the totality of medical practice, as does PSRO, but instead concentrated on the building of individual excellence. While the specialty societies have been in the act in the development of PSRO's norms, standards, and criteria, their future role as PSROs become operational is not well defined. This is generating some insecurity.

Hospitals

For the Joint Commission on Accreditation of Hospitals (JCAH), PSRO has to look like a major competitor. With PSRO, and with DHEW's apparent move through the validation surveys to discredit JCAH, we may have the seeds for JCAH's ultimate destruction. Also threatening to JCAH is the fact that hospitals and their medical staffs will tolerate only so many surveys and evaluations, and some are convinced that they have too many already. Once PSRO is fully operational, and the ground rules on delegated status are clearly defined, it is an open question whether hospitals will really need JCAH, or at least be willing to pay the steadily rising prices of JCAH surveys. JCAH is now trying gamely to redefine its turf in the new PSRO world, while attempting to maintain an image of a voluntary organization with an educational emphasis. Their new interests in outcome audits, in performance evaluation procedures (PEP), and their continuing push to improve institutional performance through TAP (Trustee-Administrators-Physicians) Institutes, does serve to identify a supplementary function to PSRO. When Dr. John Porterfield, director of JCAH, said recently, "We will continue to relate to hospitals, not directly to PSROs, helping hospitals meet PSRO standards," he also revealed, by implication, his dependency upon hospitals. Whether hospitals will continue to depend upon JCAH remains to be seen.

For hospitals, which must absorb all the economic impact of PSRO at least in its early years, the feelings are ambiguous, to say the least. The hospital administrator's sense of insecurity because he doesn't have a guaranteed seat at the table has already been described. His position is like that of a bystander at a high stakes poker game watching the players (in this case, doctors) lose, with his money. Hospitals, among other things, are an economic enterprise. A primary motivation is to keep the census high and cash flow stable. Without some security and predictability on the income side, the essential public service functions of the hospital are soon threatened. This hard reality becomes more pressing in tight economic times in states like New York and Massachusetts where major cuts in Medicaid are taking place. Hospital administrators in these and some other states are desperately trying to keep their ships afloat, financially speaking.   In this environment, realistically, they cannot be expected to regard PSRO as anything but another government threat to their institution's security.

There is a curious and possibly contradictory sidelight of the hospital administrator's attitudes towards PSRO.   He would just as soon not talk about it and, if this is possible, would prefer not to know very much about it either.   I think this relates to the long lead time on getting PSROs started, and to a deepening conviction that nothing as complicated as this can ever be made to work.   Also the fact that the hospital administrator doesn't have much input into the PSROs themselves makes the poker game seem rather tedious despite the fact that the hospital's money is in the center of the table. This attitude is, in most instances, a fair reflection of prevailing attitudes in the medical staffs, who would just as soon not talk about it either.

Perhaps this administrative ennui is general across the country and is the basis for the generally "hands off" approach to PSRO taken by organized hospitals, as represented by the American Hospital Association (AHA).   AHA has not been a conspicuous partisan in any of the main skirmishes that have been fought out through the PSRO developmental period.   Perhaps out of political prudence, it has usually stayed clear of the internecine struggles within medicine that PSRO has triggered.   However, it can not stay out much longer because vast hospital interests are at stake beyond the economic insecurity already described.   The most important one relates to whether, under PSRO, the hospital field can continue to move towards a merging of board-administration-medical staff effort and purposes so that there is unified and publicly accountable response to all the public pressures hospitals are now getting.   There continues to be, in other words, a very strong movement to make the hospital the mechanism for assuring "quality of care," "full access," "continuity of care," "comprehensiveness," etc., in its service area. These words are in quotes because they are part of the rhetoric of the continuing discussions on national health insurance, and nobody knows yet how and to whom to assign responsibility.   The reason this is pertinent and crucial to the future of PSRO (and of hospitals) is that practically you can not vest this responsibility in too many different places.   The inevitable result is that nobody does it.   The question is whether we can even have hospitals, as good hospitals have come to be known, if outside organizations gain full control of their quality assurance.   Once this happens, the hospital loses both initiative and accountability, without it being realistically possible to make the controlling agency, in this case the PSRO, truly accountable on its side.

THE ACCOMMODATION OF BUILT-IN CONFLICT

My attempt to characterize the diverse interests affected by PSRO is certainly imperfect and incomplete. We could talk at length about the professional concerns of nursing, medical record administrators, dietitians, and social workers, on whether they can get input into what has so far been defined as mostly a medical province. Enough diverse input has been identified, though, to make some points. The first is obvious. Dr. Michael Goran, director of the Bureau of Quality Assurance, has a difficult political assignment. There seems to be no way of changing very soon the concerns ascribed to the different groups who are the major players in the PSRO game. Currently, the level of paranoia is high in the voluntary sector. The reasons seem to be well based. The track record on federal health programs over the last several years has not been reassuring. Partly it has been a foggy conceptual base, as exemplified by CHP and the health component of the Office of Economic Opportunity. Partly, it has been the persistent failure to fund programs with sufficient generosity to give them a chance to prove much of anything. We are already seeing this part of the scenario unfold with the starvation-level funding proposed for PSRO in the new fiscal year. From the outside, this undermines the credibility of any program. Also, there is a growing feeling, shared by hospital people and physicians alike, that the federal commitment to health programs and health needs is sagging on all fronts and that PSRO is nothing more or nothing less than another effort to hedge on this commitment.

From my present vantage point, all these concerns have validity and credibility and deserve respect—from the fears of the private practitioner committed to the welfare of his patients to a government now trying to reconcile the reality of limited resources with ever-mounting medical care costs. The real problem for PSRO, apparently, is how to accommodate, if not to balance, all of these diverse attitudes long enough so that the program will have enough time to prove whatever it has to prove.

THE DIMENSION OF QUALITY CARE

There is another dimension to my theme of the diversity of interests that surround PSRO and the need to accommodate them. It relates to who is in charge of future efforts to advance quality of care. The leading promoters of PSRO, personified by Dr. Henry Simmons, former director of the former Office of Professional Standards Review, sound as if they are the vanguard of a new crusade. In Dr. Simmons' resignation letter to Secretary of DHEW Caspar Weinberger, he said, "I believe more strongly than ever that the Administration's support of the PSRO program will have a more favorable impact on the nation's health care system than any other effort in which we are engaged." We don't know yet whether Dr. Simmons is right, but it does seem important that PSRO be considered in clear perspective with all other efforts, past, present, and future, relating to quality of care.

I hesitate to even discuss the subject of quality of care. Over my 25 years as a representative of hospitals, quality of care was something I always have been in favor of. But I am still looking hopefully for someone who can define it, not to mention measure it. Despite extensive exposure to discussions of this subject, I retain a simplistic layman's perception of quality—it is the knowledge and skills of the physician who is taking care of me. To paraphrase, I want my brain surgeon not only to have the best available education, graduate and postgraduate, but I also hope he has had a lot of practice and is up-to-date on technique. I tend to take for granted that his backup—i.e., the hospital and its nurses and its aseptic operating rooms—will be adequate. I also relate quality to what is now talked about a lot as outcome. Beyond my brain surgeon's education and credentials, I am even more impressed with him if I survive my surgery.

Simplistic as this may seem, I still believe that the high qualifications and capabilities of the attending physician are still the *sine qua non* of quality. These qualifications are the result of a lot of effort by our medical schools and teaching hospitals, the multitude of agencies involved in continuing education, and by well-organized hospital medical staffs. Given the persistence of scientific advances in medicine and the many breakthroughs in technique, it is obvious that we can never have enough continuing education if quality is to be sustained.

Influences that are not literally educational do affect quality. For example, all the work that has been done by JCAH, Dr. Wes Eisele and the Estes Park Institute of Denver, and others, aimed at improving the hospital as a medical care environment, has had some influence. What is really involved here is creating intra-organizational relationships so that all of the organizational components, particularly the medical staff, will function in an effective and accountable fashion. The outcome here, hopefully, is more medical practice that is good within the hospital and less that is bad. I also accept the fact that standards can have some impact on quality, though we know that in themselves and when left to themselves standards are merely abstractions that may not affect much of anything. As Dr. Warren Nestler, medical coordinator of Overlook Hospital in New Jersey, said recently, "The purpose of having standards is to make measurements; the purpose of making measurements is to safeguard quality; and the way to safeguard quality is to change behavior when the measurements show performance out of compliance with the standards."

This leads us to audits, or medical care evaluation (MCE) studies, now required under the PSRO law but already functional in most hospitals because of the JCAH requirements. Over time, it can be assumed that the MCEs will improve quality.

My attempt to convey my own limited conception of quality of care is to give a frame of reference for what PSRO is and isn't. Its stated purpose in the statute is ". . . to assure, through the application of suitable procedures of professional standards review, that the services for which payment may be made under the Social Security Act will conform to appropriate professional standards for the provision of health care." This is measured, and not ringing, statutory language which places clear emphasis on assuring adherence to appropriate standards and doesn't say anything about raising them. It is essentially a modest statement with no implication that it will dominate or override or control the other activities aimed at improving quality.

PSRO is already firmly anchored in process review methodology. Prototype Medicaid concurrent monitoring programs, like those in Illinois and Massachusetts, which are also process review-oriented, have not yet been able to document results that relate to improved medical performance. They may never be able to do so. In the context of all of the efforts that have gone before to improve quality, and will certainly continue, PSRO is Johnny-come-lately on the scene. The worst mistake to make at this time would be to assume that this program will or even can have a dominant role in the improvement of quality of care. It is hoped that it will have a constructive influence. Last year's report on PSRO by a 12-member committee of the Institute of Medicine of the National Academy of Sciences supports this point. The Committee found that full achievement of PSRO's national goals "lie[s] beyond the present capabilities of either the health professions or society-at-large." It did conclude, though, that "with modest expectations consistent with current techniques, the willingness of most providers to improve when better information is provided about their performance, and through partnership with the consumer, improvement in the quality of medical care can be accomplished. The PSRO is a step along this road to better quality of health care and better health."

EXPECTATIONS ON FISCAL IMPACT

As stated earlier, we wouldn't even have PSRO if there hadn't been high expectations in Washington that the program would save a lot of money. Three years later, there are still high expectations. Dr. Henry Simmons, former director of OPSR, talked about saving $30 million a year (300,000 days of care × $100 a day) if all cataract surgery could be done as one-day surgery, implying of course that PSRO can establish such a norm. Dr. Clement Brown, director of medical education at South Chicago Community Hospital, says, with proper use of antibiotics that could be imposed by PSRO, the government would save $600 million a year in drug costs. Dr. Alan Nelson, of the Utah Professional Review Organization, points to the millions that will be saved if Boston's average length-of-stay on myocardial infarcts (23 days) could be made to conform to the 10-day norm in Salt Lake City, assuming of course that Salt Lake City is right and Boston is wrong.

There also are some extravagant expectations on the expense side, too. When DHEW staff costed out the potential expense of reimbursed physician time needed to make PSRO function, they came up with a total of $600 million a year. This calculation was derived from analysis of the initial contract submissions from the PSROs, counting up the time needed for criteria development, committee activities, reviews, policy development, etc., and multiplying it by $35 an hour. Beyond this cost, we must consider the costs that will inevitably be incurred within the hospital as a consequence of the program. Partly as a result of CHAMP (our external Medicaid monitoring program that will presumably be phased into PSRO when it becomes operational) most hospitals in Massachusetts have hired their own coordinators, just to cope with the administrative demands of CHAMP (and Blue Cross and Medicare requirements on UR) on an internal basis. Add to that the increasingly persistent demand from physicians on hospital UR committees to be paid for their time. The physicians are saying they cannot justify the increasingly heavy demands on their time for this committee activity unless they are paid for it. More and more hospitals are acknowledging the validity of this point and paying.

THE LONG-TERM CARE DIMENSION

There is another sleeping giant on the expense side that ultimately will have to be dealt with. It is what seems to lead to inevitable increases in the cost of long-term care when PSRO begins to set norms, standards, and criteria in this important area. The deficiencies of these institutions, particularly those giving skilled nursing and extended care services, are well known and widely decried. They relate in large degree to persistent underfinancing, which in turn relates to wide-spread state budgetary problems with Medicaid, which now pays a heavy proportion of the long-term care bill in most states.

One of the major deficiencies in most of long-term care, is physician services. There are hundreds of thousands of patients in these facilities who need constant medical supervision and aren't getting it. As we know, this isn't just a result of underfinancing but also an expression of widespread physician disinterest. A lot of patients in these facilities are there, we also know, because there is no place else to put them. On the face of it, medically developed norms, standards, and criteria seem somewhat irrelevant in this setting. There is reason to seriously doubt whether they can accomplish much in reducing length of stay.

What I am trying to suggest is that any kind of system like PSRO designed to get patients out of hospitals as soon as possible and into less expensive patient care settings must, if it is going to work at all, effect basic improvements in these alternate settings. Improvements always cost money.

As this is written, we are having a crisis in Massachusetts because our nursing home organization, enraged by chronically low Medicaid reimbursement rates, is boycotting all new Medicaid admissions from hospitals. Our CHAMP program, costing $1.7 million a year, goes along pronouncing Medicaid patients as ready for discharge, and then a large proportion of them are staying in the hospital anyway. Meanwhile, under the pressure of a state budgetary crisis, the legislature and the welfare department are trying to cut eligibility in the medically indigent category (many of whom are old people in nursing homes), the Rate Setting Commission is persisting in its stand of refusing to allow a promised inflationary increment in the nursing home rate, and the Public Health Department is still pushing to enforce its standards and close substandard facilities.

Whatever else this little story says about controls as they function in Massachusetts, it cannot be claimed that any of them, including the utilization controls, are cost effective. When PSRO gets seriously into long-term care, a very sophisticated consideration of this kind of problem will be needed. For example, and relating to our Massachusetts experience, I think there are substantial arguments for keeping certain categories of older patients—post-stroke, coronary, amputee, for example—in the hospital longer than any existing norm would indicate. In Massachusetts we have an alarmingly high readmission rate of these kinds of patients from skilled nursing facilities back into hospitals. Overall, I don't think getting them out fast is saving very much money.

One important basis for the high hopes that PSRO will save a lot of money relates to this category of patient. Many of our hospitals, particularly the smaller ones in nonmetropolitan areas, are filled with old people on Medicare who no longer really need the services of an acute general hospital. The privately expressed fears of PSROs conveyed to me by the administrators of these institutions relate to this reality. But it isn't just Medicare coverage that is keeping them there—it is the cold truth that in many areas the local nursing home is simply unacceptable. What merit is there in hurrying the patient out of the hospital and into a setting where the nursing service is professionally inadequate and a physician is seldom even seen on the premises? A strong push through PSRO to force the issue of prompt discharge is certain to have a strong backlash in many areas.

I am suggesting, in other words, that—just as in the case of the quality of care—high expectations of what PSRO can save in federal expenditures in long-term care do not seem justified and in fact may be self-defeating.

PSRO RELATED TO OTHER CONTROLS

As with quality of care, the interrelationship of PSRO (and other utilization monitoring) to the other major thrusts in cost control need to be clearly established. There are four main controls, all of them more or less functional in Massachusetts.

1. *Utilization controls.* The CHAMP program, the Medicare UR regulations, and soon PSRO. The purpose here, of course, is to reduce admissions and length of stay and ultimately redundant tests and medications.

2. *Fiscal controls.* There are all kinds of ways to do this—controls on hospital expenditures, controls on the hospital budget through a review process, controls on income, controls on allowable costs. At present in Massachusetts there is a control on income through our Rate Setting Commission's capacity to approve both the Medicaid per diem reimbursement rate and our Blue Cross contract. More recently, our legislature has enacted a bill authorizing controls on all hospital charges. This category of controls is frequently but inaccurately called cost controls. None of them literally control hospital costs—they merely control what a hospital is paid for its services.

3. *Controls on supply of services.* This is certificate of need and what is at least contemplated under the new federal health planning and development act—decisions on whether services already established are appropriate and still needed. The concept here is that use of services is best constrained by limiting the supply of these services.

4. *Controls of covered health benefits.* We have always had benefit controls because the benefits in any and all insurance packages, governmental or voluntary, are always limited. The uncovered service is less frequently offered and less abundantly used. The present irony of our times is that benefit controls have been working in reverse—that is, the big push has been to expand benefits, which, inexorably, is increasing hospital usage and expenditures. The best contemporary example of this is the dialysis entitlement under Medicare. The generous Massachusetts Medicaid

program is another. Since the state is almost broke, our legislature now is trying to cut benefits. These cuts will help control our state's expenditures for health, but we aren't so sure it will control the hospital's costs. We think a lot of people will continue to demand the benefits, covered or not. They are now used to getting them.

Even though the above-cited controls are quite distinctive, one cannot really function without affecting the other. For example, if PSRO carries out its mission of reducing hospital admissions and length of stay, it can't fail to increase hospital per diem unit costs. There are two elements at work here—the compression effect of putting the same volume of services into fewer days; and the elimination of the admissions that, if they weren't necessary anyway, probably weren't very expensive and therefore brought down the hospital's per diem average.

Another example is that limitations on the supply of beds and specialized services, where they are effective, will in themselves decrease utilization, the PSRO notwithstanding. Another way of making this point is that, if the PSRO is the powerful force some people think it will be, it can knock into a cocked hat all planning formulations about appropriate bed-population ratios for an area. Yet another example relates to fiscal controls. If the advocates of this category of controls make them really effective, we may not even need utilization controls and controls on the supply of services. What will happen here is that severely constrained limits on hospital income will force limitations on services offered and their usage. This is what happens, and it's happening right now in Massachusetts, when a state legislature cuts the mental health budget. Our mental hospitals aren't full. Many are not even admitting patients because they can't afford the staff to provide an adequate service. Some don't even have the funds to replace essential equipment. Everybody knows about this inadequacy and will always choose, if they have a choice, to seek the care they need in the private sector.

What is being done to our state hospitals is an example of benefit controls of the worst sort. Generous benefits adequately financed can have an opposite effect. I am only suggesting that the level of benefits in any program will have a much more fundamental impact on utilization than anything a PSRO can do. Over-utilization was never a problem before we had health insurance. What happens in the future concerning benefits and entitlements can make PSRO's job rather perfunctory or totally impossible. I, at least, am convinced that a comprehensive benefit package under National Health Insurance, such as Senator Edward Kennedy's model, will create unstoppable pressures for more utilization all through the system.

My second observation, a corollary of the first, is that it will be very difficult to measure the impact of PSRO because of what will certainly be a variable impact of other controls that will be applied to the system. One example of this is the current situation of the backup of nursing home cases into hospitals.

My third observation is that the interrelatedness, or interdependence, of the four controls I have described underlines the need for some overriding authority that coordinates and gives broader purposes to what is being attempted. Limitations on the supply of medical services and on their use can never be allowed to become ends in themselves. The need for this overriding authority is critical in Massachusetts and in Washington and must encompass in some fashion PSRO. Otherwise, the risk is that the system won't really function as a system at all and will still cost too much.

THE BIG FORCES GENERATING COST INCREASES

After our Massachusetts temporary hospital charge control legislation was passed in June of 1975, we convened a task force of the most sophisticated professionals that could be assembled from within our membership to examine our options on long-term solutions. The bill that passed mandated the development of a permanent system of controls, with a deadline of October 1 to submit a proposal to the legislature. The hospital association was guaranteed full input into the decision-making process.

The temporary legislation that was passed required that all hospital rate increases be subject to Rate Setting Commission approval and be justified on the basis of the hospital's budget, which was also made subject to the commission's scrutiny. The legislation was justified and passed on the basis of two premises. One was that, by eliminating overcharging (charge schedules that produced income substantially in excess of costs), a lot of public and private health insurance monies would be saved because hospitals wouldn't have the incentive to spend up to the limits of their allegedly inflated income. The second premise was that, by obliging hospitals to subject their budgets to public scrutiny, they would be stimulated to be more efficient, though measures of efficiency were not and still are not defined.

Soon after our task force was convened, it quickly came to one unanimous conclusion—public justification of hospital charges can't and won't save significant amounts of money for anybody, assuming there is honest recognition on the regulatory side that legitimate costs must somehow be reimbursed. There just isn't that much overcharging in the Massachusetts hospital system. Our task force knew this, and initial experience with administering the temporary law has supported this conviction.

From there, our task force embarked upon a fascinating discussion of what the root causes of our incremental increases in hospital costs were. It identified six major pressures that were generating these increases (quoting from my own summary of the deliberations):

1. *The pressure for universal entitlement.* There can be no question that all the talk about national health insurance, equal access, comprehensive care, etc., has fueled the demand for health care. The collection experience in our emergency rooms and outpatient departments suggests that an unmeasured proportion of the public has already decided, with their elected political leadership, that adequate medical care is indeed a right. In Massachusetts, this movement is further down the trail because of the extraordinary development of neighborhood health centers and a truly comprehensive Medicaid benefit schedule. Our point here is that continuing increases in demand for care, generated out of the political process, have produced equivalent large increases in costs and therefore in public expenditures. The demands and expectations are now an inescapable reality. They won't go away just because the state now wants to disavow them as a responsibility. There is an ironic current example to reinforce this point. The state law mandating private health insurance coverage for psychiatric services, alcoholism, and drug detoxification becomes effective January 1, 1976. We are now trying to anticipate its effect. One certain result will be more community based psychiatric services, inpatient and outpatient, and of course more costs, more usage, more expenditures, and higher insurance premiums. The example is ironic because the legislature, right now with its budget cutting, is pulling away from these commitments, particularly in services to alcoholics.

2. *The pressure for community health security.* After you leave the city of Boston, with its abundance and diversity of medical resources, we are confronted with another inescapable reality—having your own hospital is regarded as an essential element in health security for the community. It is also a symbol of community status. Every chamber of commerce seeking to attract new industry has two main talking points as a starter: the school system and the availability of medical care. There can be no question that this phenomenon produces a lot of expense for the system. But it is also something that won't change very soon, given the deeply engrained town meeting psychology in the Commonwealth. The experience with our certificate of need program supports this point. Attempts to close small hospitals or even terminate certain specialized services such as obstetrics have produced strong community backlashes, always supported by locally elected members of the General Court. Witness the bills passed in the last session overriding certificate of need decisions and then overriding the Governor's vetoes of these bills. All the evidence suggests that local citizens are not swayed by bureaucratic judgments about their hospital's

effectiveness or efficiency. They think their hospitals are just as essential as the police or fire departments.

3. *The pressure for patient security.* It is not generally understood that hospital regulation has done more to increase costs than to control them. This is particularly true in Massachusetts, which is the most regulated hospital state in the union. In a study we are now doing, we have identified 32 separate avenues of regulation, mostly uncoordinated, that are impacting our hospitals. There are many more of these that are what we call cost provocative rather than cost suppressive or cost preventive. Our upward hospital expenditure curve has been steeper here in Massachusetts than in our northern neighbors, Vermont, New Hampshire, and Maine, which have had much less regulation. The list of cost-provocative controls is a very long one, and does not need to be detailed. The most important is hospital licensure which, in combination with professional licensure, has been the avenue for generating extraordinarily high payroll costs. The numerous professional lobbies, including medicine, nursing, medical technology, social work, etc., have been extremely successful in mandating, through hospital licensure, rich staffing patterns in our nursing units and specialty services. Out of all of this we have created some extremely high standards but also high expense. In a time when most of the public concern is focused on high costs, it is not generally recognized that the forces creating even higher costs are still very powerful and active. The lobbies for patient rights, clean air, equal employment opportunities, fire prevention, etc., all have significant impact on hospital costs.

4. *The pressure to relieve the shortage of health manpower.* Within the last year, our member institutions, especially the teaching hospitals of Boston, have been under heavy pressure to control that proportion of costs that is represented by the costs of graduate medical education, nursing schools, X-ray, and lab technician training, etc. These costs have indeed become .formidable. The irony here is that all of the commitment is a response, quite impressive in Massachusetts, to a nationally proclaimed goal, enunciated 20 years ago, to beef up our production of health professionals. It is a fact that high production of health manpower creates its own pressure for more hospital jobs, and our hospitals have not been particularly resistive to this pressure. It is also accurate to say that more medical graduates generate more costs in the system. Cost concerns notwithstanding, the crusade for more medical manpower continues. We still hear a lot about the doctor shortage, even in Massachusetts. The Boston area is a national supplier of health professionals. Prestige notwithstanding, the bureaucrats don't like that either, because it costs too much. Even so, we have yet to hear anybody suggest a certificate of need program for nursing schools or medical residency programs.

5. *The pressure to extend longevity.* Every good nursing home or home for the aged is organized, medically speaking, to keep old people from dying of pneumonia. The reality here is that keeping people alive is very expensive. It is not generally recognized that long-term custodial cases need a lot of acute hospital care. The common pattern is admission and readmission to a hospital when a chronic condition becomes acute. My father, Daniel Kinzer, in a home for the aged two years before he died, had two hospital admissions during this period, costing about $3,000 apiece. Without the hospital care, he would have died sooner. He had congestive heart failure and emphysema, neither of which was basically affected by the hospitalization. He was only stabilized. Another example under this general heading is terminal cancer care. With medical and sometimes surgical intervention, the lifespan is extended for a few months or a few years. But the cost is very high. It can be said that what goes into keeping people alive a little while longer is one of the most important elements in hospital costs, particularly in teaching centers. Nobody knows how to control this. By the turn of the century we will have 28,842,000 people over 65. Their potential for generating health care expenditures is staggering.

6. *The pressure for medical innovation.* This overlaps the pressure described above, but it is essentially distinct. What we are talking about here is the absolute certainty of a technological breakthrough, at least one of them every year, which triggers a demand from the medical staff for new capital or personnel expenditures. A contemporary example is the CAT scanner, which costs about $500,000, but which has already demonstrated its diagnostic effectiveness. There are endless examples under this heading, some of which are controversial but popular in medicine just the same. The problems encompassed in this area are best documented by Dr. Howard Hiatt in his article "Who Shall Guard the Medical Commons" (*New England Journal of Medicine*, July 31, 1975). He talks about the implications of coronary bypass surgery, pointing out that if the manpower and facilities resources were available and if everybody who could benefit from the surgery would get it, the total costs would amount to $100 billion a year, which is a little less than what this country spends annually for all health services. The point under this heading is that we are in a situation where our capability is now outstripping financial resources, and we are into the uncomfortable business of making choices on who gets the services and who doesn't and on what is cost effective and what isn't.

We did not identify inefficiency or the lack of an integrated health delivery system as root causes of our cost problem. We didn't blame it all on doctors, either, though there was a lot of agreement on the need to involve physicians more directly in resource allocation decisions within the hospitals. Specifically, we talked about how to get them interested in decisions on what new medical services or innovations will not be provided, as well as those that must. We also talked, without conclusive result, about the necessity of giving physicians the incentives to make some tough decisions that might restrain cost increases.

Pertinent here is the fact that we did not consider wasteful, or irresponsible, or exploitive, use of hospital services by either physicians or their patients as a major root cause of our cost problem, at least not on the scale represented by the six pressures listed. The consensus seemed to be that health insurance policies and practices had an overriding impact on decisions on where to get care, and you really can't blame a patient for wanting to go to a patient care setting which he knows his insurance will cover.

An examination of our six main pressures generating cost increases, as they might relate to PSRO (and as PSRO might relate to them), does give a different perspective to our cost control problem. I have already suggested that PSRO will not and cannot be the be-all and end-all in controlling waste in the system. Looking at the six pressures, it is clear that PSRO doesn't even have the potential for affecting most of them. It won't control the public appetite for medical care, fueled by the continuing discussions of national health insurance. It won't change the feelings of isolated communities about the need to have a hospital. It won't even consider blunting the continuing drive, often spearheaded by committed physicians, to improve standards (and increase costs) in the clinical divisions of our hospitals. The manpower supply issue is not within its purview. It does in fact impose important new time demands on the medical talent pool we now have. It potentially can only impact on the last two pressures, the one about extending longevity and the one about applying medical innovations. At this time, no one can be sure how PSRO will function in these areas. I think the physicians involved in PSRO now haven't even seriously considered the kind of negative decisions that PSRO might have to make as we face the reality of limited resources. Forget the norm on length of stay for a 75-year-old man having coronary bypass surgery. Should he even have the surgery? How many hospital admissions can be allowed for a woman dying of cancer? The example of Karen Quinlan is now in the courts, but the broad implications of these kinds of decisions will certainly involve the PSROs.

What I am suggesting is that PSRO faces a risk. It will be a convenient place to put some unpleasant decision-making powers. In an economic environment where there is not, nor ever will be again, enough money to pay for everything we can do in medicine, the important decisions will not focus on appropriate utilization but on the option of who gets the service and who doesn't. I personally think the hospital will have these decisions dumped on it, but the PSRO may be involved, too.

THE LEGAL DIMENSION

My commitment to PSRO tends to concentrate on the potential of delegated status for hospitals for improving in-house medical performance. The position has some legal foundations. Court precedents, from Darling *vs.* Charleston Community Hospital up to Gonzales *vs.* Nork and Mercy General Hospital, seem to firmly establish hospital responsibility and accountability for the performance of members of its medical staff. The PSRO law does nothing to change this. Section 1167, the waiver of liability, says no provider shall be civilly liable for any action taken "in compliance with or reliance upon professionally developed norms of care and treatment," but then it goes on to say that he still must exercise "due care in all professional conduct taken or directed by him and reasonably related to, and resulting from the actions taken in compliance with or reliance upon such professional accepted norms of care and treatment."

What this says to hospitals and to the attending physician, translated, is that all of the potential liability of medical decision making still falls upon them, not the PSRO. More explicitly, due care means you better not release the patient just because the norms say he is ready, if there is any basis for the belief that there is risk to the patient's health and security by virtue of this action.

The law says the PSRO and its individual physician members incur no liability by virtue of their actions, which clearly implies that it stays where it is—on the physician and the hospital. This raises some awkward questions which are certain to come up later in the courts. In the nondelegated hospital threatened by frequent no-pay decisions on the basis of PSRO norms, there is more than a likelihood that it will be unduly swayed by the norms and incur liability as a result. That hospital will not be easily persuaded that the liability should not be shared by the PSRO. Regardless of what the federal law says, these issues will be settled in state courts under state law. This explains why some PSROs already are examining their needs for liability protection and inquiring as to whether this cost will be paid for by the federal government.

I am not suggesting that the declared legal immunity of the PSRO is bad public policy; I am only saying that the PSROs must be very scrupulous in recognizing the reality of the attending physician's and the hospital's ultimate responsibility for the welfare of their patients. It seems to be in the PSROs interests to have as much delegated status as possible. It avoids the risks of remote control decision making affecting individual patients and places this responsibility where our courts say it is, and where I think it belongs.

THE DIMENSION OF THE HOSPITAL
INTERNAL ORGANIZATION

One of the constructive outgrowths of the Darling-Nork trend in court decisions has been the persistent effort to meld the hospital into one legally accountable entity, instead of what has often been described as "a three-legged monster without a head." The hard part of this has been to get members of medical staff to believe that they function as an integral (and accountable) part of the hospital organization, and not as a separate power block functioning within the hospital walls. Progress in this area has been slow but steady. I call it progress because the melding of responsibility into functional unity is the only way the movement can go, given the main thrust of the court decisions referred to.

The internal melding of the hospital has important implications for PSRO. One is that the PSRO, by virtue of its considerable authority and discretion, has the capacity to frustrate this development or facilitate it. We have already heard from some PSRO leaders who are adamantly opposed to any delegation of hospitals. I think this is mostly an expression of the interest, strong in certain segments of medicine, to use PSRO as their own instrument for controlling hospitals. If this succeeds, it will be exceedingly damaging to our hospitals and ultimately backlash on the physicians involved. The hospital will be in the awkward position of still having the public account-ability (and the liability) without having the real capacity to control what goes on inside its doors. I don't think efforts by individual PSROs to stonewall delegation will succeed, if only because of a practical reality—it doesn't appear that PSRO will ever have enough funding to do all the monitoring required under the law on an external basis.

The board-administration-medical staff melding process has some impor-tant internal implications. For example, if we are to accept the point that the medical staff and its utilization committee are to be made accountable to the hospital board and through the board to the public (and the PSRO), then it seems to follow logically that the internal organization of the hospital involved in utilization review and quality assurance activities must be made accountable to the medical staff. Specifically, the UR coordinators can't function very effectively if they work for outside masters. This seems to be a controversial point. In Illinois, Massachusetts, and some other states Medicaid monitoring got started with the external monitoring agency hiring the coordinators and planting them in the hospital. PSRO will also have to hire coordinators for their nondelegated hospitals. As little of this as we can have, the better. The external coordinator is at best in an awkward position with the established hospital organization and usually has more difficulty than the hospital employee in getting the cooperation of staff physicians. In both Illinois and Massachusetts the coordinators have been poorly trained—mostly because of the strained atmosphere surrounding the coordinator function. Turnover has been high. This has produced some real problems in maintaining continuity for the monitoring program within the hospital.

There are some physician leaders of monitoring agencies who feel just as strongly as I do on the other side—that they must hire the coordinators and make them accountable to the external monitoring agency; otherwise they can't control their own program. They also feel that the coordinator, when an employee of the hospital, is in no position to raise the uncomfortable questions and thus quickly becomes the apologist and defender of the status quo in medical practice within the hospital.

My response to that is, yes, the coordinator can be easily pre-empted by a self-serving, self-protective medical staff. And there will always be some of these. But this misses the main point and the main need of making the medical staff and its utilization committee responsible and accountable for its performance. I think this can be accomplished to a substantial degree through sufficiently challenging standards for delegated status. Then, given the achievement of delegation, it seems insupportable that any employee of an external organization should be involved in the internal process.

We face real dangers if this principle gets lost in the PSRO shuffle. I don't believe it will be possible, for example, to have utilization committees that are any more than paper organizations carrying out perfunctory functions if they are subjected to substantial second-guessing, overruling, or too much policing from the outside. The physicians involved, already complaining about excessive demands on their time, will give up in disgust. Then the whole system will be the loser.

THE DIMENSION OF DATA REPORTING AND ANALYSIS

The continuing hassle about data policy under PSRO is just one expression of a general paranoia, described in an earlier section, which surrounds PSRO itself. The fears don't need to be explained or discussed; I'll only try to identify what I believe are some points of principle.

1. First and most important, the patient's medical record is the core document for all of the activity we have been talking about. It must be accurate, informative, instructive, and private. The privacy thing is, first of all, representative of an obligation to the patient. It is also a protection (but not so much anymore) to the hospital and the attending physician, because

the record won't be much use as an instrument for staff education and improvement if it is subject to wide public scrutiny. The record is hospital property, though the law in some states gives the patient the right of access. Given the fact that the record is hospital property, it isn't any other agency's property. This point deserves emphasis because there seems to be some misconception among PSRO leaders that reporting requirements in the PSRO law change this property right and give the PSRO rights to use of this information that override the rights of the hospital. They don't.

2. Given my first point, the PSRO not only has obligations to the hospital to be protective of the privacy doctrine (under the rules, the PSRO does have the right to know the identity of physician and patient, but this information isn't supposed to go to Washington), but to feed back to the hospital aggregated information in some meaningful and useful form. We have had an absurd situation in Massachusetts with our CHAMP program, under which it never occurred to anybody that the individual hospitals might be assisted by reports that compared their Medicaid UR experience with those of other hospitals.

3. The issue on data under PSRO is not who does the data processing but who does the analysis and whether the hospitals and their medical staffs will be allowed to have meaningful input in this process. A different way of stating this point is that the data aren't nearly as important as the sophistication and depth of their analysis. I believe it will be an unusual situation when the staff and the leadership of individual PSROs will have the capacity to do this job alone. There has to be meaningful involvement by the hospital utilization committee, some of which in Masschusetts have impressive capabilities, and by qualified professionals in data analysis and interpretation. Under PSRO we must avoid the problems of any system, such as the Commission on Hospital Professional Activities (CHPA) and the Utilization Information Service (UIS) of the Massachusetts Hospital Association, that feels it must limit its services to the cold reporting of statistical information. The big problem is that such reports are boring and therefore often unread by UR committee members. Nothing happens as a result.

4. At least in the more populous states, there is a strong case for pooling highly qualified staff resources in data analysis and interpretation, because it seems certain that the dollars available for data services under PSRO will be limited. This builds a case for the creation of independent data consortia. They can function not only as a central resource for the PSROs but for all the third party purchasers, governmental and voluntary, who use utilization data and for the hospitals themselves. While these consortia probably will never have decision-making prerogatives, they can greatly improve the quality of the decisions of the agencies charged with making them. They can

make the important contribution of protecting the whole system against the risk of superficial or totally dollar-oriented decision making.

5. Because of the interrelatedness of financial, utilization, and planning data in making good planning decisions, it seems necessary that these consortia also involve the new HSAs and hospital rate-setting or budgetary review commissions where they exist.

6. The quality of data input is, of course, a crucial consideration. This has to be made a hospital responsibility. This presents another argument for delegated status. If the hospital organization is responsible for making the system work internally, it will have an incentive for accurate input. Otherwise the PSROs won't get accurate output, and the hospitals won't be able to learn anything from the feedback. One of our problems with our CHAMP coordinators is that too few of them have understood how to fill out the form, and we have a "garbage in—garbage out" situation.

In summary, I am suggesting that the essential issue on data under PSRO is whether it will have any scientific credibility so that it can have an educational effect. If hospital data input is used crudely to justify no-pay decisions, it will kill the program.

THE DIMENSION OF HOSPITAL VESTED INTERESTS

As a representative of hospitals, I am frequently obliged to speak for their vested interests. This is the real world of trade associations. You represent your members, or try to, on what they want. There is a different perspective here, which is a protective one. The hospital is a responsible, accountable instrument for carrying out public policy. In that frame of reference, the following would be a kind of hospital platform for living (and surviving) in the new world of PSRO.

1. Fight to protect the rights of privacy of the patient. By doing this you also protect the rights of hospitals.

2. Push to put the physician at risk on PSRO decisions. Now only the hospital loses financially if the attending man fails to adhere to the norms, standards, and criteria. There has to be some financial incentive for the physician to play by the new rules of PSRO.

3. Push for an amendment to the PSRO law that would require significant hospital representation on the boards of PSROs. Support consumer representation also.

4. Insist that PSRO, as a cost control mechanism, be linked with other cost control mechanisms and be related to broad goals, objectives, and priorities in health. In other words, become aggressive on the point that utilization control should not become an end in itself.

5. Support common boundaries for PSROs and HSAs. Their decisions and activities are interdependent, so they must operate in the same territory.

6. Support public control of all control mechanisms. This implies giving the HSA a superordinate role over the PSRO.

7. Push for adequate reimbursement for hospital costs incurred as a consequence of the PSRO law.

8. Direct a maximum effort for hospitals to achieve delegated status under PSRO.

9. Work for open PSRO data systems—i.e., systems where the hospitals and their UR committees can participate as equals in data analysis and interpretation.

10. Push for the articulation of financial, utilization, and planning data input into the HSAs. Planning decisions that relate to only one of these three inputs probably won't be good decisions.

11. Push for scientific, documented, objective reporting of results of PSRO monitoring, not only to DHEW but to the citizens in the area the PSRO services.

12. Push for an adequate appropriation for PSRO. It is not in hospitals' interest that this program fail.

CONCLUSIONS

Because of the number of established interests that are threatened or feel they are threatened by PSRO, it seems imperative that the program not, at least in its early stages, assume many threatening or power-conscious postures. There is plenty of power out there with the capacity to kill the program, in spite of its legal mandates. It also seems a wise course that the program not promise too much, either in improving quality of care or in saving money. As a relative newcomer on the cost control and quality scenes, it must have time to earn its spurs.

The greatest potential for PSRO for improving quality of care lies in its power to stimulate quality assurance activities within the hospital using the numerous resources and tools already available. An inescapable corollary of such an effort is that the PSRO should push for as much delegated status for hospitals as possible, but with standards that are meaningful and demanding on the hospital organization. The hospital is legally and publicly accountable to its patient and its community in a manner the PSROs can never be. Accepting this point, it would seem to be in PSRO's interest to do everything possible to improve this accountability.

Perhaps the most hazardous aspect of PSRO is its status as a physician organization. This has already triggered consumer challenges with more certain to come. In view of this, it seems to be a wise course that PSROs give meaningful representation to nonphysicians on their governing boards, without indulging in the hypocrisy of trying to look like a consumer-controlled organization. It also seems necessary to give more representation on these boards to hospitals, since they are the agency most vitally affected by PSRO decisions.

Not far down the trail, the need must be faced for the articulation and coordination of the several approaches to cost control that are now operational. Good policy decisions are impossible to make with single-tracked approaches to control methodologies—whether they be on utilization, unit or aggregated costs, or resource allocation.

Part III

Quality Assessment Information: Management of Data and the Question of Public Access

Chapter 6
Policy Alternatives on Hardware and Software in Health Care Data Storage and Retrieval

James J. Baker

INTRODUCTION

My point of view is that of an outsider looking at the Professional Standards Review Organization (PSRO) record-keeping. In seven years with Cullinane Corporation, in the proprietary software field, I have seen a great deal of commercial data processing in banks, insurance, and manufacturing, some in federal, state, and county government, but almost nothing in hospitals and medical care. Most of my experience has been with companies that were satisfying their own data processing needs with their own money. I have had very little experience with needs mandated by law to be paid for by external funding. In this chapter I can begin to do four things:

1. Examine PSRO data processing needs from the ground up.

2. Suggest parallels with commercial data processing experience.

3. Suggest an advocacy approach as the best means of getting further information.

4. Advocate one approach that currently has no effective spokesman: the use of minicomputers for commercial data processing.

My method will be to pose certain questions and then to give my tentative answers and conclusions plus a supporting discussion.

PSRO DATA PROCESSING NEEDS

Who needs computer hardware and software? Not everybody. Someone with a record-keeping need has at least five choices.

1. Do it manually.

2. Ride piggyback on someone who is already doing what you want for himself. An example here is bank processing of checking accounts; a large bank will very often do the checking account processing for its correspon-

dent banks as well as for itself. Or a bank trust application may include, on a service basis, processing for an investment management firm.

3. Subscribe to a commercial service. We recently signed up with Automatic Data Processing to do our payroll, for example; it costs about $1.00 per employee per pay period for about 50 employees. For payroll processing, the crossover from manual to service bureau seems to us to be about 25 employees.

4. Buy package software and run it on your own or rental hardware. No shop that I know of does all its processing with package software, but for a manufacturing firm payroll, accounts payable and accounts receivable could well be packages; for a bank, it might be check processing, savings, and one or more loan applications.

5. Custom-write your own software and run it on your own or rental hardware.

The best choice for a particular PSRO would have to be determined by an on-the-spot study.

What seems rather clear now is that it is not necessary, convenient, satisfactory, or economical to force everyone into the same mode of computer application. I rather think that a pluralistic approach to PSRO data processing needs will prove to be the best solution—i.e., some PSROs will be perfectly happy with a manual operation; others will be able to justify their own hardware and software; some in the middle would be best serviced by a correspondent relationship with one of the larger processors.

How urgent are the acquisition decisions? Not very. Acquisition decisions are very often confused with decisions regarding objectives or financial aims. For PSRO record-keeping it seems to me the really important decisions are what data is to be kept and what the purpose is of keeping such data. In other words, how does health care data storage and retrieval support the business purpose of a PSRO? The parallel here between PSRO and commercial organizations is not as clear as if both were profit-making organizations. The record-keeping functions of a commercial organization are designed to support customer records, record proper sales, keep inventory, and make sure that orders are filled. As review organizations the PSROs have different problems and different objectives. Still, until these problems and objectives are clearer, the acquisition of computer hardware and computer software cannot be intelligently carried out. Anyone in a position of authority in directing a PSRO's search for health care data storage and retrieval must, therefore, be on guard against the bogus urgency towards acquisition used by some computer service vendors to get the customer to make a decision in their favor. It is a truism in the computer area that customers very seldom have anything drastic to lose by delaying an acquisition decision for a month or two months—even six months, or one year. Vendors of computer hardware and software, therefore, are often in a position of having to interject a note of urgency into a situation where basically no urgency exists.

Sometimes this is done by announcing a price increase; the prospective customer is made fearful of losing a bargain. Now the reality is that if a service is not really necessary at $10,000 per year, it does not suddenly become a bargain because the price will go to $15,000. If you don't need it, you don't need it regardless of the price. But time and again a prospective customer will feel that he is going to miss his chance at getting a bargain if he does not move. Computer hardware and software vendors will often play on this fear.

In the case of health care data storage and retrieval, the PSRO's decision to acquire is so tied up with questions of objectives, goals, aims, and methods, that the correct decision cannot be made until the person who is going to use all this data knows what he wants it for. If, then, there is a certain urgency in this whole matter, the urgency would seem to come from the necessity of deciding what it is all about, rather than from the urgency of acquiring a specific piece of hardware or software or the services of a particular vendor.

COMMERCIAL DATA PROCESSING EXPERIENCE

Historically, computer record-keeping has been approached in three major ways. The first was the do-it-yourself approach in which a company bought hardware, hired programmers, designed applications, and wrote computer programs to do its own computer processing as an entirely inhouse effort. The main examples of this approach were scientific and nonprofit organizations (mainly government funded), insurance companies, and some banks; the first round took place during the late fifties and early sixties, the second round during the middle sixties after the introduction of the IBM S/360 models in 1965 (the so-called third generation machines).

The reason for this approach at the time was that almost everything was a pioneering effort; the companies wanted computer power to do things difficult or impossible to do by hand. There was no precedent to follow, however, and no work of anybody else's to take over. Also, there was plenty of money to work with and plenty of time to get the job done. Custom programming remains today a common way of getting things done. The main plus is an exact fit: you can have exactly what you want, within limits imposed by the hardware. The main minuses are cost and time. For most recognizable commercial applications, the cost would range from 10 to 100 man-years of effort, and the elapsed time somewhere around two years. Also, the management of programming projects tends to be notoriously optimistic, and overruns of 50-100 percent are common. Someone contracting for a custom-written program, either with his own programmers or with an outside programming contracting firm, would be well-advised to allow for at least a 50 percent overrun; a job scheduled for completion in one year might—with some luck—be producing reliable results in 18 months.

The second approach was the industry cooperative approach such as occurred in banking in the late sixties and early seventies. Banks wanted to attract deposits through checking and savings accounts and extend credit through installment loans and charge cards like Master Charge. This meant, from a paper-handling point of view, processing a large number of rather trivial individual transactions, for which the use of the computer was mandatory. For a variety of reasons, some banks were more entrepreneurial than others; some went ahead while others hung back. The banks that went ahead and wrote the first banking application programs—installment loans, for example—didn't just benefit themselves. They learned things that were generally useful to the banking industry as a whole, and that knowledge was used as a starting point by other banks, which, in turn, followed the pioneers and sought to avoid some of their more costly mistakes. The pioneers themselves could profit in at least two ways: they might do the processing for other banks, in return for some consideration such as compensating balances or outright payments of a processing fee; or they might sell the application programs to those banks just getting started. Thus the package program industry was born.

The main advantages of a software package are: minimum time to be up and running; relative solidity from the moment it comes up (because the bugs have been worked out at the originating shop); and economical price (a rough rule of thumb would be 10 percent or less of development price). The main drawbacks are relative inflexibility of the package (it may not have the features you want, and if you plan any but the most minor modifications you are back to case one—development programming), and operating cost. You have trimmed start-up costs, but you still have operating costs, including equipment rental and provision of operations personnel. If you are just getting into computer data processing, you may botch the operations end of it for awhile. The other alternative mentioned above—a pioneer operating his system for a client as well as for himself—is probably the most risk-free of all the alternatives. The client knows exactly what he is getting, he has no operational investment whatever, and the amount of coordination necessary with the host or with other clients is generally very small. A bank which is doing installment loan processing for 10 other banks, for example, will generally simply require them to each have a different two digits as the first two digits of the account number, and all must of course have an account number of the same length—seven digits, or nine, or whatever.

The main drawback is extreme inflexibility. If the client wants to provide a 48-month car loan and the host system only allows for 36 months, there is no recourse. If the client wants to keep his branches open until 6 P.M. and the host begins daily processing at 5 P.M., the client must obviously gear his operations to suit the host. Surprisingly, to some who might sense a monopoly situation, costs tend to be moderate—much less than those of a straight-out service bureau. The host organizations generally absorb most of the overhead, instead of allocating it among the clients, and they tend to absorb all of the direct costs of writing the programs in the first place. For a small PSRO, which has outgrown the do-it-by-hand stage, some sort of correspondent relationship with a larger organization doing its own processing could well be a best buy.

The third approach is that of a service bureau or a facilities management firm that would take over the complete data processing job and take care of all of the user's data processing problems. (The big difference is that a service bureau maintains a central computer and you bring your data to it; a facilities management firm sends in people to run your equipment at your site.) The biggest name here is Ross Perot's Electronic Data Systems. I have never worked for them or been at a shop they serviced, but in talking with people who have been in both positions, I conclude that in many cases the biggest thing they had to sell was their management approach. The data processing content—the hardware, the software, the daily operations—were, in many cases, no different than a good installation could have achieved on its own. But an installation that did not know what it wanted to do, did not know what its objectives were, or did not know how to go about achieving objectives once they were defined, found that many worrysome management problems and hard management decisions could be shifted over to the service bureau by giving the service bureau a completely free hand in supplying needed data processing services. In fact, in many cases it was the service bureau that decided which data processing services were needed. Instead of being presented with a list of computer needs, it was invited to study the business and do whatever was necessary to keep it running. Used in this way, a service bureau is simply a substitute for effective management and decision-making power. If that happens to be a particular need of a business organization, then the use of a service bureau to fill it is a perfectly good commercial proposition. But, if the organization has enough management talent to decide what it wants to do, there will almost always be more economical ways of obtaining the strictly computer-related services desired.

Vis-a-vis correspondent or piggyback processing, which is also a form of service bureau, a "for profit" service bureau will generally have the drawbacks of greater cost, and sometimes of lesser competence. It will have greater cost because it must cover all its expenses and earn all its profit —sometimes a high profit at that—from the services it provides the user. There are no programs that it would have to have for its own use anyway. It would have lesser competence because the service bureau doesn't always know the business. If one bank goes to another to have its installment loans processed, it is pretty sure that the other bank knows something about installment loans. But if Ross Perot comes in to run a bank on a facilities management contract, it is possible that he knows nothing about banking.

THE ADVOCACY APPROACH TO GETTING FURTHER INFORMATION

General papers and general surveys are apt to be unsatisfactory because they are not detailed enough and they do not present the alternatives sharply enough for the PSROs to make an intelligent choice. People who need health care data storage and retrieval processing service are going to have to adopt an advocate approach in which the various vendors that have something special to offer will be allowed to state their case and press their advantages. The PSROs that are listening to the individual advocates will have to be careful not to be so swayed by the completeness of an answer that they forget that it is not the answer to their problem. So, in looking for more information and listening to various advocates, the PSRO personnel should look at both what problem was solved and how it was solved. Further, they should take full opportunity of the presence of various vendors to get the information they need on both these issues. The vendor himself may want to focus on how he solved the problem since, in many cases, he had no particular option as to which problem he solved. Economically, of course, he is far better off if he can sell an existing solution than if he has to develop a new one.

The five alternatives listed in the section "PSRO Data Processing Needs" will not attract a uniform distribution of advocates. To redress the balance, some means of enlisting advocates for options like "do it manually" must be found. My suggestion is to obtain the cooperation of a data processing class in a university or business school. If a sympathetic professor were to give such a class the problem of investigating the various options open to a PSRO, or were more specifically to ask certain teams to play "devil's advocate" for certain of the economically unpopular options, the result could supply information that would not otherwise be produced and lead to a much higher quality of decision making.

THE USE OF MINICOMPUTERS
FOR COMMERCIAL DATA PROCESSING

It looks to me right now as if the industry-cooperative approach would offer the best combination of flexibility of response, security of data, and results for the money. I would see the more advanced PSROs writing their own software and providing correspondent-type servicing for adjoining smaller PSROs. Furthermore, if that software could be run on a minicomputer, significant hardware cost savings could likely be achieved.

It is taken for granted that the more advanced PSROs will write their own software. In any undertaking as ambitious as the setup of the PSRO program, the likelihood that existing software will be a good fit is pretty small. Some of the review work already being done, however, may come close, and the natural extension would be to rewrite some of the existing software for the new needs. What I would like to advocate here is that the applications be rewritten for minicomputers, rather than the traditional IBM or other hardware. The reason for this is that some recent experiences, both with our corporate products and on a consulting assignment, point out the possibilities in minicomputers of dramatically reducing the hardware cost component of a data processing application. So far these indications are only straws in the wind, and it is not at all clear that the expected economics can be achieved. But the indications are promising enough so that the possibility ought to be checked out, especially since by the time any specific software is to be written for PSRO needs the available evidence on minicomputers will be much more voluminous. The following are two examples which point out the possibilities.

1. Cullinane Corporation has as one of its proprietary software products a database called IDMS, which competes with IBM's IMS, Cincom's TOTAL, and others. IDMS presently runs on IBM 360/370 hardware. Cullinane Corporation is working on a version of IDMS for the PDP-11 machines available from Digital Equipment Company (DEC), and the work is far enough along so some capability and timing figures are available. Results so far show that the full IDMS capability can be implemented on a PDP-11/70, and that the running speed will be about equal. The hardware cost of the PDP-11/70 would be on the order of $100,000—that of the 370/158, several million dollars. It is not clear that DEC will ever supply the software to let the PDP-11 service a large number of jobs held in core at once, which is how most 370/158s are used, but it does seem as if the average user could replace a share of a 370/158 with a dedicated PDP-11/70 for database applications and still come out way ahead on money.

Since running a database is a relatively demanding task for a computer, I think these cost indications would be valid for a wide variety of business data processing. I think that this replacement—of a share of a large machine by a dedicated mini—is the most significant thing that will happen in data processing over the next four to five years. It promises dramatic cost reductions for data processing applications that are relatively fixed and well understood. (For those that aren't, the cost of the software and of the analysis that goes into the software probably will exceed the hardware cost by enough to negate substantial savings.)

2. I recently did a consulting study for a Boston investment counseling firm to investigate the economics of replacing service bureau data processing with an in-house PDP-11. An investment counseling firm (as distinguished from investment management) gives advice but does not have custody of the assets or do the actual trading. Thus, the data processing function needed is mainly to keep track of the clients' portfolios. When the client buys and sells, the records are updated; when buy or sell recommendations are made, a record is kept of them. Several times per year, for the average client, the portfolio is priced and counsellor and client meet for advice. The size of the job is about as follows: roughly 1,000 portfolios under advice, with the average holding about 25 items; about 50 transactions (buy and sell recommendations or actions) per day; portfolios priced and reports generated both when any change is made and as needed for the counsellor-client meetings.

The complete job, as handled by a service bureau, runs about $100,000 per year. The dedicated mini replacement—feasible only because there is commercially available existing software for a similar application written for a PDP-11—would have the following estimated costs:

$80,000—one time cost for hardware and software

$25,000/yr.—costs for hardware and software maintenance, pricing service, paper, etc.

Moreover, the system would probably accommodate double the business with no additional hardware and very little additional operational costs. It will not be clear until the system is actually built and operated whether these economics can in fact be achieved, but it looks promising enough for my consulting client to be going ahead with his plans.

Chapter 7
Public Access to Health Care Information: PSRO Data and Its Availability to Patients and Consumers

George J. Annas

Energy and production now tend to fuse with information and learning. Marketing and consumption tend to become one with learning, enlightenment, and the intake of information ... electric automation unites production, consumption, and learning in an inextricable process.

Marshall McLuhan
Understanding Media, 1964, p. 358

As the importance of information increases, the central issue that emerges to challenge us is how to contain the excesses of this new form of power.

Arthur R. Miller
The Assault on Privacy, 1971, p. 274

INTRODUCTION

The purpose of this chapter is to outline the law as it currently relates to medical records in general, and to Professional Standards Review Organization (PSRO) data in particular, and to summarize the arguments in favor of patient access to their own medical records and consumer group access to PSRO profile information on both institutional and individual providers. It should be emphasized at the outset that regulations interpreting the confidentiality and access provisions of the PSRO statute have not yet been promulgated, and only one case directly challenging the PSRO statute has been litigated. Moreover, even in the general area of medical records, there have only been a couple dozen cases that have reached the appellate courts regarding confidentiality, privacy, and patient and third party access to medical records. Thus, the law in this area must be considered to be in its infancy, and much resort must therefore be made both to public policy and to arguments by analogy.

This chapter is divided into two sections. The first section outlines the pre-PSRO law concerning medical record access. The second reviews the PSRO statute as it applies to medical record data and its interpretation by DHEW to date, and outlines public policy arguments favoring patient and consumer access to PSRO-generated data.

THE LAW REGARDING MEDICAL RECORDS

Confidentiality and Privacy: Third Party Access to Individual Medical Records

Preliminary Definitions and Distinctions[1]

Almost all of the existing law concerning third party access to medical records can be placed under the headings of confidentiality, privilege, and privacy. In common speech, to tell someone something in confidence means that the person will not repeat what you said to anyone. *Confidentiality* thus presupposes that something will be told to someone. The presumption is, however, that the information disclosed will not be repeated. Relationships like attorney-client, priest-penitent, and doctor-patient are said to be confidential relationships. When one uses the term "confidential" in the doctor-patient context, it is descriptive of an express or implied agreement that the doctor will not disclose the information received from the patient to anyone not directly involved in the care and treatment of the patient. This obligation is generally considered to be an ethical one imposed on the members of certain professions, rather than a legal one.

A communication is said to be *privileged* if the person to whom the information is given is forbidden by law from disclosing the information in a courtroom without the consent of the person who provided it. In short, privilege is a legal rule of evidence, applying only to judicial proceedings. It is also important to recognize that the privilege belongs to the client and not to the professional. Unlike the attorney-client privilege, the doctor-patient privilege is not recognized at common law, and therefore exists only in those states which have passed a statute establishing it. Twelve states do not have such statutes.

There are at least two senses in which the term *privacy* is generally used. The first describes a constitutional right of privacy. This right, while not found directly enunciated in the Constitution, was the basis for decisions by the U.S. Supreme Court limiting state interference with birth control and abortion. This right is said to be one of *personal* privacy and involves the ability of an individual to make decisions regarding her/his body.

In the more traditional sense the term has been defined as "the right to be let alone, to be free of prying, peeping, and snooping," and as "the right of someone to keep information about himself or access to his personality inaccessible to others." [2] In both of these, the privacy concept is based more on property interests than on bodily control interests. As a property right, it usually requires a state statute to recognize it before it will be enforced.

Public Policy Reasons for These Doctrines

Confidentiality. The doctrine of confidentiality applies to all third party communications by a physician about his patient, whether in or out of court. It is based mainly on medical ethics and implied contract in the doctor-patient relationships rather than on statute (although some state physician licensing statutes provide penalties, including license revocation, for disclosure of confidential information).

The Hippocratic Oath first set out the duty of confidentiality in the following words:

> Whatsoever things I see or hear concerning the life of man, in any attendance on the sick or even apart therefrom which ought not to be noised about, I will keep silent thereon, counting such things to be professional secrets.

This oath has been reinterpreted in the current formulation of the American Medical Association's Principles of Ethics:

> A physician may not reveal the confidences entrusted to him in the course of medical attendance, or the deficiencies he may observe in the character of patients, unless he is required to do so by law or unless it becomes necessary in order to protect the welfare of the individual or the community.

The rationale for this doctrine is generally stated in terms of encouraging candid disclosures by patients to their physicians:

> Since a layman is unfamiliar with the road to recovery, he cannot sift the circumstances of his life and habits to determine what is information pertinent to his health. As a consequence, he must disclose all information in his consultations with his doctor—even that which is embarassing, disgraceful, or incriminating. To promote full disclosure, the medical profession extends the promise

of secrecy. The candor which this promise elicits is necessary to the effective pursuit of health; there can be no reticence, no reservation, no reluctance when patients discuss their problems with their doctors.[3]

Most cases alleging violation of confidences against physicians involve one of the following situations: disclosure to a spouse (involving either a disease "related to the marriage" or a condition relevant in a divorce, alimony, or custody action); disclosure to an insurance company; or disclosure to an employer.[4]

Because disclosure issues usually arise in cases involving either litigation or the possibility of litigation, understanding of the doctrine of privilege is important. As mentioned, it is this doctrine which restricts the ability of the physician to reveal medical confidences in judicial proceedings.

There are generally said to be two competing values wrapped up in this doctrine. The first is that certain types of relationships are potentially so beneficial to individuals and society that they should be fostered by forbidding in-court disclosure of the informational content of the relationship. In this view, a privilege is granted to encourage the employment of professionals by individuals who need their services and to promote absolute freedom of communication. The contrary principle is that the courtroom is a place for the discovery of truth, and no reliable source of truth should be beyond the reach of the court. At common law the court's interest in the truth routinely won out, and physicians were forced to testify to the matters disclosed to them by their patients.

The great majority of courts currently agree that the principal reason for the privilege is to encourage a patient to freely and frankly reveal to his physician all the facts and symptoms concerning his condition so that the physician will be in the best possible position to correctly diagnose and successfully treat the patient, and most states have adopted the privilege by statute. Nevertheless, the statutory adoption of the privilege has been highly criticized by the revered John Henry Wigmore, late dean of Northwestern University Law School and perhaps the leading legal expert on evidence. He argues that in most cases it only serves to frustrate the ends of justice by denying truthful information to the courts. He contends, for example, that most information communicated to a physician is not intended to be held strictly confidential since most of one's ailments are both immediately apparent and openly discussed, that even when information is intended to be maintained as confidential it would be disclosed to the physician even if no privilege existed, and finally that in litigation involving personal injuries it is absurd that the physician not be required to disclose the true extent of the litigant's injuries.[5]

Privacy. In his book *Privacy and Freedom,* Alan Westin defines privacy as "the claim of individuals, groups, or institutions to determine for themselves when, how, and to what extent information about them is communicated to others."[6] He goes on to argue that, as thus defined, the concept has its roots in the territorial behavior of animals, and its importance can be seen to some extent throughout the history of civilized man. In the modern context specific protections of privacy were built into the U.S. Constitution by the framers in terms that were important to their environment. With the subsequent inventions of the telephone, radio, and instantaneous photography and the introduction of mass communications, more sophisticated legal doctrines were developed in an attempt to protect the informational privacy of the individual. One such approach was suggested by Warren and Brandeis in the *Harvard Law Review* in 1890. Their approach, directed toward private rather than public or governmental invasions, suggested that there be developed a legal remedy for individuals whose privacy was invaded by the press or others for commercial gain. As a result of this and other arguments, a number of states passed statutes making such invasions actionable at law.

While many diverse acts may be said to come under the heading of privacy violations that may give rise to a cause of action, most involving medical records would fall in the area generally described as the "publication of private matters violating ordinary decencies."

No statute is necessary, however, for a court to find the unauthorized disclosure of medical records an actionable invasion of privacy. As an Alabama court put it recently in a case involving disclosure of medical information to a patient's employer:

> Unauthorized disclosure of intimate details of a patient's health may amount to unwarranted publicization of one's private affairs with which the public has no legitimate concern such as to cause outrage, mental suffering, shame, or humiliation to a person of ordinary sensibilities.[7]

The policy underlying the right is that certain information about individuals should not be repeated without their permission. In the words of one legal commentator: "The basic attribute of an effective right to privacy is the individual's ability to control the flow of information concerning or describing him."[8]

Most of the cases which have arisen in the doctor-patient context alleging violation of the right to privacy have involved actions in which personal medical information has been published in some manner, and often the suit is against the publisher rather than the physician.[9]

Exceptions to Nondisclosure Duty

While the doctrines of confidentiality and privacy are, on the surface, very powerful legal tools, their effect in the day to day practice of medicine is considerably diluted by the statutory exceptions and defenses physicians can raise to a charge of unauthorized disclosure. There have been no reported appellate decisions in the United States, for example, where any physician or hospital has ever had to pay any money damages to any patient for the unauthorized disclosure of medical records. A number of problems with the enforcement of these rights, therefore, merit specific discussion.

Implied Consent. This is probably the major cause of leakage from the current medical records system. When one is in a hospital, for example, one impliedly consents to the viewing of one's medical record by all those concerned with one's care. This may include the nurses on all three shifts, the ward secretary, all medical students, interns, and residents in the hospital, the attending physician and any consultants called in, and perhaps social, psychological, medical, or psychiatric researchers. All of this may, of course, take place without the patient being made aware of it, and it is said to be a matter of "custom." One also impliedly consents to review of one's record by utilization review committees.[10] Initial PSRO chart review, of course, adds very little to current third party access problems in hospitals.[11]

Public Reporting Statutes and Supervening Interest of Society. Almost all states have a wide variety of conditions and diseases which must be reported to the public authorities when discovered by the physician. These fall into four major categories (vital statistics, contagious and dangerous diseases, child neglect and abuse, and criminally inflicted injuries) and state a public policy that takes precedence over both privilege statutes and the physician's ethical obligation to maintain a patient's confidences. PSROs should not be required to make any disclosures under these statutes since their purpose is mainly data collection and evaluation and because they should be able to assume that the physician or hospital in question has made the appropriate report.[12]

General Release Forms (Consent). Upon entering a hospital a patient may be asked to sign a wide variety of forms. One of these is likely to be an authorization which says essentially that the hospital may release medical information concerning the patient to anyone it thinks should have it. This will include such persons as insurance companies, the welfare department (if they are paying all or part of the bill), and other agencies or individuals monitoring cost. No restriction is generally placed on the amount of material that may be released or the use to which many of these third parties may put the information so received. Arguably, however, receivers would be liable for an invasion of privacy action if they used the medical information for other than the specific purpose for which the hospital released it. As will be discussed in more detail later, the PSRO statute provides for stiff criminal penalties for misuse of confidential medical information obtained in the PSRO review process.

While I am not aware of the argument ever having been made, it would seem that most of these general release forms could be attacked as unduly broad and so vague that the patient could not reasonably and knowingly have signed them. (e.g., if he understood the form, he would not have signed it; therefore, his signature is evidence either of his incompetence or of his misunderstanding of its significance.) [13] The cases regarding the invalidity of blanket surgical consent forms, which give the doctor and hospital authority to perform whatever procedures they think necessary, would support this line of reasoning. Another argument that could be made is that the patient's lack of bargaining power made the form ineffective (e.g., a sick patient may need admission and cannot afford to forego it by refusing to sign a required form). [14]

Private Interests of the Patient. The general rule is that courts will afford physicians wide latitude in making disclosures that physicians believe are in the best interests of their patients. This rule, for example, is used to justify many disclosures to spouses and near relatives without the patient's consent. While this rule has been criticized on the grounds that when only the patient's individual welfare is involved, only the patient should have the right to decide when confidential information should be released, [15] courts will probably continue to give physicians and hospitals much discretion in this area. [16]

Legitimate Public Interest. This particular exception applies more to the press than to individual physicians. It states the general circumstances under which a newspaper or other medium may publish private medical information. Two leading legal commentators have argued that:

> The fact that the patient is not a "private" person, but rather a celebrity who customarily feeds on publicity, usually thought to be a defense in cases involving relatively innocuous information, will probably be considered of no consequence where intimate medical data, covered by explicit legal and ethical requirements of confidentiality, are involved. The fact that medical data are newsworthy or will advance sciences is likewise not controlling. [17]

The authors go on to argue that one exception to this would probably be the condition of the president of the United States since the public has a right to this vital information, although government officials in all high policy-making positions should arguably be required to disclose medical conditions that might affect their ability to perform their tasks.

The events surrounding the release of medical data in the newspapers concerning Senator Thomas Eagleton and District Attorney Frank Hogan raise another issue: Does the manner in which the press obtains private medical information matter? The case law seems to indicate—following rather technical logic—that so long as the press did not themselves commit a crime in obtaining the information, they can publish it with impunity so long as there is a legitimate public interest in it.[18] The press will not even be held liable as accessories after the fact for receiving stolen goods because the courts will generally find that what they received was "information," the actual documents having been copied and replaced.[19] The publication of stolen or surreptitiously obtained materials is actionable on the civil side, however.

While the courts have had some difficulty in deciding between two competing public goals, the maintenance of privacy and freedom of the press, one can predict that future cases will continue to develop the definition of "legitimate public interest" as the only viable exception to the general rule of personal privacy. At least one commentator has expressed the opinion that "it is hard to believe that [physician and patient profiles] will remain unavailable to the press."[20] While no one can guarantee their confidentiality, the PSRO statute does contain a section which makes the leaking of confidential medical information to the press a crime punishable by a fine of "not more than $1,000, and imprisonment for not more than six months, or both, together with the costs of prosecution."[21] This provision should deter most would-be press sources.

Judicial Process. When someone makes his own physical condition an issue in a lawsuit—e.g., a personal injury claim—most courts will permit examination of his physician under oath either before or during the trial. Even in states which have privilege statutes, there are generally many exceptions which would permit bringing medical information into court. For example, medical information is often available in criminal cases, and almost always in malpractice cases. It remains to be seen whether or not PSRO norms or individual practitioner or institutional profiles will be admissible in court (although the latter will probably not be since it could only prove past conduct, something not necessarily relevant to conduct in a particular case).

The PSRO profile data on individual patients, however, will probably never be admissible since it is a summary only and not the best evidence. The patient's actual medical record will be the relevant document for the courts.

One way to increase the confidentiality of medical records is to specifically protect them against the various possible exceptions by statute. As has been noted in a number of instances already, this is the approach taken by the PSRO statute.

Patient Access to Medical Records. Like other consumer-citizen movements, the quest to obtain more information from persons or institutions which control various aspects of one's life is of relatively recent origin. Indeed, a search has revealed no United States cases on point prior to the 1930s. The probable explanation is that, until relatively recently, medical records were not well enough defined for patient access to make much sense. Also, organized medicine has consistently argued that the medical record is the exclusive property of the physician or hospital which has absolute discretion in determining whether or not the patient shall be permitted to view it.

A small number of states have passed special access statutes which enable patients treated in hospitals within those states to view and copy their medical records. (Some statutes limit this right to the patient's attorney or authorized representative.)[22] Perhaps the most liberal of these statutes is that of Massachusetts, which grants patients an absolute right of access both during their hospital stay and after discharge.[23] A 1973 study of the effect of this 1945 statute on hospital practice in the Boston area by the Center for Law and Health Sciences of Boston University School of Law revealed, however, that nine of 10 major hospitals routinely denied patient requests for information, most on the basis that this was a medical decision that had to be made by the patient's physician. Only one followed the statutory language. Typical of the hospital's response was that from Dr. Mitchell T. Rabkin, Director of Boston's Beth Israel Hospital, who argued, "We would prefer to send the chart to a physician so that he or she might interpret the information to the patient ... [I]n order to make a reasonable judgment on the request that the patient directly receive the chart."[24]

While legal commentators almost all agree with Attorney Leon L. Wolfstone that "It needs to be said—the patient *is* entitled"[25] to see his medical record, the fact is that hospital practices almost universally discourage such access. Therefore, as a practical matter in the absence of a special access statute, the only way a patient may legally be certain of obtaining the information in his medical record is by commencing a lawsuit against the doctor or hospital involved (usually alleging malpractice in the course of treatment), and obtaining the record through court-sanctioned discovery procedures. This fact was noted by the Commission on Medical Malpractice of the Department of Health, Education and Welfare (DHEW) in early 1973, which found that "the unavailability of medical records without resort to litigation creates needless expense and increases the incidence of unnecessary malpractice litigation."[26]

The Commission's background report specifically concluded that "the most serious impediment to obtaining access to hospital records can be the policies of individual hospitals."[27] Contrary to such restrictive policies, the few cases that have reached appellate courts have almost uniformly found that while the physician or hospital may own the paper on which the record is written, the interest of the patient in the information on the record is so vital that he has a right to a copy of it.[28]

POLICY ARGUMENTS SUPPORTING PATIENT AND CONSUMER ACCESS TO PSRO DATA

The PSRO Statute and Current DHEW Interpretation

Regarding the disclosure of data, the PSRO statute provides in relevant part:

> (a) Any data or information acquired by any Professional Standards Review Organization, in the exercise of its duties and functions, shall be held in confidence and shall not be disclosed to any person except (1) to the extent that may be necessary to carry out the purposes of this part [the PSRO statute] or (2) in such cases and under such circumstances as the Secretary shall by regulations provide to assure adequate protection of the rights and interests of patients, health care practitioners, or providers of health care.
>
> (b) It shall be unlawful for any person to disclose any such information other than for such purposes, and any person violating the provisions of this section shall, upon conviction, be fined not more than $1,000 and imprisoned for not more than six months, or both together with costs of prosecution.[29]

When the PSRO statute was challenged on the basis of its constitutionality, and in particular as a violation of the rights of privacy of patients and physicians, the court pointed to this section in upholding the law and noted that it ". . . does limit access to the information under the penalty of criminal sanctions . . . [and] contains provisions that properly balance the plaintiff's right of privacy with the government's interest in maintaining proper health care in an economical manner."[30] The report from the 1974 Conference on Confidentiality of Heath Records quite properly concluded that "The PSRO program—controversial from the beginning—may serve as a testing ground for confidentiality. . . ."[31]

It remains to be seen how these issues will be resolved. DHEW contends that it has delayed formal rule making in the form of regulations "to avoid being locked into premature regulations that have the effect of law . . . [and to get] maximum input from any and all interested and affected parties outside the government in the development of regulations."[32] In the meantime, and subject to some criticism,[33] DHEW has been "making law" for the PSROs by contract, in the form of periodic "transmittal letters." While proposed regulations on confidentiality of PSRO data have been promised as forthcoming for some time, they have not yet been issued. The only statement on confidentiality has come in the form of a transmittal letter, and its tentative nature warrants no more than a summary of its provisions as we await formal proposals to be published in the *Federal Register.*

PSRO Transmittal No. 16, "Specifications for Confidentiality Policy on PSRO Data and Information" was issued February 14, 1975. It enunciates the following policies on data disclosures.

1. Patients are to have access to their own medical files upon request. However, their physicians are to be given notice of this disclosure "in writing at least ten working days prior to patient access" and the physician "may be present when the patient accesses his individual files" for the purposes of clarifying information (although the physician cannot prevent access).

2. Health care facility profiles may be disclosed upon payment of a fee to cover costs, provided that the facility receive thirty days written notice "to review the information for accuracy and to provide comments to accompany the disclosed information."

3. "Medical data and information identifiable to an individual patient and information indicating patterns of health care practices identifiable to individual health care practitioners" shall be considered privileged data and shall not be disclosed."

4. Local PSRO norms, criteria, and standards are to be disclosed, but PSRO sanction reports and deliberations are to be privileged and not subject to subpoena in any civil action.

The remainder of this chapter will argue that the final version of the PSRO Confidentiality Regulations should contain no restrictions on patient access to their own files, and should provide open access to the profiles of both health care facilities and individual health care practitioners.

Policy Arguments Regarding Patient
Access to Their Own Records

Doctor's Office Records

The American Medical Association (AMA) holds a typically restrictive view on patient access to medical records:

> It is our position that the right of a patient to medical information from his physician is based upon the fiduciary relationship which imposes a duty to act in the best interest of the patient. It would be a violation of that duty to provide information which would be harmful to the best interest of the patient as a matter of sound medical judgment. It is our position that a physician has both a right and a duty to withhold information in circumstances in which he reasonably determines that it would not be in the best interest of the patient.[34]

I have been able to locate no reported cases that deal with the question of a patient's access to his medical records held by a private physician in his office. The closest analogy is access to one's X-rays. In a lower court case, in which a patient demanded copies of X-rays of his leg for purposes of litigation, the court denied the request saying that in the absence of an agreement to the contrary, common understanding of both doctors and patients is that the physician retain the X-rays. In the words of Judge Esterbrook:

> It is essential that the physician retain it as a permanent record in support of his diagnosis ... to justify its correctness in the event of challenge to his professional opinion. What the plaintiff sought was a diagnosis of his ailments and professional advice as to how to treat them to effect a cure ... [X-rays] ... were taken with his knowledge and consent and delivered to his physician for his professional aid and use and not as a work of art .... The X-rays are the property of the defendants in the absence of an implied agreement.[35]

In the only appellate decision involving this issue ever reported, the court held similarly that "in the absence of agreement to the contrary, such negatives are the property of the physician or surgeon who made them incident to treating a patient. It is a matter of common knowledge that X-ray negatives are practically meaningless to the ordinary layman. But their retention by the physician or surgeon constitutes an important part of his clinical record in the particular case."[36] The court went on to add the importance such evidence might have in defending a malpractice action.

Even though these cases involved access to a diagnostic test itself, rather than a written report about it, from them one can argue that courts will find in favor of the physician retaining absolute control over the medical records only in cases where it can be demonstrated that:

(1) the patient could not understand the material in the record;

(2) the ordinary understanding of a patient would be that the doctor would retain absolute control; and

(3) it was not possible to make a duplicate copy of the material in question.

In cases where one or more of these elements is missing, it is arguable that judicial authority supports the right of the patient to obtain at least a copy of the materials in his medical record no matter who has custody of the record. In the case of a PSRO, of course, both elements two and three would necessarily be missing and therefore access should be required.

Hospital Records

As previously noted, the courts have almost universally recognized that patients have an interest in viewing their hospital records, at least when questions of insurance or possible malpractice litigation is involved.

There are nine states that have specific statutes permitting the patient or his representative access to hospital records without resort to the courtrooms. All of the reasons doctors give for not wanting patients to see their medical records (e.g., increased anxiety, irrelevant and potentially damaging materials, misunderstandings, etc.) apply equally to hospital records. Arguably, therefore, passage of such an access statute amounts to an outright rejection by the legislature of these medical rationales for preventing access. In cases where the legislature has restricted access to patients after discharge or to their legal representatives, a compromise position has been adopted.

Patient Access to His PSRO File

Since the PSRO profile of a patient is likely to contain much less information than his actual medical record, many of the policy arguments favoring individual access to medical records do not directly apply to individual access to PSRO profiles. Nevertheless, the bits of information the profile does contain may be of interest to patients for a variety of reasons, and access can likewise be supported on a number of grounds.

The most persuasive argument favoring access is that decisions may be made concerning the patient on the basis of the data (e.g., third party payment), and therefore the patient has an interest in making sure the information is accurate. Likewise, the PSRO has an interest in spot checking for accuracy, and one way is to see how many patients who do access their profiles find mistakes in them. Moreover, the information contained in the profile is about the patient, and this fact alone should give him or her enough interest in it to mandate access. The information accessed might also help encourage the patient to become more knowledgeable about his own health care, and thus act as an important educational tool. It could also improve the doctor-patient relationship by promoting an openness regarding information that may not otherwise be present.[37]

Arguments Against Patient Access to PSRO Profiles

At least as persuasive as the positive reasons for access is the lack of any strong argument against access. The traditional arguments against patient access to medical records, such as incompleteness, alteration of the record by the patient, illegibility and incomprehensibility, and dual record systems, have little or no applicability to the type of data contained in the patient profile.[38] Perhaps the only argument that may have some merit is the contention that the patient might become unduly alarmed or apprehensive by the information in the PSRO file (e.g., a previously undisclosed diagnosis).[39]

Two things can be said about this argument. The first is that it can be accepted without denying access to the vast majority of patients. The second is that, if the doctor feels strongly about not informing his patient, he will feel strongly about it at the time the information is transmitted to the PSRO. He should, therefore, make that attitude known at that time, and only then should the 10-day notification requirement come into effect. The recently promulgated DHEW regulations under the Privacy Act of 1974 provide an additional, though questionable, alternative. Those regulations specify that a person desiring access to medical records shall name a representative. The records will be reviewed before disclosure, and if the reviewer thinks that for some reason the medical record should not be directly disclosed, it must be turned over to the named representative. The representative may be any adult named by the person to whom the record pertains, and need not be a physician.[40]

Consumer Access to Provider Profile Data

Generally

While there are some distinctions to be made between access to facility data and individual data, most of the policy arguments favoring such access apply equally to both, so they will be dealt with together.

Initially, it is worth noting that no privileged data compiled by the PSRO are required to be disclosed by any provision of the Freedom of Information Act. That act does not apply to data "specifically exempted from disclosure by statute," and the confidentiality section of the PSRO statute previously quoted is broad enough to provide such an exemption to disclosure of PSRO data unless "necessary to carry out" the purposes of the act or "in such cases and under such circumstances as the Secretary shall by regulations provide to assure adequate protection of the rights and interests of patients, health care practitioners, or providers of health care."[41]

Also, federal law would not prohibit public disclosure of physician profiles. One purpose of the Privacy Act of 1974, for example, is to limit federal agencies from divulging information it has collected so that the personal privacy of the individual is not invaded.[42] It provides in part that:

> No agency shall disclose any record which is contained in a system of records by any means of communication to any person, or to another agency, except pursuant to a written request by, or with a prior written consent of, the individual to whom the record pertains, unless disclosure of the record would be, ... (3) for a routine use.[43]

Routine use is defined by the act to mean the use of a record for a purpose which is compatible with the purposes for which it was collected.[44] Therefore, the privacy act would not prohibit the dissemination of physician profile data, because the disclosure would be pursuant to the purposes of the PSRO legislation—to assure "adequate protection of the rights and interests of patients, health care practitioners, or providers of health care."

While some have argued that the Consumer Protection Acts of individual states might be used to compel consumer access to profile data,[45] this seems unlikely in view of the Supremacy Clause of the United States Constitution which mandates that federal law take precedence over state law when the two are in conflict. On the other hand, if federal regulations provided that disclosure of profiles was optional with the local PSRO, state consumer protection acts might be used to compel such disclosure.

The most likely manner in which profile data will be made available to consumers is by DHEW Regulation based upon a finding by the Secretary that such disclosure is necessary "to assure adequate protection of the rights and interests of patients ... ," or by the amendment of the PSRO statute.

Informed Choice

The initial rationale for patient access to this information is the obvious one. Patients under treatment or contemplating treatment may want to know the type of information in the PSRO profiles before deciding which physician or health care facility to select for help. Patients may want to know about the number of times a certain physician or institution has dealt with a particular problem, what the average length of stay was, and what the typical outcome or chance of success is. Without such information, which is currently unavailable to anyone, the patient's role in the medical decision-making process is strictly limited since he or she is unable to make meaningful choices among health care institutions or practitioners prior to personal contact. With access to this data, comparisons could be made by consumers who would then be in a position to determine which physician's practices best suited their individual desires.

The doctrine of informed consent provides a more specific rationale. Prior to 1960 the general doctrine was that all a physician had to obtain from his patient was sufficient consent to protect himself from an assault and battery action alleging intentional and unauthorized touching. Since that time, however, state courts have consistently recognized that prior to giving consent, a patient needs to know a certain amount of information about his condition, the recommended treatment, and the probable results of treatment. The rationale for requiring physicians to disclose such information is that the patient has a right to self-determination—a right to refuse and choose between alternative treatments, no matter how irrational the physician may regard the patient's decision.

Before 1972, legal commentators felt safe in asserting that in deciding how much to tell a patient a physician could be guided by the doctrine that "good medicine is good law."[47] In that year, however, three separate jurisdictions held that doctors could no longer limit their disclosures to what "the average medical practitioner would disclose under similar circumstances." The new test enunciated was that the measure of disclosure was based on the patient's need to know, which was to be based not on a polling of the local county medical society, but on whether or not the patient was given sufficient material and relevant information about the nature of the treatment and its important risks (e.g., death, disability, and problems of recuperation), so that the patient was in a position to make the ultimate decision of whether or not to accept the doctor's recommendation. This duty to disclose was, somewhat ironically, based precisely on the fiduciary nature of the doctor-patient relationship that the AMA had traditionally relied upon to deny patients access to their medical records.[48]

These decisions currently represent the rule in a minority of states, but are indicative of the modern trend. That trend is for the courts to view the doctor-patient relationship as a partnership in decision making rather than as a medical monopoly. Under this view the doctor is obligated to disclose not what other doctors disclose, but what the individual patient needs to know to be able to intelligently make up his own mind concerning the proposed treatment. The major interest being protected is the individual's right of self-determination, but the promotion of rational decision making is a strong secondary goal.

While courts have, in the past, given physicians much discretion to withhold certain information if it might unduly upset the patient (the so-called "therapeutic privilege"), this exception should not apply to PSRO profile data since its source is not the individual physician and since its import is not directly on the patient's diagnosis or alternative treatments, but rather concerns the patient's physician and health care institution.

It should be noted that as applicable to any particular physician, however, one could argue that the disclosure obligation for treatment decisions should be placed on the physician himself (since he will know his own profile as well as the PSRO norms) rather than on the PSRO.

Consumer Education

Another major argument favoring disclosure is of a more general nature. It is that consumers are ignorant of medicine and the variations in medical practices and quality, and that this ignorance tends to help perpetuate substandard medical practice. Thus, as a study commissioned for the Massachusetts Consumers Council argued, "Without a deliberate policy of public disclosure, existing institutions and incentives will perpetuate unnecessary and undesirable consumer ignorance and subordination within the medical sector."[49] The Consumer's Council agreed, and in March 1975 voted 7-0 to oppose DHEW's restrictive access policies and to recommend that any contracts between the Massachusetts PSROs and state agencies include a complete disclosure requirement concerning profiles.[50] The Consumer Council was urged by the report to take the lead in supplying consumers with understandable directories and periodic reports based on PSRO profile data to promote patient choice and quality services.

A counterargument is that consumer education is not the role of PSROs. The goal is, if anything, physician education so that they will voluntarily change their practices, if necessary, to conform with approved norms.[51] This argument is unpersuasive, given the lack of effective peer review in the past and the unlikelihood that PSROs will have a major impact on unqualified physicians. If the elimination of unnecessary procedures is thought to be a major goal, consumer access to the profile data of individual hospitals and practitioners may be essential. As attorney Robert McGarrah has argued, "We would like to provide the public aggregate data on the overall performance of a given physician in a year. In surgery it would show whether normal tissue was removed, and if there was no reason for the operation to be performed. You could find out if a physician was overprescribing antibiotics for the common cold."[52]

Public Accountability

A final argument in favor of public disclosure is the need for accountability. While aggregate data will be submitted to DHEW, without public access to individual provider data, there is no way the public can know whether or not the PSRO is performing its function as required by law. It is likely that a system without such built-in accountability will fail, and therefore the mandated disclosure of profile data could be found by the Secretary as "necessary to carry out the provisions of the act" on this basis alone. Indeed, too much attention to secrecy will probably prove counterproductive, tending to confirm the public's general skepticism about the effectiveness of peer review. If, however, one is in favor of consumer-dominated medicine, rather than peer review, this may be precisely the effect desired.

Health Care Planning

Even if one rejects all of the above arguments, profile data should nevertheless be made available to a health systems agency (HSA). These agencies, which must be consumer-controlled by law, will need such data as they work out their local health care plans and provide input to the state plan. To have a realistic plan, the HSAs will need to know the type of information the PSRO is compiling. For example, they will have to know if doctors in one area or at one particular institution admit patients more frequently, keep them in longer, order more diagnostic tests, or perform more surgery, both to work out their plans and to make reasonable recommendations regarding Certificate of Need proposals.

The act which mandated the formation of HSAs requires them to coordinate with PSROs.[53] However, that same act provides that HSAs shall "make [their] records and data available, upon request, to the public."[54] If this provision is read to require public disclosure of any information made available by PSROs (and it probably does), then it is unlikely that PSROs will make such information available unless the statute is amended or unless regulations clearly exclude information provided by PSROs. Of course, if this is the result, cooperation between these two organizations will be impossible unless DHEW permits profile data to be available to the public.

CONCLUSION

The major objection to making PSRO data available to consumers seems to be that physicians and hospitals will not cooperate voluntarily in this program if the data are made public. This reason should not be seen as sufficient because, as has been argued, unless the public has access to this data, the program will have no public accountability and is unlikely to directly benefit the health care consumer. Moreover, any moratorium on releasing data until the standards, norms, and criteria are completely worked out and agreed upon will probably result only in a perpetual denial of consumer access. If relevancy or accuracy of the data is in question, the institution or physician to whom it pertains should have the opportunity to formally rebut the data or its implications, but not to suppress it. If the entire PSRO process turns out to be so inexact or arbitrary that no conclusions can or should be drawn from the data, the answer is to abandon the program, not to restrict access to the data that would prove it a failure.

NOTES

1. G. J. Annas, *The Rights of Hospital Patients* (New York: Avon, 1975), pp. 121-135.

2. Ervin, *Civilized Man's Most Valued Right, 2 Prism* 15 (June, 1974); *cf.* A. Westin and M. Baher, *Data Banks in a Free Society* (New York: Quadrangle, 1973), pp. 17-20; A. Miller, *The Assault on Privacy* (New York: New American Library, 1972), pp. 184-220.

3. *Hammonds v. Aetna Cas. & Sur. Co.,* 243 F. Supp. 793 (N.D. Ohio 1965).

4. In *Curry v. Corn,* 227 N.Y.S.2d 470 (1966), for example, the physician disclosed information to his patient's husband who was contemplating a divorce action. In *Schaffer v. Spicer,* 215 N.W.2d 134 (S.D. 1974), the wife's psychiatrist disclosed information to the husband's attorney to aid him in a child custody case. Representative of the insurance cases is *Hague v. Williams,* 181 A.2d (N.J. 1962), where the pediatrician of an infant informed a life insurance company of a congenital heart defect that he had not informed the child's parents of, and *Hammonds v. Aetna, supra* note 3, where the physician revealed information to an insurance company when the insurance company falsely represented to him that his patient was suing him for malpractice. Cases involving reporting to employers include *Beatty v. Baston,* 13 Ohio L. Abs. 481 (Ohio App. 1932), where the physician revealed to a patient's employer during a workman's compensation action that the patient had venereal disease, *Clark v. Geraci,* 208 N.Y.S.2d 564 (S. Ct. N.Y. 1960), where a civilian employee of the Air Force asked his doctor to make an incomplete disclosure to his employer to explain absences, but the doctor made a complete disclosure including the patient's alcoholism, and the recent case of *Horne v. Patton,* 287 So.2d 824 (Ala. 1973), which involved the disclosure of information not specified in the opinion.

5. 8 Wigmore on Evidence § 2380a. Retention of the privilege was also the most controversial item in the new Federal Rules of Evidence. While initial versions eliminated the privilege entirely, the final version provides that the privilege shall "be governed by the principles of the common law as they may be interpreted by the courts of the United States in the light of reason and experience." Where, however, state law governs a case, the privilege shall be "determined in accordance with state law." Rule 501.

6. A. Westin, *Privacy and Freedom* (New York: Atheneum, 1967), p. 7.

7. *Horne v. Patton,* 287 So.2d 824 (Ala. 1973).

8. Miller, *Personal Privacy in the Computer Age,* 67 MICH. L. REV. 1089, 1107 (1968).

9. In 1939, for example, *Time* magazine published a story in its "medicine" section with a photograph of the patient, a young woman who was receiving treatment for uncontrollable

gluttony apparently induced by a condition of the pancreas, *Barber v. Time, Inc.,* 159 S.W.2d 291 (Mo. 1942). Other cases, like *Horne v. Patton, supra* note 7 however, indicate that publication is not necessary to sustain an invasion of privacy action. For example, having unauthorized persons in a delivery room, *DeMay v. Roberts,* 9 N.W. 146 (Mich. 1881), or, by analogy, permitting unauthorized persons to view confidential medical records, may also be an invasion of privacy.

10. *Klinge v. Lutheran Medical Center,* 518 S.W. 2d 157 (1975).

11. Rabinow, "Privacy—A Measured Right," *PSRO Update,* Sept. 1974, p. 4.

12. A physician does not need a statute to release confidential medical information while a danger to the public exists. The leading case enunciating this exception, *Simonsen v. Swenson,* 177 S.W. 831, was decided by the Supreme Court of Nebraska in 1920. In that case a fellow who was visiting a small town was seen by a physician who was also the physician for the hotel in which he was staying. The physician diagnosed syphillis and advised the patient to "get out of town" or he would tell the hotel. When the patient remained in town the doctor notified the landlady who disinfected his room and removed his belongings to the hallway. The court decided that the doctor had the right to reveal just as much information concerning a contagious disease as was necessary for others to take proper precautions against becoming infected with it and that his actions under the circumstances were justified. The California Supreme Court has recently extended this reasoning to the psychotherapist whose patient threatens serious bodily harm to a named individual. The court goes one step further, however, in actually finding a *duty* on the part of the therapist to warn the named "victim." *Tarasoff v. Regents of Univ. of Calif.,* 529 P.2d 553 (1974). The general rationale for this exception is that at some point the interests of society outweigh the individual's interests in maintaining privacy concerning his medical conditions. From the cases, one can gather that physicians will be granted a large measure of discretion in making such disclosures so long as they are made in good faith in an effort to protect third parties.

13. *See, e.g., Commonwealth v. Wiseman,* 249 N.E.2d 610 (1969). This case involves a finding of invasion of privacy of the rights of mental patients in the filming and showing of the documentary "Titicut Follies."

14. Under a similar theory, clauses by which the patient has agreed not to sue the hospital for negligence have been ruled invalid because the patient really had no choice but to sign the form. *Tunkl v. Regents of Univ. of Calif.,* 60 Cal.2d 92, 383 P.2d 441 (1963). One could also argue that it is impossible to give consent for release of medical records before they are in existence (*e.g.,* at the beginning of a hospital stay rather than at the end) since at that time one may have no reasonable idea of what they might contain.

15. Note, *Medical Practice and the Right to Privacy,* 43 MINN. L. REV. 943, 960 (1959).

16. Even though there has been little judicial explication of the content of this exception, one can deduce that such cases as telling a spouse of a patient's heart condition or impending death, or telling an employer of a roofer that the roofer is subject to blackouts would probably qualify (since the patient would be endangering his own life by continuing in this trade).

17. J.R. Waltz and F.E. Inbau, *Medical Jurisprudence* (New York: The Macmillan Co., 1971), pp. 275-76.

18. *See generally, New York Times v. Sullivan,* 376 U.S. 254 (1964); *Rosenblatt v. Baer,* 383 U.S. 75 (1966); *Curtis Publishing Co. v. Butts,* 388 U.S. 13 (1967); *Rosenbloom v. Metromedia, Inc.,* 402 U.S. 29 (1971); *Time, Inc. v. Hill,* 385 U.S. 374 (1967).

19. *Dodd v. Pearson,* 279 F. Supp. 101 (D.D.C. 1968).

20. Welch, "Professional Standards Review Organizations—Problems and Prospects," 289

New Eng. J. Med. 291, 294 (1973).

21. This provision is discussed in more detail later in the chapter.

22. A summary of the laws of all 50 states is set forth in Helfman, *et al. Access to Medical Records* in Appendix, Report of the Secretary's Commission on Medical Malpractice, (Washington, D.C.: 1973), U.S. Government Print. Office, pp. 186-213.

23. Mass. Gen. Laws Ch. 111, § 70.

24. *Boston Evening Globe,* March 1, 1974, p. 1.

25. Wolfstone, "Patient's Right of Access to Inspect and Obtain Copies of Medical Records," ed. C. Wecht, *Legal Medicine Annual: 1971,* (New York: Appleton-Century-Crofts, 1971), p. 379.

26. Secretary's Report, *supra* note 22, p. 75.

27. Appendix, Secretary's Report, *supra* note 22, p. 186.

28. *Wallace v. University Hosps.,* 164 N.E.2d 917, *aff'd and modified,* 170 N.E.2d 261 (Ohio Ct. App. 1960), *motion to dismiss granted,* 171 Ohio St. 487, 172 N.E.2d 459 (1961). This case involved a patient whose lawyer wanted her records to determine if filing of a malpractice action was indicated. In another case where an insurance company sought access upon patient authorization the court said the hospital is only the custodian of the record and the patient has a property right in it sufficient to allow him access to it and to copy it without resort to litigation. *Pyramid Life Ins. Co. v. Masonic Hosp.,* 191 F. Supp. 51 (W.D. Okla. 1961). A New York court has also held that a hospital cannot withhold a patient's medical record for the purposes of concealing the identity of a physician who may have committed malpractice on the patient. *Matter of Weiss,* 47 N.Y.S.2d 455 (1955).

In a District of Columbia federal case a dispensary and a private physician were ordered to hand over medical records to a surviving son even though the statute of limitations for a wrongful death action had expired. The court specifically rejected the argument that the filing of a lawsuit should be a prerequisite to access: "We are unwilling to hold that one to whom a duty to disclose medical data is already owed is compelled by the rule of reasonable diligence to engage in legal proceedings to attain a loftier status." *Emmet v. Eastern Dispensary & Cas. Hosp.,* 396 F.2d 931 (U.S. App. D.C. 1967). This case was followed in a recent Illinois case which directed the handing over of pertinent medical information upon request. In the court's words: "It is our opinion that the 'fiduciary qualities of the physician-patient relationship' require the disclosure of medical data to a patient or his agent on request. . . . " *Cannell v. Medical and Surgical Clinic,* 315 N.E.2d 278 (Ill. App. 1974).

In the area of disclosure of mental health records, however, the case law is not unanimous. In a Texas case, for example, a patient was able to obtain access to records of a mental institution on the basis that the institution was "public" and that they were open to inspection by patients. *Morris v. Houster,* 377 S.W.2d 841 (Tex. Civ. App. 1964). Taking the contrary position, a recent New York Federal District Court case decided against a patient's access to mental hospital records on the very narrow view that "neither the statutory, administrative nor decisional law of New York recognizes a former patient's entitlement to his medical files in the absence of pending litigation." *Gotkin v. Miller,* 379 F. Supp. 859 (1974); *cf. Shikara v. Commissioner of Mental Health,* 227 N.E.2d 477 (Mass. 1967). The case involved a woman who wanted her records to help her write a book about her experiences. The logic of this lower court decision is not persuasive since it simply encourages the filing of a possibly unfounded malpractice action to gain records access. While the case was affirmed on appeal, the higher court noted that the plaintiff was "not undergoing or contemplating treatment" and implied that if she had been, the physician might have had an obligation to disclose her records on request. *Gotkin v. Miller,* 514 F.2d 125, 130 (1975).

Some physicians argue that there may be circumstances under which it would affirmatively harm the patient to see his medical record and that under these circumstances access might properly be denied. The state of the law was summarized by one leading legal commentator as follows: "Generally, the law will make information from the record available unless it is contrary to the best medical interest of the patient." Hagman, "The Non-Litigant Patient's Right to Medical Records Medicine *vs.* Law," 14 *J. Forensic Sci.* 352, 366 (1969). A medico-legal text has taken this exception one step further to argue that in the absence of clear case or statutory dictate "the decision to allow or not to allow the patient or his authorized agent to see the record can be made on the basis of administrative considerations, taking into account the circumstances of the particular case." Health Law Center, *Hospital Law Manual* (Germantown, Md.: Aspen Systems Corp. Medical Records, May 1973), p. 16.

29. 42 U.S.C. § 1320(c)-15 (1972).

30. *Association of Am. Physicians & Surgeons, Inc. v. Weinberger,* 395 F. Supp. 125 (N.D. Ill. 1975).

31. Spigarn, *Confidentiality: Report of the Conference on Confidentiality of Health Records,* Key Biscayne, Florida, November 6-9, 1974 (1975), p. 29.

32. Simmons, "PSRO Today: The Program's Viewpoint," 292 *New Eng. J. Med.* 365 (1975).

33. Willett, "PSRO Today: A Lawyer's Assessment," 292 *New Eng. J. Med.* 340, 343 (1975).

34. Letter from Richard P. Bergen, Director, American Medical Association Legal Research Dept., to Boston attorney Garrick F. Cole, June 18, 1974.

35. *Cited in* Fleischer, The Ownership of Hospital Records and Roentgenograms, 4 Ill. Cont. Legal Ed. 73, 82 (1966); and see *In Re Culbertson's Will,* 57 Misc. 2d 391, 292 N.Y.S.2d 806 (Sun. Ct. Erie Co., 1968) (directing records of deceased physician not to be destroyed but refusing to compel their delivery directly to former patients on the basis that they were "property" of the physician. The executor was directed to make the records available to succeeding physicians at the patient's request.)

36. *McGarry v. Mercier,* 272 Mich. 501, 262 N.W. 296, 297 (1935).

37. *See* Shenkin and Warner, "Giving the Patient His Medical Record: A Proposal to Improve the System," 289 *New Eng. J. Med.* 688 (1973).

38. *See, e.g.,* Hagman, *supra* note 28.

39. Letters to the Editor, 290 *New Eng. J. Med.* 288 (1974).

40. Implementation Regulations, Department of Health, Education, and Welfare (DHEW) Privacy Act of 1974, *Federal Register,* Oct. 8, 1975, 47406, 47411. (These regulations would not, of course, apply to PSROs unless they were found to be so subject to DHEW control as to make them "federal agencies.") On the other hand, the recently passed Education Amendments of 1974 specifically enumerate "scores on standardized intelligence, aptitude, and psychological tests, interest inventory results, and health data" among the items which educational institutions must make available to parents of students under 18 and to the students themselves if aged 18 or over. This is a direct repudiation of the persuasiveness of the previously noted medical reasons for denial of access to such "sensitive" and "potentially disturbing" data. 20 U.S.C. 1232(g); Sec. 438(a)(1) of P.L. 93-380.

41. *See, supra* note 29. The act would also be inapplicable unless PSROs were considered federal agencies for the purposes of the Administrative Procedures Act.

42. 5 U.S.C.A. § 552a.

43. 5 U.S.C.A. § 552a(b).

44. 5 U.S.C.A. § 552a(a)(7).

45. Kirsch, et al., *PSRO Information and Consumer Choice: The Case for Public Disclosure of Health Services Data,* Harvard Univ. Center for Community Health and Medical Care, Feb., 1975.

46. *Natanson v. Kline,* 186 Kan. 393 (1960).

47. Hagman, *The Medical Patient's Right to Know,* 17 U.C.L.A. L. REV. 758, 764 (1970).

48. *Canterbury v. Spence,* 464 F.2d 772 (D.C. Cir. 1972) (duty to disclose 1 percent risk of paralysis in laminectomy); *Wilkenson v. Vesey,* 295 A.2d 676 (R.I. 1972) (duty to disclose risks of radiation treatments); *Cobbs v. Grant,* 502 P.2d 1 (Cal. 1972) (duty to disclose risks of operation for a duodenal ulcer). *See generally* Annas, "Informed Consent: When Good Medicine May Not Be Good Law," 1 *Medicolegal News* 3 (1973).

49. *See, supra* note 45, at 97.

50. *Boston Globe,* March 17, 1975, at 3.

51. *See, for example* Jessee, *et al.,* "PSRO: An Educational Force for Improving Quality of Care," 292 *New Eng. J. Med.* 668 (1975).

52. Spivak, "Medical Care Review Stirs a Fiery Debate Among U.S. Doctors," *Wall St. J.,* June 24, 1974, at 1.

53. The National Health Planning and Resources Development Act of 1974 (P.L. 93-641) provides that "each health systems agency shall coordinate its activities with—(1) each Professional Standards Review Organization—...." § 1513(d).

54. *Id.* § 1512(b)(3)(B)(viii)(III).

Chapter 8
Confidentiality and Quality of Care

Steven B. Epstein

PATIENT DATA AND COMPUTERIZATION

The increasing trend toward computerization of individual health data has generated enormous concern for the potential risks to confidentiality of patient data. The purpose of this section of the chapter will be to examine the current thinking on computerization of health data and then to analyze the effect, if any, of the computerization-confidentiality controversy on quality of health care.

The Extent of the Problem

Third party payors of health care (insurance companies, Blue Cross/Blue Shield and federal and state governments) collect individual health data (patient data) as a necessary part of the claims paying process. After claims processing, patient data are maintained by the third party payors in retrievable form through the use of computers. It has been estimated that Blue Cross/Blue Shield has 25 million individual patient files in retrievable form, while the Social Security System, which maintains a similar volume, receives Medicare information on five million people annually. The Medical Information Bureau (MIB), a shared data bank used by 700 insurance companies representing 90 percent of the nation's life insurance policies, contains 12 million records and 15 million requests for information each year. Information is obtained for MIB both during the investigative process for life insurance (blanket authorizations for release of medical information is generally required) and when a health insurance policyholder applies for health benefits (blanket release of all relevant medical information is required). MIB information is available to all participating insurance companies.

Computerized collection of patient data on the scale described above clearly indicates a formidable problem.

Advantages and Disadvantages of Computerization

Advantages to computerization often cited include legibility of records, quick retrievability in case of emergency, complete storage of information in one place or facility, prevention of loss of records, and facilitation of research, statistical and epidemiological studies. In particular, in the health insurance field, it is argued that computerization reduces the costs of processing health claims and enhances speed and efficiency. Furthermore, computer advocates argue that there is no greater danger to privacy by storing information in one centralized place than in leaving such information where it presently resides unprotected in doctors' offices and hospitals.

Opponents of computerization contend that computerization facilitates unauthorized disclosure to unauthorized persons, such as employers, banks, health insurance companies, and the press. In addition, inaccurate information may be recorded and remain on file for an indefinite period of time with no opportunity for correction. Moreover, information collected for one purpose may be matched (i.e., using computer programs to compare two different data systems, such as medical records with military or internal revenue service records) or linked (i.e., using a series of computer programs which bring together the records on the same individual, such as data originating at different times and in different clinical settings) with other data, to the detriment of the individual. Although it is admitted that both matching (useful for new sociogeographic epidemiological correlations) and linkage (useful for medical research, longitudinal, and genetic studies) information may be helpful for certain kinds of research, it nevertheless presents a real danger to the privacy of an individual and may result in serious abuse.

Privacy and Due Process Questions

The continuing debate on computerization has created a series of due process and right to privacy questions which private and governmental entities are just beginning to resolve. As to due process issues, certain principles are being developed which entitle an individual to basic rights in the data collection process. These principles include:

1. The right of the public to know that a data system exists;

2. The right of an individual to know that a data system includes information on him;

3. The right of an individual to have access to the information maintained on him in such system; and

4. The right of an individual to challenge the quality and accuracy of the information maintained on him.

Right to privacy questions include:

1. What information should be collected about an individual through compulsory means?

2. Should information be linked and matched with other information and, if so, on what terms?

3. What judgments should be made on the basis of this information?

The solutions to the above raised questions will vary depending upon the nature of the data being collected—i.e., the balance between individual rights and data collection needs may shift depending upon whether the data being collected are for health purposes, tax purposes, or criminal purposes. Each different area of concern may produce a result unique to the needs of that area. Let us therefore examine the type and purpose of data collection as it relates specifically to the health field.

Health Data Collection

Health insurers routinely collect three types of information during the claims process: patient identification, clinical information, and financial information. This information usually includes the following items:

Patient Information

Name
Address
Name of Subscriber
Patient's Occupation/Employer
Birthdate/Age
Sex
Relationship of Patient to Subscriber
Group Number

Clinical Information

Attending Physician
Referring Physician
Accident/Emergency/Onset:
    Date
    Time

History
Final Diagnosis and Complications
Operations/Procedures (Dates of Each)
Disposition of Patient (Alive or Dead)

Financial Information

Date/Time of Admission
Date/Time of Discharge
Length of Stay
Charge per Day
Accommodation
Charge Information

Insurance companies utilize this information for administrative, actuarial, claims and utilization review, and research purposes. As long as insurance companies and other third party payors are responsible for the payment of health claims, information must be provided to such companies and payors to enable them to properly and efficiently carry out this function. Furthermore, without the necessary health data, an insurance company would not be able to formulate sound fiscal policy. It is argued that most patients would probably not object to the release of information to a health carrier contained in the basic claims form. However, objection would probably be forthcoming if a patient realized that an insurance company had access to his entire medical record and that such access could result in the subsequent sharing of this information with other insurance companies through the mechanism of a shared data bank. (The question of informed consent to the release of patient data has created a controversy as to whether an individual fully understands the consequences of signing an insurance company release of information form, since the individual neither knows the fate of the information released, that it may be taken out of context, nor that it may be matched with other data or released to other companies. It is also unclear whether such consent is truly voluntary since failure to sign a consent form may result in an inability to receive health care.)

As in other data areas, the computerization of patient data must be resolved by a balancing of interests. The necessity of a third party payor to require certain information to perform its function effectively and the needs of legitimate research to improve the health system must be weighed against the necessity of providing adequate safeguards to the privacy rights of individual patients. In attempting to analyze this balancing of interests, it is important to review the necessity of mandating patient identification.

Patient Identification

Patient identification is required almost exclusively to varify benefits and eligibility. If neither eligibility nor extent of benefits is at issue, patient identification becomes surplusage. A patient's medical record is generally obtained from a hospital only when information on a claim form is erroneous or incomplete. This information is usually for benefits determination purposes and is generally not necessary for any other health purpose. (In this connection, it would seem more appropriate for an insurance company to inform the hospital of the problem and allow the hospital to correct the error or supply additional information to justify the claim, rather than to request the patient's entire medical record. It would also seem more appropriate for the insurance company to return the file to the hospital or destroy it rather than maintain such medical record for its data files.)

In actuality, should a comprehensive system of national health insurance (NHI) be adopted, it would appear to be unnecessary to collect patient identification at all, assuming no copayments or deductibles were required. For example, if national health insurance covered all United States citizens regardless of age for all health services (i.e., no copays or deductibles), then a provider would merely have to determine citizenship eligibility through the use of an identification number or social security number. Once eligibility was determined, he would only have to report clinical and financial information to a fiscal intermediary for payment purposes. It could be argued that patient identification would still be necessary to prevent fraud, for certain research purposes, or to identify patient abusers of the health care system, but such arguments may not be able to withstand an overriding desire for confidentiality and the protection of a patient's privacy rights, especially in light of the fact that alternative mechanisms (such as field audits for fraud detection) may be available to accomplish the competing goals.

Patient Identification and Quality of Care

Since, as stated above, patient information becomes part of the computerized data set of a health insurer for claims purposes, it becomes necessary to examine the impact, if any, that computerized patient data has on quality of care. Upon reflection, it appears that computerized patient data have little direct effect on quality. Identifiable patient data have no direct connection with the evaluation of inpatient or ambulatory quality of care by a third party payor. Such a review can be undertaken quite satisfactorily without knowledge of the patient's identity. Certain research studies may find it helpful to have access to identifiable patient data (e.g., a study concerned with multiple hospitalization), but such research could well be undertaken on a special study basis and would hardly justify the capture of substantial patient identification into a computerized system in the name of quality assessment.

We should therefore recognize that confidentiality of patient data, although an acute problem for the third party payor for cost and eligibility purposes, is not an essential consideration for quality purposes since quality of care review does not require disclosure of identifiable patient information into a centralized computer data bank. Moreover, quality of care review undertaken internally by a facility would not require disclosure of patient data to a centralized data bank.

The Professional Standards Review Organization (PSRO), on the other hand, is charged with the responsibility of reviewing institutional quality of care in a nondelegated hospital and monitoring quality in a delegated hospital. Patient information will necessarily be disclosed to a PSRO. At the same time, the PSRO, which is not an internal component of a hospital, will maintain a computerized data system which will contain patient identifiers. Let us therefore examine the protection afforded to patient data by PSROs as mandated by the Department of Health, Education, and Welfare (DHEW).

PSROs and Patient Data

DHEW has provided in Transmittal 16 for the protection of patient data which must be submitted to a PSRO. Identifiable patient data are defined as privileged data and information. Privileged data are subject to protection against disclosure outside the PSRO and must be maintained in coded form with personal identifiers purged as soon as such identifiers are no longer necessary. Transmittal 16 also addresses the due process data principles discussed above: (1) notification of the existence of the PSRO data system must be mandated; (2) procedures must be established and implemented to inform individual patients that data is being collected on them; (3) an individual must be allowed access to the information on him to ascertain the accuracy of such information; and (4) procedures must be established and implemented to verify the accuracy of the data.

Transmittal 16 recognized the pitfalls and problems which face an entity establishing a computerized data system containing identifiable patient information, and attempts to establish a balance between the PSRO's need to collect such information and adequate protections for the public to provide for the continued confidentiality of such information. Although continuing modification will be necessary as the PSRO data system is implemented, the transmittal represents an intelligent attempt to balance difficult conflicting interests.

Policy Determinations by the Judicial System

A final matter of discussion involves the role the courts are presently playing in matters of policy concerning patient data confidentiality. Issues of confidentiality most frequently arise out of context in the judicial system. Determinations by a court which may have wide policy implications occur frequently as a discovery issue in a malpractice action. The court must view the discovery issue in the context of the action and parties immediately before it. This procedure would appear ill-suited to deal with the complicated ramifications of computerization and confidentiality. Further, an individual with a legitimate grievance against an institution which may raise a significant policy question concerning confidentiality may not be able to afford to litigate his case unless substantial damages are involved. Such damages are often extremely difficult to prove. Because of these factors it would appear incumbent upon the legislature and not the courts to provide for a resolution of many of the difficult confidentiality policy issues facing the health field.

PROVIDER DATA

Unlike the plethora of information and papers which accompanies the patient data problem, comparatively little has been written about the confidentiality of provider data. Provider data can be defined for our purposes as data which are identifiable to an individual institution or health professional. In particular, we are concerned about the creation of patterns of practice or profiles which are identifiable to a given provider.

Provider data are collected by all third party payors of health care. These data are, however, overwhelmingly used for non-quality-of-care determinations such as cost (e.g., length of stay), actuarial, fraud control, and determination of fee schedules. Some third party payors have developed provider profiles (e.g., MADOC for Medicare and some state Medicaid programs), but generally do not use such profiles for quality purposes. This attitude can probably be traced to the fact that third party payors have a clear incentive to review cost issues, but have little incentive to concern themselves with areas involving matters of professional judgment.

PSROs, however, are specifically and statutorily charged with probing into the actions providers are taking with regard to medical matters. PSROs will also be creating provider profiles for both institutions and individual health professionals.

PSROs (and their predecessor foundations for medical care) can therefore be considered unique in the health care industry and have consequently raised new issues concerning the confidentiality of provider data.

Confidentiality of Provider Data

The crucial question facing provider data is whether full disclosure should be made to the public of the quality of care that a provider is rendering to the public. As is the case with the issue concerning patient data, any decision as to confidentiality of provider data must take into consideration two conflicting viewpoints.

Proponents of disclosure argue that provider patterns of practice and profiles of care should be public information if the consumer of health services is to make a rational decision in the marketplace as to choice of provider. Furthermore, it is felt that full disclosure will force providers into a higher level of quality of care by focusing public attention as to problem areas.

Mitigating against this position is the relatively poor state of the art regarding quality of care. Is it possible for a PSRO to effectively determine through the mechanism of a profile whether a provider is in fact delivering care of high or low quality? In addition, if provider data are made public, will such data be misinterpreted or misunderstood by a potential consumer? Will the publication of a morbidity rate or the percentage of appendectomies per 1,000 patients have any real meaning to a consumer or, even worse, be a subject of misinterpretation by him? Finally, there is some concern that data submitted by a provider may not be as candid if publication is anticipated. This may be especially true in the case of hospital medical care evaluation (MCE) studies. The crux of the issue simply stated is will it do more harm than good to disclose provider data?

PSRO Disclosure

DHEW through Transmittal 16 has determined that PSRO-generated data and information indicating patterns of health care practices identifiable to individual health care practitioners are privileged data and information. However, PSRO information which is uniquely identifiable to a given health care facility may be disclosed (to the public) upon request and payment of a fee to cover the expense of copying the requested information. Because institutional provider data are being disclosed to the public, DHEW recognized the possibility of such data being either inaccurate or misunderstood. As a compromise, Transmittal 16 requires that a facility must be notified in writing 30 days prior to disclosure and be permitted an opportunity to review the information for accuracy and to provide comments to accompany the disclosed information. Moreover, Transmittal 16, in recognition of the potential problem this disclosure may create for hospital MCE studies, has determined that data and information collected and/or generated for MCE studies (as defined in regulations) are privileged data and information.

As the transmittal clearly indicates, DHEW has determined that health care facility data and information, except MCE studies, should be disclosed to the public, but data and information on health care practitioners should not be disclosed. If facilities provider data are to be disclosed, then it is essential that the interpretation of such data be carefully explained. The transmittal is unclear as to whether a PSRO is to release basic facility data or to provide an interpretation of such data. If interpretation is to be offered, who at the PSRO will make the necessary evaluation and analysis and on what basis will such interpretation be made? Considering the present monetary problems facing PSROs, and consequently the likely unavailability of sufficient staff to perform adequate interpretation, it may be necessary for a PSRO, as an alternative, to provide raw data to a hospital and allow a hospital to prepare a report acceptable to the PSRO (perhaps in a manner similar to a prospectus filed in the securities field). In any event, it is almost certain that if any controversial hospital data are released by a PSRO, the hospital will provide a detailed explanation of such information for public purposes. Such explanation will probably be far more comprehensive in scope than the PSRO will initially prepare.

Nevertheless, the decision to require disclosure of facilities information and not to allow disclosure of health professionals information appears to be a sound one. First, in general, much more analysis concerning the quality of hospital care (which the PSRO is initially charged with reviewing) is available. Second, an institution such as a hospital is in a much better position to respond to the publication of a PSRO profile than an individual practitioner, both from an economic and a time consumption point of view. Third, disclosure of data about an institution (especially an institution which is considered in many cases to be publicly oriented with public advantages such as tax-exempt status) does not offend the sensibilities to the same degree as disclosure of data about an individual. An inherent concept of fairness mandates that we move much more slowly toward disclosure of information which through inaccuracy or misinterpretation may ruin a professional's livelihood.

Finally, further analysis must be undertaken with respect to the mechanism for the creation of individual health professional's profiles, even if such profiles will not be disclosed to the public. At present, it is unclear how such profiles will be developed, but almost certainly a review of raw data will have to be undertaken by a committee of PSRO physicians (in the case of physicians) to interpret such data. Careful procedures will have to be created to both allow the physician to have input into the formation of his profile and to assure the confidentiality of his profile within the physician community. A health professional may in many cases be more seriously damaged by peer reaction to an incomplete or misleading profile than to disclosure of such a profile to the lay public.

In general, the DHEW transmittal appears to be an excellent first step in resolving many of the developing confidentiality problems facing provider data. Nevertheless, actual implementation of the procedures in developing individual health professional provider profiles will have to be carefully analyzed by DHEW as individual PSROs develop these procedures as an internal matter. Further, procedures concerning interpretation of institutional profiles must be developed to provide the public with access to accurate and meaningful information.

Part IV

Licensure and Hospital Privileges

Chapter 9
Professional Licensure and Hospital Delineation of Clinical Privileges: Relationship to Quality Assurance

Claude E. Welch

PROFESSIONAL LICENSURE

Definitions

At the outset, certain definitions will be made since they will be used frequently in the discussion.[1]

Licensure is defined as "the process by which an agency of government grants permission to persons meeting predetermined qualifications to engage in a given occupation."

Certification is defined as "the process by which a non-governmental agency or association grants recognition to an individual who has met certain predetermined qualifications specified by that agency or institution." In the present discussion certification is confined to specialists, and is given to an individual by any of the American specialty boards recognized by the American Medical Association (AMA) and included in the American Board of Medical Specialties (ABMS) (Table 9-1).

Certification usually has been awarded on the basis of competitive examinations. Recertification theoretically could either be compulsory or voluntary, depending upon whether or not such examinations were required or taken at the option of the practitioner. Relicensure, on the other hand, can only be compulsory and never is voluntary.

Licensure is subject to several modifications. It can be limited so that a doctor can practice only in one area—e.g., a specified hospital or a single state. In the United States a license qualifies an individual for the unlimited practice of both medicine and surgery. Theoretically, at least, it could be granted also at a specialist level.

Thus, there are many possibilities and many combinations of certification and licensure. What is the history and what is the present situation? For

179

Table 9-1: Specialty Boards

Surgical	Medical	Other
Surgery	Dermatology	Anesthesiology
Colon & Rectal Surgery	Family Practice	Nuclear Medicine
Neurological Surgery	General Practice	Ophthalmology
Obstetrics-Gynecology	Internal Medicine	Pathology
Orthopedic Surgery	Pediatrics	Physical Medicine
Otolaryngology	Preventive Medicine	& Rehabilitation
Plastic Surgery	Psychiatry & Neurology	Radiology
Thoracic Surgery		
Urology		

historical details the author has drawn chiefly from Rosemary Stevens' admirable study.[2]

Licensure

Despite the definition given above, licensure has had a checkered career in America. In 1760, governmental licensing of physicians was adopted first by the state of New York. However, somewhat later, medical societies were organized throughout many states; the Massachusetts Medical Society was granted powers to license physicians by its own examinations. This innovation was followed elsewhere so that several state medical societies carried the functions of licensure by 1825. This then was countered by the advent of educational institutions which also demanded similar power. Beginning in 1803 in Massachusetts, either the Harvard degree or a license granted by the Massachusetts Medical Society qualified a man for practice. When Yale established a medical school in 1810, after long arguments it was decided that it would give degrees, while the Connecticut Medical Society would give licenses.

However, in the first half of the 19th century, proprietary medical schools began to proliferate. The first one was set up in Castleton, Vermont, by three physicians. These schools diluted and weakened the authority of the university medical schools. Professional regulation was weakened even further, according to Stevens, by attacks on elitism that were characteristic of Jacksonian democracy at all levels of the American society. As a result, medical legislation was repealed by many states. By 1890 the tide had turned again, and control of licensure at this time passed to the individual states rather than to medical societies or universities. By 1893 18 states required an examination for licensure, and in 17 others a school diploma was considered to be adequate only if the school had been approved by the state. Ever since that time, licensure has remained under the control of individual states.

Thus, in the United States licensure at various intervals has been under the control of medical societies, medical schools, and the various states. The federal government (as another possible agent) had not been suggested at high governmental levels until the recent bills introduced by U.S. Senators Edward M. Kennedy and Daniel K. Inouye gave impetus to this possibility which had been considered frequently by many others in the past.

It is interesting to note that licensing has followed an entirely different pattern in England. There, the Royal Colleges were established several centuries ago, and either they or the major hospitals acquired the power of licensure. There was another major difference—namely, that American licensing permits the practice of medicine *and* surgery, while in Great Britain individuals were licensed either as physicians *or* surgeons. Furthermore, British physicians who practiced in hospitals were many steps ahead of general practitioners both in prestige and in financial rewards. These same differences persist today except that financial returns have tended to become more equal between general practitioners and specialists in very recent years.

It should be noted that the doctrine of elitism *vs.* egalitarianism is still sharply in focus throughout the world. Elitism is extremely prominent in England. In the Peoples Republic of China, egalitarianism erased elitism in 1949. These conflicting trends exist today in America. Thus the AMA has striven historically for an egalitarian approach indicating that one doctor is equivalent to another. To some extent, however, this attitude has been belied by the institution of the American Specialty Boards by the AMA which do, in themselves, confer an elitist attitude. As an example of equal privilege, most licensure now allows physicians unrestricted powers to carry out medical therapy or surgery. On the other hand, a recent study of the surgical services in the United States conducted by the American College of Surgeons (ACS) and the American Surgical Association (ASA) demands that surgery be done by qualified surgeons. This issue must be faced squarely in the development of any future plans, and should not be considered to be snobbery if it is in the best interest of the public.

To summarize, historically, power of licensure has been acquired by several bodies. Even some other organizations could be included as present possibilities in view of the British experience—e.g., hospitals, or the United States counterparts of the Royal Colleges—the Specialty Societies, of which the ACS is a prime example. However, in the United States even other possible bodies could be added, including the ABMS and the Coordinating Council on Medical Education (CCME).

In this complex mélange of voluntary and governmental agencies, many have served or could serve as agents of government as licensing bodies.

Therefore, there is nothing immutable in the present picture of licensing by states.

If changes are to be made, what are the possibilities? At this time it seems entirely reasonable that licensing be a governmental function so that the voice of the public can be heard and a proliferation of guild-like organizations prevented. If it is to be a governmental function, it necessarily must have to be done primarily either by individual states or by the federal government. However, it is obvious that if licensure of physicians is to have any reasonable base, the state must accept the advice of the medical profession. Licensing boards must at least contain a preponderance of physicians to be effective.

Qualifications for licensure in nearly all states at the present time include only a few essentials; they are graduation from an approved medical school, qualification by an examination, and often a year's internship. Examinations are of different quality; in some instances it has been suggested that they were designed to restrain professional competition and to keep doctors out of specific states. Licensure of physicians at a federal level is attractive in many ways. Standardization would occur and probably at a level higher than that which it attains in many states at present. National licensure would remove irregular practices such as mentioned above. However, other effects might follow. For example, it could promote migration of physicians from one state to another. Conceivably for example, South Dakota might lose physicians and Florida gain them, at least in the depths of winter.

Limited Licensure

After the M.D. degree has been acquired, interns or residents in training are given licenses that permit them to practice only in their parent institution. Usually, licenses are given for periods of one to five years. An extension of this type of licensure is visualized in the recent Report of the Committee on Goals and Priorities, of the National Board of Medical Examiners.

Licensure as Specialists

Separate licensure of physicians and surgeons, as mentioned above, has been the rule in Great Britain, but it has never attracted support in the United States. Not only is it conceivable that these two large classes of practitioners could be separated by licensure, but that each of the other medical specialties could be given separate licensure. Let us first consider the separation of physicians and surgeons.

From the historical point of view, attempts to separate licensure in the United States have failed. According to Rosemary Stevens, associate professor of public health at Yale University, specialist licenses were considered by Alberta in 1926; a specialist would need to show that he had completed one year of general internship and two and a half years of hospital specialty training. In 1929 a bill to regulate general surgery, all of its subspecialties, and the fields of radiology, pathology, and anesthesia was introduced in New Jersey. This was fought by the state medical society and narrowly failed to pass the N. J. State Assembly in 1930. Since that time there has been relatively little interest in the procedure in any state, though a somewhat similar bill was introduced in California two years ago.

On first sight, major advantages seem to follow such a method. Specialists could be identified easily, would be well trained, and in the long run improve public welfare. Major difficulties, however, are encountered in the legal definitions of specialties, particularly since they overlap in many respects. Such a plan also could succeed only if there were an adequate supply of specialists throughout the country. With the problems of distribution of medical care in the United States, it would seem unfortunate to require sharp legal restrictions of practice. Medico-legal problems would escalate if doctors stepped outside their specialty. The medical profession has been strongly opposed to any such actions because of the inflexible nature of legal definitions that could reduce the availability of medical care rather than improve it. It seems logical to agree with Stevens who stated, "the days of endorsing licensing of specialists are long over; the problem of doing so today would be even more complex than when licensing was seriously considered in the 1920s."

The GAP Report

In 1973 a Committee on Goals and Priorities of the National Board of Medical Examiners submitted a report to the parent board. This report, the GAP Report, described a prospective evaluation system for certification and licensure that is of great interest in this context. The report, needless to say, engendered a great deal of attention—both favorable and unfavorable; it has not been adopted by the parent organization, but it does indicate an alternative policy toward licensure.

It was proposed that medical educational institutions would grant an M.D. degree to an individual; this degree would indicate that an individual should be competent to assume responsibility for patient care under supervision. An examination carried out by the National Board of Medical Examiners (NBME) then would confirm competence at this level. Assuming that the individual passed this examination, a state medical board would then grant a limited license which would allow the individual to practice in a supervised setting. After an unspecified period (which theoretically could last anywhere from one to 15 or even more years), the director of the institution could then state that the individual was capable of caring for individuals in an independent environment. This would be confirmed by a second examination. Licensure would then be granted by the state for independent practice outside of the hospital walls. Whether or not this competence would be limited to one specialty or extend across the whole field of medicine is not clear, but it is probable that it would be at a specialty level since the report states "certification at the level of independent practice should be concerned with professional and personal qualifications that predict competence in a chosen specialty including the primary care specialties of family practice, internal medicine, and pediatrics."

Relicensure

The concept of relicensure is based upon the fact that medical knowledge has been expanding at such a rapid rate that it has been estimated that at least 50 percent of one's basic medical knowledge will be outmoded five years hence. Needless to say, this topic has been discussed very thoroughly by physicians and has, in general terms, been quite unpopular. For example, in one questionnaire submitted to surgeons by the Study on Surgical Services for the United States (SOSSUS) only 2.1 percent of all M.D.s were strongly in favor of periodic relincensure, and 6.3 percent favored it; 15.1 percent were not sure; 28.7 percent were opposed; and 47.1 percent were strongly opposed.[4] There was relatively little difference in opinion regardless of the date of graduation of these persons. In a similar poll, 65.4 percent of AMA members declared themselves opposed to relicensure.[5]

However, there are many trends that point in the opposite direction. In 1967, the President's Commission on Medical Manpower recommended that "the professional societies in state government should explore the possibility of periodic relicensing of physicians and other health professionals. Relicensure should be granted either upon certification of acceptable performance in continuing education programs or upon the basis of challenge examinations in the practitioner's specialty."[6]

New Mexico was the first state to require relicensure. Its law became effective in June 1971. At the present time, five states have granted authority for relicensure to the state boards of registration (Kansas, New Mexico, Maryland, Kentucky, and West Virginia). Three have implemented the law (New Mexico, Maryland, and West Virginia).

Besides the states in which it is now required, the possibility of relicensure has been raised in several others where bills have been introduced into the legislature. They include California, Virginia, and Maine. Annual registration, but not relicensure, is required in Colorado, Minnesota, Ohio, and South Carolina. Reregistration for the practice of osteopathy is required in 12 states (Arizona, Florida, Maine, Maryland, Michigan, Nevada, New

Mexico, Ohio, Oklahoma, Tennessee, Vermont, and West Virginia). Relicensure for D.O.s is required in Florida, New Mexico, and West Virginia on the basis of post-graduate education.

Experience with these methods is not great enough yet to indicate whether the medical profession approves them or whether there has been any significant gain in patient care. Dr. Robert C. Derbyshire, a Sante Fe surgeon and past president of the National Federation of State Medical Boards, has reported recently that relicensure has been accepted favorably in New Mexico. It is of interest, on the other hand, that professional malpractice problems (which theoretically should be partially alleviated by the fact that doctors have agreed to this method of improvement of their own standards) have become severe recently in Maryland, where relicensure has been accepted.

Relicensure is thus a fact of life in several states. It is important to decide whether or not this denotes a developing trend for, if it is so, it would be wise either to fight the trend or to find methods by which relicensure could improve the position of medicine and not develop into a political ploy. It should be noted that the great attention placed on the Professional Standards Review Organization (PSRO) in the past three years has led to diminution of interest in relicensure.

One disadvantage of either relicensure or reregistration is that it involves an assessment which could form an unjust tax on physicians. In most states in which reregistration is required, the charge is $5 or $10. Larger amounts could be confiscatory unless it could be proved that this amount would be necessary for the exact purposes of the legislation.

The following arguments in favor of relicensure may be listed.

1. Medical knowledge increases at an astonishing rate so that continued re-education is necessary to maintain competence.

2. Lifetime education is a goal that is important for all citizens as well as for medicine.

3. Because of the enormous responsibilities upon the medical profession, it is incumbent to maintain the highest possible standards. Relicensure will help to secure them.

4. There is evidence that the public is demanding more evidence that the profession is cognizant of current knowledge than it ever has been in the past. Otherwise, the laws that approve relicensure would never have been written nor would other prospective bills have appeared in the legislatures.

If relicensing is to be carried out, there are several other features that would require consideration. What agents should carry out the relicensure? At what level should the relicensure be done? What methods should be employed for relicensure?

It would seem that only two agencies concerned with relicensing would need to be considered—individual states and the federal government. At the present time reciprocity occurs between many states so that passing one state examination will allow practice in many others. However, this practice is not universal, and if some states require relicensure, they almost surely would not wish to accept physicians from other states in which these examinations were not required.

The possibility of federal rather than state licensure and relicensure has gained considerable impetus in recent years. A sudden overriding of state laws could occur if the federal government decided that national licensure and relicensure were necessary. The passage of a national health insurance act will increase the chances for national licensure and relicensure.

The next question is to decide the level at which relicensure should be applied. Three possibilities exist. It could be done at the M.D. level; it could be, as in the British system, as physicians *or* surgeons; or it could be at a level which could require separate licensure of each specialty. The first of these alternatives is the only one in use at present. The second would be difficult to establish in the United States. The third, licensure at the specialist level, requires further discussion. This would mean, for example, that orthopedic surgeons would be licensed as such, urologists as urologists, and pediatricians as pediatricians. Bills introduced into the last and present Congress also would establish the necessary requirements for training of specialists, indicating that there will be increasing pressure for relicensure as specialists.

Certainly the procedure has merit if quality control is the reason. For example, except in emergencies, operations would have to be done by certified specialists. On the other hand, if every specialist required licensure in his specialty, there could be no more certain way to fragment medicine, make doctors unavailable, or increase costs. At the present time, an enormous amount of primary care is carried out by specialists; it would be unwise to eliminate this type of care. If relicensing of specialists occurs, it would be very wise to be certain that every specialist could act as a primary physician as well. Legal details should not be drawn so tightly that malpractice could be defined solely on such a basis. Ultimately, relicensure could serve as a basis for compensation as well as quality control.

The third question is that if relicensure is to be carried out, by what means should it be effected? At the M.D. level it could be done in one of three ways. First, it could be done on the presentation of credits for post-graduate study and continued medical education. This has been the popular method because it has been comparatively easy to specify the number of hours spent in post-graduate study. A yearly total of 25 hours is the usual present level, though it perhaps might not be unreasonable to consider not over 50 hours of such work during the course of the year. However, communities with few doctors hardly could afford to lose each of them for a week's post-graduate study. The second method would be by repeated examinations. This is a very unpopular method and introduces the difficult consideration that many doctors would fail to pass such examinations. Should they be declared incompetent and removed from practice, it would seem that this would be unfair both to physicians and to the communities in which they serve. Particularly in the United States, which tolerates medical quackery in the form of chiropractic, it would seem totally unjust to remove a doctor from practice because he failed an examination in basic science.

A third method by which relicensure could be maintained would be by an elaborate system of peer review combined with an examination of an applicant's record in practice. This would require the cooperation of medical and specialty societies. Such a concept is visualized in the Medical Disciplinary Board recently established in Massachusetts, which has powerful statutory provisions that will allow introduction of peer review mechanisms. An insurance company set up in Massachusetts now requires 50 hours yearly of post-graduate education and 50 hours of peer review for the physicians who are insured. The introduction of members of the public on such boards could mitigate the criticism that such boards would be entirely favorable to doctors.

Each of these methods has advantages and disadvantages. The simplest method—evidence of continuing medical education of 25 to 50 hours yearly—has been the one adopted by all states in which relicensure is required either for M.D.s or D.O.s. It is the method used by the only specialty organization (American Academy for Family Practice) with continuing requirements for membership. This is almost certainly the best available way at present. The mechanism is easy, and certainly some value should accrue from continuing medical education even if the participants sleep through most of the lectures.

The AMA has advocated continuing medical education as well as expanded peer review. In approximately 1970 it established a Certificate of Competence based upon the compilation of credits from continuing medical education, presentation of papers, demonstrations, teaching, etc. This is known as the AMA Physicians Recognition Award. Meanwhile, by this continued approval of post-graduate medical education courses given by a variety of organizations, it thus has become a de facto certifying agency to place a stamp of approval on programs given by medical schools, specialty societies, community hospitals, large private clinics, and federal government facilities.

At least nine state medical societies have moved to make continuing medical education a requirement for continuing membership (Arizona,

Florida, Kansas, Massachusetts, Minnesota, New Jersey, North Carolina, Oregon, and Pennsylvania). In Oregon, several physicians have been removed from the medical society since they have not carried out these requirements. The AMA has carried out the staff work in Oregon, and in Pennsylvania the Physicians Recognition Award of the AMA is acceptable evidence of continuing medical education.

Certification and Recertification

The last few decades have seen an astonishing improvement in the education and definition of specialists. Even family practice has become a specialty so that now it is estimated that about 85 percent of physicians in the United States consider themselves to be specialists of one type or another (Table 9-2).[7] True specialist qualifications are determined by the medical specialty boards (Table 9-1). The percentage of board-certified specialists is considerably lower and average from 91 percent for American-born radiologists to 5.9 percent for foreign medical graduates in general practice (Table 9-3).[8] These boards originated in 1915 with the Board of Ophthalmology. The American Board of Surgery was instituted in 1937. These boards are united into an organization known as the American Board of Medical Specialties. This organization started as a loose organization of all boards but has gradually assumed more executive power in recent years. With the development of the Coordinating Council on Medical Education another organization has been superimposed, but the authority on the boards has been and will remain substantial. By granting certificates the boards now have the primary function of certifying specialists. These certificates until recently have been permanent. They carry no legal power and have not served to restrict the individuals to the procedures specified by the specialty board, nor have the diplomates of boards been specified or advertised to any appreciable degree outside the medical profession itself. There is no question but that the boards have elevated the standards of medical practice in a very important way. Failure rates for their examinations have been high, averaging in the neighborhood of a quarter to a third of all applicants who take the examinations.

It must be admitted that there has been no thorough study of individuals who have taken the examinations and failed. Under permissive practices in this country, it is still possible for them to carry on the work of specialists even though they are not certified by the boards as such.

The influence of boards upon medical practice is very impressive. Recent figures collected by SOSSUS showed there were 50,454 board-certified surgeons in the United States on January 1, 1973. At the same time, approximately 30,000 practitioners were carrying out surgical procedures but were not certified by surgical boards. Twelve thousand residents were

Table 9-2: Specialty Distribution of Physicians—1973*

Specialty Group	Number	Percent
Total Physicians	366,379	100.0
Anesthesiology	12,196	3.3
General Practice	53,946	14.7
Internal Medicine	61,735	16.8
Obstectrics and Gynecology	20,494	5.6
Pathology	11,498	3.1
Pediatrics	20,849	5.7
Psychiatry	25,063	6.8
Radiology	15,345	4.2
Surgery	71,055	19.4
Other	32,186	8.8

* Source: *Socioeconomic Issues of Health*[7]

Table 9-3: Board Certification of
Office-Based Physicians by Specialty*

(Percentage of Physicians Who Are Board-Certified)

Specialty	Foreign Medical Graduates [a]	U.S. & Canadian Medical Graduates [b]
All Specialties	35.4%	56.2%
General Practice	5.9	14.0
Internal Medicine	15.3	56.0
Surgery	52.7	76.7
Pediatrics	62.7	78.5
Obstetrics-Gynecology	49.3	78.1
Radiology	52.8	91.3
Psychiatry	46.3	54.8
Anesthesiology	43.5	63.4
Other Specialties	36.7	57.8

[a] Based on 945 observations
[b] Based on 3,777 observations
* Source: *Profile of Medical Practice*[8]

employed at the same time in surgery and the surgical specialties. It is estimated that in 1978 there will be 57,000 board-certified surgeons; this almost surely will be accompanied by a decrease in the number of non-certified practitioners of surgery (Table 9-4).

Table 9-4: Number of Board-Certified Surgeons*

Specialty	Counted		Estimated	
	1968-69	Jan. 1, 1973	Jan. 1, 1976	Jan. 1, 1978
General Surgery	13,175	14,203	14,703	15,638
Neurosurgery	1,353	1,516	1,566	1,779
Obstetrics-Gynecology	9,786	10,905	11,195	12,528
Ophthalmology	5,853	6,430	6,630	7,156
Orthopedic Surgery	6,011	6,216	6,417	7,637
Otolaryngology	3,674	4,241	4,391	4,333
Plastic Surgery	828	944	979	1,177
Thoracic Surgery	2,178	2,111	2,186	2,624
Urology	3,289	3,565	3,690	3,953
Colon-Rectal Surgery	322	323	334	326
Total	46,449	50,454	52,091	57,151

* Source: *Surgery in the United States*[4]

Certification by a board generally has required graduation from an approved medical school, an educational program in an approved hospital for a specified period of time, and the successful passing of one or more examinations. In addition, some boards have required a year or two of practice after the examinations have been passed before certification is granted. Failure rates as noted above have been relatively high. However, there always has been a large number of individuals who apply for examinations and never expect to pass. It has become quite apparent in recent years that many hospitals have large resident staffs; when these institutions are approved for residency training, an enormous supply of potential candidates are eligible for board examinations. This has led to over production of specialists in many areas. The SOSSUS has pointed out that this excess is particularly apparent in general surgery. It is probably so in neurologic surgery, perhaps in urology.

The problem also is compounded by the fact that many foreign medical graduates enter the system and can become certified by the board if they fulfill the essentials. Two large groups are trained in foreign schools. One consists of the natives of foreign countries who, graduating from their native medical schools, come to the United States for further training. The other is composed of the native Americans who go to foreign schools, graduate from them, and then return to this country for further training. At the present time, the country is heavily dependent upon these individuals for medical manpower. In 1972 there were seven states in which the proportion of physicians who were foreign medical graduates (FMGs) exceeded 30 percent

(Connecticut, Delaware, Illinois, New Jersey, New York, and Rhode Island). In four other states, one-fourth or more of the total physicians were FMGs (Maryland, Michigan, Ohio, and West Virginia). In many hospitals foreign-educated physicians represent more than three-fourths of the available house staff. On December 31, 1973 there were 71,335 FMGs in the United States; the major countries represented were the Philippines (9,533), India (7,244), and West Germany (3,402).[7]

One facet of this problem that needs careful consideration is the fact that nearly all specialties have unfilled positions in residencies in hospitals throughout the country. This has led, therefore, to a ready acceptance and increasing number of FMGs who enter specialty training. For example, approximately a quarter of all the individuals who pass the American Board of Surgery examinations are FMGs, though their failure rate is very high.

The policy of unlimited certification by boards, while it has improved surgical standards, has introduced other difficulties. Thus the overproduction of surgeons has led in many areas of the country to an oversupply and lack of patients, so that the skills of the operating surgeon are maintained with difficulty. Specialty boards also are exceedingly chauvinistic, and there has been an internecine warfare between various boards when it comes to the mapping of certain geographic areas of the body. However, it is possible for corrections to be made in these defects by the boards themselves. For example, if residency approval committees (which certify the institutions available for training) tighten their standards, many institutions that are now listed as educational facilities, but actually only provide services through their resident system, would be eliminated. Such a course would seem far more desirable than the imposition of strict legal or statutory limits on the number of specialists who are to be trained in this country. Nevertheless, the issue remains; it is this: should the number of individuals who enter specialties be controlled by voluntary organizations such as the specialty boards or should they be specified by the government as suggested in various bills by Congressman Paul Rogers of Florida?

Certification by boards therefore has great advantages, but it also has some disadvantages. Flushed by success, the boards have moved to recertification; the concept has become increasingly popular in the last few years. Despite the minor disadvantages above, it is clear that there is extraordinarily strong support for the boards among the profession and every indication that the voluntary-state partnership which is so necessary in the practice of medicine in the future should be promoted on this basis.

The arguments for recertification are exactly the same as they were for relicensure. However, there has been a great deal more approval of recertification than of relicensure. The American Board of Medical Specialties in March 1973 urged voluntary periodic recertification of medical specialists. The American Board of Surgery (ABS) approved this principle very rapidly but then shortly proceeded even further so that by 1985 certificates will be valid only for a five-year period, at which time they must be renewed. At the present time, all of the boards have expressed interest in this principle. A number of them have developed periodic voluntary examinations, and others are contemplating only a limited length of certification.

The method to be chosen for recertification is of great interest. Either continuing education, outcome analysis (peer review), formal examination, or a combination will be required.

If continuing medical education is to be the main avenue, there is great need for coordination of the many organizations now engaged in this process. The American College of Surgeons holds the largest and most effective postgraduate courses in the world. The AMA has been effective in cataloging available courses and in the development of a system of credits. Universities, specialty societies, hospitals, and medical societies (AMA and state) have developed courses. It would be unfair and undesirable from the point of view of propagation of knowledge to exclude any of these agencies.

If outcome analysis or peer review is to be considered, specialty societies with their peer review mechanisms will play a prime role. If examinations are required, the boards themselves will develop the system.

It is not unreasonable to consider a combination of the above methods, and a cooperative effort between boards and specialty societies is needed in this venture.

HOSPITAL DELINEATION OF CLINICAL PRIVILEGES

Delineation of clinical privileges is a complex problem and is a most important consideration in the assurance of quality care. It requires interaction of boards of trustees, clinical staffs, administrators, the Joint Commission on Accreditation of Hospitals (JCAH), the government, and the community. The quality of care also is closely dependent upon the hospital itself. Some of the important features of these relationships will be outlined in the following paragraphs.

In the United States essentially all office-based practitioners have hospital privileges. In addition, many physicians practice only in hospitals; they include both professional staff and interns and residents (Table 9-5). The approximate 35,000 hospital-based physicians have their clinical privileges delineated by terms of their contracts. It is with the approximately 200,000 office-based physicians who may practice in one or more hospitals that this section primarily is concerned. All of these individuals have been licensed by

Table 9-5: Federal and Nonfederal
Physicians in United States
and Possessions by Specialty and Activity*

(December 31, 1973)

Specialty	Total	Office-Based Prac.	Hospital-Based Practice		
			Interns	Residents	Phys. Staff
Total	295,257	201,435	11,953	46,299	35,570
General Practice	52,918	47,908	0	1,805	3,205
Medical Specialties	77,598	48,689	4,593	14,740	9,576
Surgical Specialties	88,050	63,483	1,801	15,807	6,959
Other Specialties	76,691	41,355	5,559	13,947	15,830

* Source: *Profile of Medical Practice*[8]

the state as physicians and surgeons. The problem is to decide whether or not they are capable of practicing in all fields of medicine and surgery or whether restrictions should be imposed.

At the outset it must be emphasized that there is almost universal agreement that this delineation of privileges must be placed at the local level. The large number of hospitals, the available medical personnel, and community demands are important factors that contribute to flexibility that could not be assured by the imposition of strict outside controls.

That friction exists in this system is supported by many observations. As an example, in one hospital in Massachusetts a few years ago the board of trustees summarily dismissed all of the clinical staff without due process by which the physicians could defend themselves. In another situation, one physician threatened with loss of his privileges by the chief of staff attended meetings with a loaded revolver on his hip. Such incidents are rare; they do not lead to a peaceable solution of a difficult problem.

These relationships were the subject of an extensive *Report on Physician-Hospital Relations 1974* that was approved by the House of Delegates of the AMA in June 1974.[9] This 100-page document outlines many controversial points, with suggestions for alleviation of the difficulties.

The influence of the community in which the hospital is located may be extremely significant. For example, in the Lincoln Hospital, New York City, the community recently forced the resignation of a highly qualified professional staff and replacement by physicians who were more closely oriented to the community and to the ethnic groups served by the hospital. Pressure is felt not only from these groups but also from doctors practicing in the community who frequently request hospital privileges.

Boards of trustees exercise the legal powers and are directly responsible for the activities of the hospital, including those of clinical staffs. This authority generally is exerted through executive or administrative committees. Many of these committees have not had physician representatives among them; strong requests for such membership have been made by many organizations, including the AMA and the ACS. These various boards then must approve any appointments that are made within the hospital.

Administrators of hospitals occupy important positions. The Darling case, in which a hospital was held liable together with the attending physicians for malpractice, has accentuated the importance of the hospital and its direct responsibility; administration and staff are partners in medical care. On the other hand, administrative officials are the agents who must hire or dismiss full-time hospital employees so that members of clinical staffs or even chiefs of staff are not immune from such actions. The right of all aggrieved persons to follow the legal steps outlined in due process has been emphasized by the AMA.

There are many decisions about clinical privileges that therefore must be made at the local level. For example, in the field of surgery, board-qualified surgeons will be in competition with older self-trained surgeons or even younger general practitioners who wish to carry out surgical procedures. Specialists in various fields, such as plastic surgery or otorhinolaryngology, may compete with plastic surgeons, general surgeons, and dentists. Podiatrists may invade the field of orthopedics. The primary consideration has been made essentially on the personnel who are available to carry out these various duties. When competing specialists wish to cover the identical anatomic area, some means of accommodation must be found. Attempts to do this at a national level until the present generally have led to the issuance of many pious platitudes, but actual decisions have remained at the local level. It is doubtful that any specific legislation could be any more successful in the solution of this problem.

Let us now assume that all of these problems have been solved at the local level. Even when this has been done, the hospital has become responsible only to itself. This still does not guarantee patient care of high quality. There must be control from other agencies. Governmental control has been exerted primarily through the state boards of public health with their power to license hospitals. Cooperation with other medical peer review groups has led to beneficial results in certain areas. For example, the Commonwealth Institute of Medicine set up by the Massachusetts Medical Society has been able to exert in certain hospitals corrective measures that were unpalatable to the physicians. However, the impact was less than if these measures had been imposed by the Public Health Department.

Governmental control in the future may be replaced by or exerted through PSROs, provided that Congress continues the necessary financial support. They have the power to overview all hospital activities and have the opportunity to improve all aspects of medical care. Other peer review groups such as are active in Blue Shield in many areas of the country can also exert important influence.

However, by all odds, the most important regulating agency in the country is the Joint Commission on Accreditation of Hospitals. The history of the JCAH was recorded by Schlicke under the title "American Surgery's Noblest Experiment."[10] He characterized a number of hospitals in the year 1910 as "walk-in garbage cans which people entered reluctantly as a last resort before death." The American College of Surgeons began a system of standardization of hospital equipment and hospital work in 1912. The program was a great success but became exceedingly costly. By 1952, 2,390 hospitals were on the approved list. In 1951 the JCAH was incorporated in Illinois. Authority is vested in a Board of Commissioners composed of three members of the American College of Surgeons, three from the American College of Physicians, seven from the AMA, and seven from the American Hospital Association (AHA). In 1964 because of the cost of surveys, a fee was charged for the first time, and this has been continued in order to maintain financial stability.

Of 7,123 hospitals in the United States, 5,075 (or 71 percent) were accredited by the JCAH in 1972. The other 2,000 hospitals either have not been surveyed or have been refused accreditation. However, for the most part, they are small hospitals and often proprietary. The JCAH surveys practically all hospitals with more than 100 beds, 75 percent of the 1,713 hospitals with 50 to 100 beds, and only 12 percent of the 447 hospitals with less than 25 beds. Of the surveys conducted in 1970, 78 percent received a two-year accreditation, 19 percent a one-year, and 3 percent failed accreditation. Of those undergoing initial survey, only 45 percent received full accreditation.

The economic import of the JCAH is immense. Hill-Burton funds are given only to hospitals that are accredited. Any intern and resident training program is endangered if a hospital is discredited. Seventeen of 74 Blue Cross/Blue Shield plans include accreditation provisions for payment. After the advent of Medicare in 1965, JCAH accreditation, together with an acceptable utilization review plan, made the hospitals eligible for Medicare payments.

Since all of these philosophic, economic, professional, and governmental forces impinge directly on the JCAH, it is no wonder that there have been serious criticisms from all parties. Interestingly enough, despite recent governmental criticism that JCAH standards were said to be too low, 1,010 nonaccredited hospitals have been certified by the government for Medicare payments.

The JCAH has also been subjected to spot checks by representatives of DHEW to see whether or not standards are maintained. At least half of the hospitals that had been certified by the JCAH were considered to be in default by these investigating agencies. However, a great deal of criticism has arisen from this inspection. In most instances, the difficulties that were pointed out were with hospital plants, particularly in regard to safety regulations. These regulations are not specified by national requirements and have changed drastically in various states in the recent past. In addition, they are not uniform. The validity of this secondary investigation has therefore been questioned, and political motives have been suspected.

To return to the delineation of clinical privileges, Schlicke has stated that the JCAH "has made the hospital by virtue of its delegation of clinical privileges the most powerful standard setter and police agent for the medical profession completely superceding the token requirements of legal licensing agencies." It is needless to say that if the JCAH takes a firm stand in the delineation of clinical privileges, some members of the medical profession will be unhappy. A most serious point of controversy arises in the delineation of surgical privileges, since many self-styled specialists may wish to carry out surgical operations despite the fact that there are other board-certified surgeons available for such care. Approximately two years ago the JCAH requested that each member of the surgical staff be certified by his respective chief concerning the type of operations he could perform. These "laundry lists" led to great resentment. The result is that now they are not required. However, chiefs of surgery, when they deal with unqualified surgeons, must in individual cases limit surgical privileges for the good of the patient. Diplomates of boards are allowed great latitude, particularly when they are allowed to carry out what has been specified in the training program of the boards.

The attitude of the JCAH to delineation of hospital privileges is expressed in their *Accreditation Manual for Hospitals*.[11] Standard VIII states: "The governing body shall delegate to the medical staff the authority to evaluate the professional competence of staff members and applicants for staff privileges; it shall hold the medical staff responsible for making recommendations to the governing body concerning initial staff appointments, reappointments, and the assignment or curtailment of privileges." Standard X states: "The governing body shall require that the medical staff establish controls that are designed to insure the achievement and maintenance of high standards of professional ethical practices."

Policing by Other Organizations

The only logical alternative to the voluntary concept of the JCAH is an extension of governmental control either at the national or state level. Such power would immediately encompass all of the hospitals that have not joined the voluntary organization of the JCAH. This would be, in my opinion, essentially the only advantage. Certainly medical practitioners would be far less happy with strict governmental control than with the JCAH. Even though they fume and fret under voluntary control, the attainment of accreditation universally is regarded as an important goal, and any hospital that loses it is in severe difficulty. The quality of JCAH inspection is clearly visible through the detailed reports that are written to hospitals. In this respect one might ask under what circumstances these 1,010 nonaccredited hospitals that were certified by Medicare were inspected and whether a re-inspection by the JCAH would not have shown many deficiencies.

The delegation of the police power—to JCAH or government—is an important issue. The writer agrees with Schlicke, who stated that "if the concept of a self-regulation is untenable, the very concept of self-government is at stake."

There are certain other comments that must be made on the subject of hospital delineation of clinical privileges. At the present time, it is possible for a doctor to have his clinical privileges revoked in one hospital because of professional incompetence, but he then may go to a neighboring community and carry out exactly the same practices. This certainly is a mistake. It can be rectified in several ways, preferably by certification of all hospitals by the JCAH, or by PSROs or peer review organization of medical societies.

Hospital staffs may be either "open" or "closed." The open staff permits all doctors from the community to practice in a hospital. Clearly, it will be much more difficult to establish standards under such circumstances than if the staff is closed, so that the qualifications are well known to the hospital staff.

Another problem occurs when a surgeon has patients in many hospitals so that he operates only occasionally in a given institution. The net result is that his qualifications are not well known; he is relatively unfamiliar with the local territory, and in many respects he is playing ball in a foreign field. The chief of service, likewise, will know nothing of the activities of this surgeon in other hospitals. For these reasons, the surgeon who operates only occasionally in a given hospital must be looked upon askance. It is far more satisfactory from the point of view of delineation of privileges if essentially all of a surgeon's work is carried on in one or two hospitals. Similar, but less serious problems, arise with physicians.

A word of caution should be raised concerning the delegation of strict limitations of privileges in written documents. Such statements may become the basis for legal suits but, even more important, tend to pigeonhole clinical practices so strictly that patient care may suffer.

The dimensions of the problem of delineation of clinical privileges for osteopaths either in osteopathic hospitals or in hospitals that accept them with M.D.s are still an unknown.

The following guidelines are suggested in order that hospital care may be maintained at a high level:

1. Whenever possible, clinical privileges should be accorded to specialists on a basis of certification by respective boards of membership in corresponding national specialty societies. Operative procedures, unless dictated by emergency considerations, should be performed by qualified specialists. Strict interpretation of this guideline, specifying that *only* those specialists can serve, may act in restraint of trade and be illegal.

2. The hospital should provide adequate supporting services—e.g., anesthesia, X-ray, pathology, laboratory facilities, blood banks, ICUs, respiratory units, nursing care, social service, and adequate professional consultation.

3. Hospital activities should include provisions for continuing education and peer review. Utilization review committees, audit, and tissue committees shall be supplemented by medical care evaluation studies. Aid may be secured from other organizations such as the JCAH, the Commission on Professional and Hospital Activities (CPHA), and PSROs.

OTHER MEANS TO SECURE QUALITY ASSURANCE

The relationship of licensure and of hospital delineation of clinical privileges has been explained in the previous pages. The writer, in this section, will comment on several other items of quality assurance that are not easy to classify but are important, and which may be overlooked. They include distribution of M.D.s and limitation of the number of specialists, if licensure should be regulated other than by supply and demand; professional attitudes; the influence of length-of-stay on quality care; the performance of surgical procedures by qualified surgeons; and legal considerations.

Distribution of Physicians and Specialists

It has been suggested in recent legislation introduced in the Congress that the number of primary care physicians or specialists who are licensed should be specified to provide the proper type of primary and specialist care in all sections of the country, and to prevent an oversupply.

Opinions differ as to whether or not there will be a sufficient number of physicians in this country in a target period of approximately 10 years. Former Assistant Secretary of Health Charles E. Edwards' belief, based on long acquaintance with this problem, is that there will be enough doctors and perhaps even an oversupply. Distribution of primary physicians has been spotty, although not as serious as may be suggested by some figures. For example, the *National Health Insurance Resource Book* listed the counties without an active physician in patient care as of December 31, 1972.[12] There were 140 counties, but they comprised only 0.2 percent of the total population. Thirty-two of these counties were adjacent to standard metropolitan statistical areas, and 35 of these counties had an estimated population of only one per square mile. The point is that in most of these areas rapid transportation of ill patients to doctors is the most reasonable way to attack the problem. Airplane and helicopter evacuation are being employed in some states.

Corresponding studies of distribution of specialists by Francis Moore of Harvard Medical School show also that the distribution of general surgeons is quite uniform throughout the country. Clearly areas of shortage do exist, but they can be pinpointed. If this knowledge is available to prospective practitioners, they would be more likely to settle in such areas. The distribution of the surgical specialists likewise has been found to be quite reasonable throughout the country. Comparable studies of other specialty groups are not available.

It should be noted that distribution of physicians in countries with state medical systems always has been imperfect. This criticism applies to Sweden, England, and Russia, where the outlying districts are poorly served by the medical profession.

Most observers believe that there must be some control. Thus, the important issue remains—can the number and distribution of primary care physicians and specialists be done by voluntary methods, as the medical profession believes, or will governmental action be required?

It is not inappropriate to state here that the public often is poorly informed about doctors or specialists who are ready to give patient care. Attention should be given to methods by which this information can become easily available.

Professional Attitudes

The professional attitudes of physicians is an important feature in the delivery of medical care. For example, in the British system, highly qualified surgeons and reasonable facilities for medical care exist. Yet, the extremely long waiting lists of patients waiting for elective surgery remain a blot on their national health system. It is very difficult to escape the impression that payment by salary has removed a very important incentive and that patient care has suffered severely as a consequence. Ready evidence is furnished by the fact that when patients "jump the queue" and are received as private patients, they are cared for almost immediately; facilities therefore seem to be adequate. In a few of the hospitals, waiting lists essentially have been eliminated by hard work of the professional staff. This, however, is not the rule. Waiting lists for hernias or varicose veins usually average one to two years.

Many American observers who have visited the British hospitals have noted that old patients, or the very ill with severe neurosurgical or pediatric diseases, may die before they can be admitted to the hospital for procedures that could be lifesaving. It is interesting to speculate whether or not this system recognizes that demands for medical care never can be met, particularly with inadequate resources. This is not a situation that is best for the patient nor one that in the long run would be tolerated in America.

Regardless of what other inducements or emoluments might be offered to the medical profession to induce it to take care of more patients, the only one, in my opinion, that is sure to work in the long run is on the basis of financial rewards. Titles or honors are nice to display but are given to few and do not lead to harder work. In salaried systems the emoluments usually are shorter work hours, longer vacation periods, or fringe benefits; none of these is likely to lead to care of more patients. If the American medical system would turn into a 9 to 5 day, with a five-day work week, it is safe to predict that demands for medical care would be unfilled and that the actual needs of the public would not be met. This does not deny that some individuals will work extremely hard in salaried positions—this is true of nearly all of the British consultants who labor inordinate hours—but in the long run financial incentives will provide more care for more people.

This, of course, resurrects the arguments concerning the compensation by salary, by salary augmented by further inducements, or by fee for service. There has been a great deal of consideration given to the fact that some of the high costs of medical care could be cut if salaries were paid to all hospital-based specialists and fee for service were abolished. On philosophical grounds I believe that this is wrong. On practical grounds, such an attitude would be repulsive to practicing physicians in this country. In the SOSSUS study, it was noted that between one-half and two-thirds of all specialists responding to the questionnaire reported their principal mode of compensation was from fee for service practice and that surgeons working on a straight salary tend to be dissatisfied with their means of payment, the majority preferring fee for service. Surgeons practicing in fee for service arrangements performed more operations than those working under other conditions.

Length of Stay (LOS)

Determinations of average LOS can represent an index of quality control. In this respect the frenetic activity in many of our major voluntary hospitals contrasts with the deliberate care in many veterans' hospitals. Inordinate LOS in many instances may be due to professional lethargy or to administrative delay—a term that includes such items as waits for special examinations such as X-ray, operating room time, etc. Too short an LOS, on the other hand, can indicate poor patient care.

In the aggregate, particularly in busy hospitals, decreased LOS acts to the benefit of the group of patients on the waiting list since more people can be treated in a briefer period of time. Hence, though it may seem cruel in many instances to discharge patients at an earlier date than might seem desirable because of their social circumstances, in the long run this is far better for the community.

There probably would be little quibbling with the above statements. The important question is how can LOS be reduced without jeopardizing the care of the individual patient. There has been a good deal of optimism that this can be achieved by PSROs because this is one of the items that is emphasized in the care of every patient. Norms of LOS are available, particularly through the CPHA, so that a hospital that is completely out of line is readily identified. On the other hand, even the hospitals whose experiences have been combined to furnish norms may be replicating the same errors, so that the LOS is not a certain indicator of hospital efficiency.

Another approach that undoubtedly will be required will be the use of analyses of records chosen at random. Such items as adequate preoperative evaluation before the patient enters the hospital for an elective operation, lack of delay for operating room facilities, lack of waiting for indicated X-ray procedures whether elective or emergency, rapid return of laboratory tests, and adequate provisions for discharge are items that can be checked in individual cases, and corrective measures can be undertaken. These specific items should be studied adequately by PSRO. Emphasis must be placed upon these very important details in the future.

Surgical Procedures

One of the most important questions facing American medicine today is concerned with the performance of surgical procedures. While there is no absolute proof, it seems logical to believe that the best surgical care will be given by the best qualified surgeons. At present, nearly a third of all the operative procedures in the United States are carried out by individuals who do not have the qualification of certification. (Table 9-6). It is assumed,

Table 9-6: Total Physicians and Those Carrying Out Major Operations*

(Summarizing Table, 1975)

All figures rounded to the nearest thousand

M.D.	Number
Total	380,000
(177 per 100,000 population)	
Retired	31,000
Physicians not active in care of patients	40,000
Physicians active in care of patients	309,000
(144 per 100,000 population)	
Board-certified surgeons active in care of patients	50,000
Board-qualified surgeons in practice	2,000
Board-certified surgeons not active in care of patients	2,000
(Board surgeons = 16.8% of active physicians)	
Nonboard-certified surgical practitioners active in care of patients	21,000
General practitioners with primary or secondary interest in surgery	9,000
Total nonboard-certified surgical practitioners	30,000
Total active board surgeons and surgical practitioners	82,000
(26.5 percent of active physicians)	
Residents in surgery	12,000
Total active in surgical work, postgraduate, and resident	94,000
(30.4 percent of active physicians)	

D.O.	
Total	14,000
Osteopathic surgeons	1,550
(11 percent of total)	

* Source: *Surgery in the United States*[4]

although again there is no absolute proof, that the great bulk of so-called "unnecessary operations" are performed by these relatively unqualified individuals.

The best interests of the country would be served by restricting surgical procedures to well-trained surgeons. The question arises as to how this can be done. Several mechanisms might be mentioned.

1. Natural attrition will lead to this end as an increasing number of surgeons now are certified by boards and by the membership in the American

College of Surgeons or other major surgical specialty societies. Older practitioners or family practitioners who perform major operations will be phased out. Counter trends, of course, must be recognized. If too many surgeons are certified, many of them will drift into family practice and again surgical skills would be lost. On the other hand, if too few qualified surgeons are produced, the vacuum will be filled by others.

2. It should be noted that financial benefits can be very important in determining the type of care that patients will receive. For example, if general practitioners are paid handsomely, they will be quite content, they will become more numerous, and the amount of primary care that is furnished will rise in direct ratio. Also, if the fee for service ascribed to various operative procedures is the same regardless of what person does the operation, there can be no stimulus for quality control. On the other hand, if certified surgeons were paid at a certain rate and noncertified practitioners carrying out surgery paid at a lower scale, surgical problems would soon migrate into the hands of those who are qualified.

3. Licensure acts could be changed so that individuals would be qualified either as physicians or surgeons but not as both. This would substitute the British approach, and would be such a fundamental change that it would be met with great resistance.

4. A highly structured method might be considered. This could be constructed somewhat similarly to the British system. For example, a general surgical post could be specified for approximately every 8,000 to 10,000 of the population, a urologist for every 50,000, etc. Areas of need could be pinpointed, areas of excess number of surgeons could be determined, and by voluntary methods adequate distribution could be met. Moore's studies would indicate that at the present time general surgeons are very well distributed throughout the entire country. Shortages appear in family practitioners rather than in surgeons or surgical specialties.

5. This same highly structured organization could be set up by the government, posts identified, and filled either by voluntary or nonvoluntary measures.

Legal Procedures

The relationship of law to medicine is emphasized in other chapters. Recognition must be made of many features. Restriction of privileges, as for example in a hospital, to certain groups may be regarded as monopolies and are illegal. Due process of law must be accorded aggrieved individuals. Voluntary systems must avoid any strict fee schedules since they are in conflict with the Sherman Antitrust Act; on the other hand, such schedules could be established by the federal government. Some lawyers believe that the medical profession has no conscience, and that it can be kept honest and effective only by malpractice actions. A definition of death, and even of the onset of life, may be established by lawyers rather than physicians. In this chapter, these considerations can only be mentioned as examples.

SUMMATION OF THE ISSUES

This section lists the major issues and possible solutions that have been discussed in the foregoing pages. The author's preference is indicated by italicizing certain alternatives.

PROFESSIONAL LICENSURE

1. Who shall issue licenses? (Individual states, *federal government,* or other)
2. What types of licenses should be given?
   a. *Limited license* (Supervised practice in hospital)
   b. *Full license to practice medicine and surgery*
   c. Full license to practice medicine or surgery
   d. Licensure as a specialist
3. Licensure: in perpetuity or *relicensure?*
   a. Who shall relicense? (state or *federal government)*
   b. Level of relicensure (*M.D.* or specialist)
   c. How often should relicensure be done? three years, *five years,* other)
   d. How shall relicensure be done?
      (1) *At the M.D. level*
         (a) *Continuing education*
         (b) Outcome analysis (peer review)
         (c) Examination
      (2) At the specialist level
         (a) *If it ever occurs to accept recertification by boards*
4. Certification: in perpetuity or *recertification?*
   a. Who will confer it? (*American Board of Medical Specialties* or others)
   b. Recertification: How often (*five years* or other)
   c. Recertification: Voluntary or *required*
   d. Recertification: How shall it be done?
      (1) Continuing education
      (2) Outcome analysis (peer review)
      (3) Examination
      (4) *Combination of above*

HOSPITAL DELINEATIONS OF CLINICAL PRIVILEGES

1. Who is originally responsible for delineation? *(Individual hospitals, state, national level)*
2. What supervisory group should be responsible for review of such privileges? *(JCAH,* state or federal government, PSROs)
3. What features should influence delineation of clinical privileges? Possible choices include:
   a. *Board qualification including recertification*
   b. *Membership in national specialty societies*
   c. *Amount of practice carried out in individual institutions*
   d. *Participation in hospital activities*
   e. Medico-legal considerations

METHODS TO MAINTAIN QUALITY ASSURANCE

1. Control of supply of primary physicians or specialists
   a. Present projections of M.D. manpower indicate adequate number in 1985 *(yes,* no)
   b. The important need is for more primary care physicians rather than specialists *(yes,* no)
   c. Supply and distribution of primary care physicians and specialists can be accomplished best by
      (1) *Voluntary methods*
      (2) Governmental control of residencies, sites of practice, number of doctors, etc.
2. Professional attitudes
   a. How may maximum efforts be achieved from physicians?
      (1) Salary
      (2) Salary plus other financial inducements
      (3) *Fee for service*
      (4) Increased fringe benefits, vacation, etc.
      (5) Distribution of honors
3. Length of stay
   a. Is it a measure of quality care? *(yes,* no)
   b. How may it be effective?
      (1) *Hospital utilization committees*
      (2) *PSROs*
      (3) Other
4. Control of surgical procedures
   a. Should operative procedures be performed insofar as possible by surgical specialists? *(yes,* no)
   b. If answer is yes, how may this be done?
      (1) *Natural attrition*
      (2) *Differential schedule of payments for specialties*

(3) Change of licensure acts
(4) A system of distribution of general surgeons or specialists (*voluntary* or governmental)
(5) Medico-legal considerations

NOTES

1. C. E. Welch "Quality Care, Quasi-care, and Quackery," *Bulletin of the American College of Surgeons,* Nov. 1973.

2. R. Stevens, *American Medicine and the Public Interest* (New Haven: Yale University Press, 1971).

3. National Board of Medical Examiners, *Evaluation in the Continuum of Medical Education,* Report of the Committee on Goals and Priorities of the National Board of Medical Examiners, Philadelphia, 1973.

4. American College of Surgeons and American Surgical Association, *Surgery in the United States,* a summary report of the study on surgical services for the United States, 1975.

5. American Medical Association, *Opinions of AMA Members 1975* (Chicago: American Medical Association, 1975).

6. *Report of the National Advisory Commission on Health Manpower,* Vol. I. (Washington, D.C.: U.S. Government Printing Office, 1967).

7. American Medical Association, *Socioeconomic Issues of Health,* ed. B. S. Eisenberg (Chicago: American Medical Association, 1974).

8. American Medical Association, *Profile of Medical Practice,* eds. J. Warner and P. Aherne (Chicago: American Medical Association, 1974).

9. American Medical Association, *Report of Physician-Hospital Relations* (Chicago: American Medical Association, 1974).

10. C. P. Schlicke, "American Surgery's Noblest Experiment," *Arch. Surg.* 106(1973)379-385.

11. Joint Commission on Accreditation of Hospitals, *Accreditation Manual for Hospitals* (Chicago, 1971).

12. *National Health Insurance Resource Book* (Washington, D.C.: U.S. Government Printing Office, 1974).

Chapter 10
The Legal Aspects Of
Physician Credentialing

Gregory Halbert

INTRODUCTION

This chapter addresses the topic of professional licensure and hospital delineation of clinical privileges and their relation to quality assurance in the acute care hospital. Earlier chapters have discussed the possible alternatives that can be taken to implement a program of limitation of medical privileges, as well as the likely effects such programs would have on the level of the quality of care that would be rendered.

Ideally, since the goal we hope to attain by delineating medical privileges is an improvement in the quality of health care, we would only want to consider such alternatives that clinical analysis tells us would have the optimal effect on the quality of care. But, one other criterion must be satisfied: the credentialing program that is selected must conform to legal requirements. In our attempt to raise the level of health care delivery, we must be careful that we do no harm to the legal rights of individuals or of institutions, nor violate any laws that pertain to the practice of medicine or to commerce. This consideration then adds a second, albeit subordinate, criterion to the selection process.

Before proceeding further I would like to define one term. The word *credential* will be used comprehensively to describe several programs to limit the practice of medicine: the limitation of clinical privileges in the hospital; the relicensing at periodic intervals of all doctors by the state; and recertification or limited certification by specialty boards.

Three sources of credentialing programs will be considered: specialty medical boards; hospitals; and government licensing authority. Each has its own legal considerations. For the boards, the major legal requirement is that the credentialing program not constitute a restraint of trade so as to violate the Sherman Antitrust Act. Hospitals must ensure that their programs observe due process of law which means that, before any credentialing decisions can be made, the hospital must give notice of the impending action to the parties to be affected thereby, must hold a fact-finding hearing at which the affected persons can present their case, and must provide for the appeal from adverse fact-finding decisions.

The government possesses broad powers to regulate the public health—the so-called "police powers." This plenary authority enables the states to establish the requirements for the practice of medicine to provide for both licensing and relicensing of practitioners.   Contrasted to the judicially recognized discretion that hospitals have in such matters as medical staff organization and membership, the states have even more all-encompassing freedom to act.   However, when a state does act, it must be in conformance with due process of law.

To illustrate the concept of due process of law, and to see just what the procedures for hospitals and licensing boards are, cases are presented that have arisen over credentialing programs, the legal reasoning is analyzed, and the standards established are given.

As these cases indicate, litigation sometimes results from credentialing programs, but it almost always is decided in favor of the hospital.   The individual physicians serving on credentialing committees are protected by common law privileges against legal liability for their acts.   This protection can be extended to cover even the danger and expense of a suit through enactment of state law, hospital by-laws provisions, and not least by insurance.

THE CREDENTIALING PROCESS

It is important to begin the legal analysis by looking at the types of credentialing programs that have been most frequently considered. As will become clear in the discussion of due process and the antitrust law, the question of whether a program is legally acceptable depends in part on the purpose or goal that it is established.   There must be a reasonable relationship between the program and the purpose to satisfy due process, and to escape condemnation as a restraint of trade.

The focus of the credentialing programs under consideration here is the acute care hospital.   Therefore, we will consider those programs that either directly or indirectly, by improving the level of ambulatory care, serve this purpose.   Because this type of program is most logically implemented by the hospital, the legal aspects of clinical privilege limitation efforts will be examined most closely.

There have been many recommendations and suggestions for hospital-based credentialing programs to delineate the clinical privileges of physicians. The Report of the Secretary's Commission on Medical Malpractice found that:

> ... all too often doctors whose staff privileges should be restricted continue to practice unrestrained either because there are loopholes in the system or because good men fear the law.[1]

The Commission went on to recommend that:

> ... states enact legislation to authorize, with due process, the appropriate committee of a hospital medical staff to suspend, revoke or curtail the privileges of a physician or hospital staff member for good cause shown.[2]

The Joint Commission on Accreditation of Hospitals (JCAH) includes among its accreditation standards the requirement that it establish and maintain a program to define and limit the clinical privileges of its medical staff. These standards are set out in Exhibit 10-1.

Programs that seek to improve the quality of hospital health care by the limitation of privileges are based on the premise that by so limiting the procedures that any one physician can perform in a hospital, he will do a better job on each of them. The validity of this proposition is a medical question that will not be considered by a court or legislature. Because it is for medicine to decide, this chapter will not argue either in favor of or against such a program, but will present legal issues that can be expected to arise if such a program is adopted.

There is, however, another reason for a hospital to limit clinical privileges—one that does have a basis in law. A hospital may be legally liable for any malpractice committed within its walls. This liability can be founded on either of two distinct legal theories. The first, and the one that does not apply to the majority of physicians who treat patients in hospitals, is the doctrine of respondeat superior. The hospital as an employer is indirectly liable for the negligence of its employees committed in the scope of their employment. This means that if a patient files suit alleging medical malpractice, he can also sue the physician's employer—the hospital. If the physician is found to be liable for damages, liability would attach to the hospital as well.

The second legal theory is the hospital corporate liability theory. This is most often associated with *Darling v. Charleston Community Memorial Hospital*,[3] where the hospital was held to be independently liable for its own negligence in connection with the negligence of a physician practicing in the hospital. This theory holds that because a hospital has the authority to set rules to regulate the practice of medicine, it has a legal duty to do so. A breach of this duty can constitute negligence independent of that of a physician who practices in the hospital.

The Supreme Court of Georgia reached the same result in *Mitchell County Hospital Authority v. Joiner,*[4] where a patient sued, alleging that his surgeon had been negligent, and that the hospital had also been negligent to allow the physician to hold staff privileges when his incompetence was a known fact. The court found liability because:

> ... a Hospital Authority operating a public hospital has authority to
> examine the qualifications of any physician seeking staff privileges
> and to limit his practice to those areas in which he is deemed
> qualified to practice or to completely bar him from such practice if
> he is incompetent, unqualified, inexperienced, or reckless.[5]

It is no defense for the hospital to assert that it is the responsibility of the medical staff to determine competence when it reviews applications for staff privileges. The medical staff in such a situation is acting as the agent of the hospital corporation, which remains legally responsible as the principal for the acts of its agents.

All jurisdictions have not adopted the corporate theory of liability. Some have expressly rejected it, such as in *Hull v. North Valley Hospital.*[6] In other states, the question has yet to be presented in a case for decision. However, some other states have enacted the principle into statutory law. In any event, it would not be advisable for a hospital in a jurisdiction that has yet to speak on this issue, or which has rejected the Darling case, to ignore this trend in the law. Cases will arise in the future where the facts will differ from the Darling case and which, therefore, could go against the hospital.

A credentialing effort by the specialty boards is also advocated by the Report of the Secretary's Commission which noted that the purpose of these boards is to "regulate and approve training programs to assure that a physician whom they certify is qualified to act as a specialist."[7]

The report points out that it is just as important to assure that the special skills are maintained and improved after initial certification and suggests that a specialist's peers "by a reasonably simple assessment, perhaps an oral examination, can well evaluate his continuing competence."[8]

The report recommends that the "specialty boards periodically re-evaluate and recertify physicians they have previously certified."[9]

This has been adopted by at least two specialty boards already. The American Board of Family Practice and the American Board of Surgery have instituted programs to measure the continuing competence of their members on a periodic basis. It is highly improbable that a specialty board would ever be held legally accountable for the conduct of one of its certified physicians on the Darling theory, so long as the established procedures were followed in certifying the physician.

The relicensing of physicians under the various state medical practice acts has been proposed and adopted by a few states. The Report of the Secretary's Commission pointed to the rapid changes that have been made in the field of medicine and recommended that states:

> ... revise their licensure laws, as appropriate, to enable their licensing Boards to require periodic re-registration of physicians, dentists, nurses and other health professionals, based upon proof of participation in approved continuing medical education programs.[10]

Kansas, Kentucky, Maryland, and New Mexico are just four states that have statutory authority for relicensing programs and have instituted relicensing programs. Several states have also passed legislation this year in response to the medical malpractice insurance crisis. Probably the most extensive such law is the California Medical Injury Compensation Reform Act,[11] which was approved on September 23, 1975 by Governor Edmund G. Brown, Jr. In addition to changes in the law, with regard to the filing and procedure of medical malpractice law suits, the law creates committees to review successful claims against physicians, investigate patient complaints that can be made directly to the committee, and require continuing medical education in cases where it is found warranted. The more drastic steps of suspension or revocation of the license to practice can also be taken.[12] The medical quality review committees are under the jurisdiction of the Division of Medical Quality.

A program of continuing medical education for all physicians and surgeons is also set up under the act, to be operated by the Division of Licensing.[13] The division has until 1977 to establish standards for continuing education, and to require certificate holders to satisfy these standards every four to six years. This latter program is in addition to the one that may be required of individual physicians and surgeons by the medical quality review committees above. This amounts to a program of relicensure, because if a physician fails to attend the requisite courses, his license will be revoked by the division.

The malpractice insurance reform laws enacted in other states specify that, among other reasons, the state's licensing authority may suspend or revoke a license to practice medicine if the license holder is found by a court of law to have caused a medical injury through negligence or gross negligence in the practice of medicine.[14]

Laws such as these are, in effect, physician relicensing acts. Whenever a physician is referred to such a committee having the authority to revoke or suspend the license to practice based on past professional conduct, the committee may always exercise its power to take lesser action in the form of allowing the physician to continue to practice on the stipulation that he complete specified continuing education courses.

The state governments have an additional purpose to institute a relicensure program. They have the authority and responsibility for comprehensive health planning under the National Health Planning and Resources Development Act, Public Law 93-641.[15] The Congressional findings in the act include a determination that there is a "maldistribution of health care facilities and manpower"[16] in the United States. The act focuses on this deficiency by setting up national health priorities that place emphasis on the development of ways to improve the delivery of health care.[17] A state could seek to meet the needs defined in the act in part through a program of relicensure of physicians, perhaps by granting a waiver from that requirement for those physicians who provide "primary care for medically underserved populations."[18]

LEGAL ASPECTS

Contrary to the concerns expressed by some,[19] the law imposes few real burdens on credentialing programs. Basically the concern of the courts is that these programs treat persons reasonably and fairly—i.e., with "due process of law."

The legal concepts of reasonableness and fairness should not require any changes to a well-designed credentialing program. The law on this subject is concerned with procedure—an accurate determination of facts followed by administrative action that is logical and goal related. These are important values to medicine as well as to law, so that one would expect a credentialing program to strive to be reasonable and fair for medical purposes even if the law did not so require.

The legal analysis of credentialing programs is presented on the basis of the organizations that can sponsor such a program. In this way the different legal responsibilities of each can be readily appreciated.

Specialty Boards

The primary legal criterion that the specialty boards will have to satisfy in their credentialing efforts is the Sherman Antitrust Act, which provides, in part, that: "Every contract, combination in the form of trust or otherwise, or conspiracy, in restraint of trade or commerce among the several States, or with foreign nations, is declared to be illegal . . . ."[20]

The act provides that a violation of its provisions is a misdemeanor, punishable by a fine and/or imprisonment.

In the 1974 term, the U. S. Supreme Court handed down a decision with far-reaching implications for all professions, and not just lawyers, which was the profession involved in the case. In *Goldfarb v. Virginia State Bar,*[21] the court held that a fixed fee system established by the state bar and enforced through the prospect of professional disciplinary proceedings constituted a restraint of trade in interstate commerce and was, therefore, illegal. The defendants had contended that it was merely an advisory schedule of fees, but the court disagreed, saying that compliance on the part of the member attorneys was compelled by the threat of the professional sanctions that could include disbarment.

Of special significance was the court's treatment of the defendant's claim that lawyers constitute a "learned profession" and, therefore, are exempt from the act. They contended that lawyers should not come under the antitrust law "because enhancing profit is not the goal of professional activities; the goal is to provide services necessary to the community."[22] The court found no merit in that argument.

Congress intended that the Sherman Act apply to trade and commerce in the broadest sense possible. An examination of the act itself and of the legislative history behind it yields no mention of a learned profession exclusion. Subsequent judicial interpretation of the law has also not produced such an exclusion. [L]anguage more comprehensive" than that used in the act "is difficult to conceive."[23] Such an implied exclusion would be totally at odds with the intent of the law, for it would allow attorneys "to adopt anticompetitive practices with impunity."[24]

The learned profession argument is not entirely without merit, however. That a particular restraint operates on a profession rather than a business is significant in determining whether the restraint violates the law, for as the Court explained: "The public service aspect, and other features of the professions, may require that a particular practice, which could properly be viewed as a violation of the Sherman Act in another context, be treated differently."[25]

This is a recognition that there still is a difference between a profession and other forms of commerce that will be judicially honored. While this difference is not sufficient to provide a total exemption for the professions, it does allow a much greater latitude for practices to improve the quality of the profession that also have a secondary restraining effect on commerce. But, in the Goldfarb case, there was no connection between a fixed price for legal services and high quality of legal advice, so the practice was struck as a violation of the law.

This opinion will permit most types of credentialing programs that specialty boards would want to consider and, therefore, not raise much fear of legal action. The board should be ready to show that there is a rational connection between their credentialing program and the benefit—improved quality of health care. However, this should present no problem, for one would expect that at least this much correlation will be developed to justify the program on medical grounds.

Recently the U.S. Justice Department filed an antitrust suit against the American Society of Anesthesiologists alleging a conspiracy to raise, fix, and maintain fees for anesthesia services. Reportedly the suit alleges that the society has adopted and circulated a minimum fee schedule to its members. The schedule was described by a member of the society as: " . . . a relative value guide to assist its members and others in developing appropriate fee schedules."[26]

The spokesman went on to deny that the guides specify or suggest a fee, or that they are illegal. The case has not come to trial, so it is not possible to comment on the merits of the government's complaint. However, this case does clearly indicate that the government will file charges against medical groups if it believes there is evidence of a restraint of trade.[27]

Hospitals

Credentialing programs to limit medical staff membership must do so with due process of law. Courts will look at both the standards that are used and the administrative procedure that is followed to make the credentialing decisions. Both must satisfy this legal requirement. The test is a reasonable relationship between the standards and procedure that are selected and the goal—improvement of the quality of medical care. A court will not strike either simply because it would have established the program differently. This would involve a medical judgment of the kind that courts defer to the medical profession.

Words such as "reasonable," "arbitrary," and "due process of law" are terms of art in law. However, their meanings are not as precise as a scientist might expect or desire, but have developed over many years of court opinions in constantly changing factual situations. In order to gain an insight into these legal precepts, it is helpful to examine some of the cases that have been decided which have construed and applied these legal terms.

Due Process of Law

This requirement comes from the Fourteenth Amendment to the U.S. Constitution, which provides in pertinent part " . . . nor shall any State deprive any person of life, liberty or property, without due process of law . . . ."[28]

The analysis to determine whether due process of law applies in a situation is a two step process. A "property" or "liberty" right must be present, and it must be threatened by state action.

The cases that follow will develop the concepts of "property," "liberty," and state action as they apply to hospital credentialing programs.

The Supreme Court spoke of the limits of property and liberty interests that qualify for due process protection in *The Board of Regents of State Colleges v. Roth.*[29] An associate professor at a state college who had no tenure rights to continued employment was informed that he would not be rehired after his first academic year of teaching. He brought suit, claiming that this action infringed on his Fourteenth Amendment rights to due process of law. The Supreme Court reversed the judgment of the lower court that had found for the professor, and held that the state action in not rehiring him did not deprive him of either liberty or of property.

The court noted that "liberty" and "property" are terms of broad meaning. The latter encompasses much more than the possession of tangible objects, and the former includes, but goes far beyond, a freedom from confinement. The principal attribute of a property right is that the person claiming it has a "legitimate" claim of entitlement to it ... (a claim) upon which people rely in their daily lives ...."[30] These rights are not created by the constitution, but are created and defined by other law—state or federal.

The right to liberty includes " ... the right of the individual to contract, to engage in any of the common occupations of life," as well as a person's "good name, reputation, honor, or integrity."[31] Whenever state action would infringe on these rights, a person is entitled to due process of law before the state can act.

Although the professor had an expectation of being rehired, and wanted to continue to teach, this was not enough to create a property right. Also, he suffered no loss of liberty because no public charges questioning his professional competence were made. Had any such charges been made, " ... due process would accord an opportunity to refute the charge before university officials."[32]

The concept of "state action" that comes under this constitutional provision has also been the subject of judicial interpretation which has broadened its meaning. As in the Roth case, where the court emphasized that it has "eschewed rigorous or formalistic limitations on the protection of procedural due process" by rejecting a "wooden distinction between 'rights' and 'privileges'," courts have continually adjusted the definition of state action to reflect the realities of a changing society.

The classification of state action has been applied to certain actions of hospitals, both private and public. There is not much difficulty understanding the inclusion of public hospitals, for the denomination "state" has long been considered to apply as well to the actions of its subordinate levels of government, city, county, or special purpose boards that are appointed by another government agency. However, on two separate theories, private hospitals have been held to constitute a "state" for the purposes of constitutional law.

The first theory involves the Hill-Burton Hospital Construction and Survey Act,[34] which provided funds to private and public hospitals for construction and remodeling projects. Receipt of such funds is "significant in determining the existence of state action in acts alleged to have violated a person's constitutional rights . . . "[35]

Under this theory, if a hospital has ever received financial assistance under Hill-Burton, its acts to limit or define clinical privileges must meet the test of due process of law.

Again, this imposes no real restriction on the range of hospital conduct, because courts are reluctant to involve themselves in the operation of medical facilities, preferring instead to defer to the knowledgeable discretion of the medical staffs and trustees of the institutions. This standard only provides that certain procedures may not be used, and that certain minimum requisites be met.

The other legal theory for finding state action in the staff deliberations at private hospitals does not consider any federal funds that may have been received. This theory holds that where a private hospital performs a public purpose it will be treated as if it were, in legal organization, a public body. One of the first cases to so hold was *Greisman v. Newcomb Hospital*.[36] There an osteopathic doctor had sought admission to the medical staff of the hospital, but was rejected. The hospital bylaws required that to be eligible for staff privileges a doctor had to be a graduate of a school of medicine that was approved by the American Medical Association (AMA), and also be a member of the county medical society, both of which conditions were not met by this doctor.

The court considered several facts in reaching its conclusion that the hospital served a public function: it had received a grant from the Ford Foundation; the construction of a new building had been financed almost entirely by a public subscription; it had received funds from both the city and the county governments for the provision of medical care to indigent patients; it had received a tax exemption as a charitable corporation; and it was the only hospital in the metropolitan area. All of these facts taken together led the court to say that the hospital had the power to determine staff membership and a corresponding fiduciary duty to the community to exercise that power reasonably and for the public good.

The court went on to say that this fiduciary duty, which is the legal embodiment of the Golden Rule, required the hospital to consider the staff application of the plaintiff doctor without regard to the bylaws requirements pertaining to graduation and society membership. These bylaws provisions were offensive, in part, because they interfered with the doctor-patient relationship. If any of this doctor's patients required hospitalization, they were faced with the equally undesirable choices of either going to a hospital some distance from their home, to one that had granted staff privileges to their doctor, or they could enter this hospital and transfer their care to a doctor who had staff privileges.[37] It is important to note that the court did not order the hospital to grant staff privileges to this doctor, but only required that it consider his application on its own merits.

Hospital credentialing programs can be divided into two components. Admission to the medical staff is governed by standards that are set out in the corporate or medical staff bylaws. The bylaws also prescribe the procedure to be followed to judge the applications for admission to or continuation of staff membership. Courts examine these components individually for reasonableness and fairness, to ensure that they do not contain arbitrary provisions. These next cases provide examples of the legally acceptable standards and procedures.

Standards for Medical Staff Membership

The discussion of the permissable limitations programs must begin with *Hayman v. City of Galveston*,[38] which held that a physician has no constitutional right to practice in a hospital. An osteopathic doctor licensed by the state of Texas sought admission to the staff of a municipal hospital, but was rejected because of the regulation adopted by the Board of Managers that excluded osteopathic doctors from the staff. The doctor claimed that the Texas constitution and laws gave him a right to practice in a hospital maintained by public funds.

The court answered his due process of law argument, saying:

> ... it cannot, we think, be said that all licensed physicians have a constitutional right to practice their profession in a hospital maintained by a state or political subdivision, the use of which is reserved for purposes of medical instruction. It is not incumbent on the state to maintain a hospital for the private practice of medicine.[39]

The plaintiff also alleged a denial of equal protection of law, also guaranteed under the Fourteenth Amendment, but again the court said:

In the management of a hospital, quite apart from its use for educational purposes, some choice in methods of treatment would seem inevitable, and a selection based upon a classification having some basis in the exercise of the judgment of the state board whose action is challanged is not a denial of the equal protection of the laws.[40] (Citations omitted.)

This decision, although almost 50 years old, is still cited in almost every opinion where suit was brought by a physician who is denied or has had his hospital privileges terminated. There can be no doubt, then, that this aspect of hospital law is unchanged. The following cases have considered challenges to various standards. First are the cases that have upheld as reasonable the setting of standards. A physician licensed to practice by the State of Illinois brought suit against the hospital in *Dayan v. Wood River Township Hospital*,[41] because he was not readmitted to the medical staff. He had been an associate member of the staff for four years, but was denied further privileges after a hearing at which charges were made against him alleging that he had a poor clinical record. He was unable to recognize proper surgical procedure, and he failed to call for a surgical consult at the proper time.

One of the issues that was presented was whether a hospital board of trustees has the jurisdiction to base its medical staff decisions on a finding of medical incompetence where the physician had been licensed by the state to practice medicine. The plaintiff contended that this license established his medical competence beyond the question of the hospital board of trustees.

In finding for the hospital, the court pointed out that the hospital trustees are vested with "regulated discretion" to decide who to reappoint to the medical staff. The grant of a license to practice medicine is a recognition by the state of the physician's competence as of the date of licensing, and does not reflect an official determination of the continuing competence of the physician. The recognition by the court of a discretionary power in the hospital trustees is a grant of broad authority. For that means a court will only reverse the action of a hospital medical staff or trustee board for an abuse of discretion, which is a very difficult standard of proof for a plaintiff physician to meet.[42]

Another case upholding medical staff requirements was *Moore v. Board of Carson-Tahoe Hospital*,[43] where a staff member was removed after he was found by the staff to have engaged in unprofessional conduct. The physician argued that unprofessional conduct was not a grounds for removal specified in the medical staff bylaws and that, therefore, the staff had acted improperly. However, it was held that the staff had acted within its allowable zone of discretion. The standard of professional care that the plaintiff was measured against was established by his peers at an open hearing that he attended, and the court found such a determination to be reasonable. While it is not possible to define "professional conduct" or to enumerate an exhaustive list of unprofessional acts, it is nonetheless a standard capable of determination in individual cases.

Dr. Moore did not complain of a denial of procedural due process, but rather of a lack of substantive due process, i.e., that the standards were not known to him prior to the filing of charges against him. However, this is the kind of technical decision over which courts will not second-guess hospitals.

This reluctance of courts to inquire into the substantive aspects of hospital decisions was explained by *Sosa v. Board of Managers of the Val Verde Memorial Hospital*.[44] There it was held that a medical staff can impose requirements in addition to those set out in their bylaws so long as they meet the same test of being reasonably related to the operation of the hospital.[45]

A unique set of facts which illustrates the breadth of allowable regulations a hospital can prescribe is presented in *Pollock v. Methodist Hospital*.[46] As a condition of practice in the hospital, the defendant asked that all physicians have their professional liability insurance carrier deposit with it a certificate showing that the physician carried at least $1 million in insurance. This condition was imposed to meet the hospital insurance company's condition for insurance that the hospital demand that all physicians on the medical staff maintain professional liability insurance.

The plaintiff refused to comply with the hospital's request. He did not claim that the amount of required insurance was unreasonable. He opposed the idea that he would have to disclose the details of his insurance coverage to the hospital. It was held that this requirement is not per se unreasonable. It does not impose an absolute bar to the physician's practice of medicine, for all he has to do is comply with the hospital's request.

Prior to his suspension the physician was granted a fact-finding hearing with the hospital officials at which his counsel was present. The court said that here, where there are no issues of fact, a hearing was not required by law before the hospital could take disciplinary action.

There is no trouble in seeing the reasonableness of the hospital's rule in this case, although it is out of the ordinary in terms of bylaw provisions. The hospital has little choice in the matter. It was told by its insurance carrier that it would not be covered unless it could prove that all the physicians who practice there carried their own liability insurance. It was essential to the operation of the hospital that it carry liability insurance. The only alternatives open to the hospital were to either comply with their insurance company's request, or close their doors. In the current state of medical malpractice insurance there was likely no other insurance company that the hospital could turn to.

Even though the law recognizes a broad zone of discretion in which hospitals can act to supervise their medical staffs, there are cases in which hospital bylaws have been held to be unreasonable. The following are representative of those cases. A medical staff rule that staff physicians must comply with the requests of other staff members for professional assistance was struck in *Findlay v. Board of Supervisors*.[47] The court felt this rule could cause a violation of the physician-patient privilege in some cases, by requiring a patient's physician to take time away from his treatment to go to the assistance of another physician.

Rules that authorize staff action denying admission or reappointment to the medical staff based on the personal relationship of the applicant to the other staff physicians have generally been held to be unreasonable and, therefore, unallowable.[48]

The requirements of membership in medical societies, and of reference letters from staff physicians were disallowed in *Foster v. Mobile County Hospital Board*.[49] There the county hospital medical staff bylaws required applicants to be members of the county medical society and to enclose two reference letters from staff members who were acquainted with the applicant and could attest to his character and general fitness. The legal issue was whether these bylaw provisions "are unreasonable or arbitrary and thus violative of the Fourteenth Amendment." The court agreed with Dr. Foster's equal protection argument, saying that:

> ... such state action demands equal treatment of members of the
> same class (i.e., physicians) is a fundamental requisite of equal
> protection of rights. Any distinctions which are drawn must be on a
> reasonable basis. Moreover the distinctions which are drawn must
> in some way relate to the purpose of the classification made.[50]
> (Citations omitted.)

The bylaw requirement that applicants belong to the county medical society discriminates between members and nonmembers, all of whom are members of the same profession, and thereby constitutes a violation of the above standard because:

> The distinctions ... are not related to the express purpose for the
> formation of the medical staff, stated in the staff's bylaws to be "to
> insure that all patients admitted to the hospital or treated in the
> outpatient department receive the best possible care."[51]

The two reference letter requirement also denies equal protection of the laws because it "may be arbitrarily and discriminatorily withheld."[52]

Procedure for Determining Staff Membership

The proper procedure for considering medical staff membership cases centers around the fact-finding hearing. This is a requirement whenever there is a question of fact which must be resolved before administrative action can be taken. Where there are no such questions, summary action is permissible as in the *Pollock* case.

The scope and formality of the hearing that must be held varies with the type of credentialing decision that is to be made. Where existing privileges are to be terminated or limited, an adversary proceeding must be held. In the case of an applicant for admission to the medical staff, a more formal hearing must be accorded an applicant who meets all of the formal criteria for admission than for an applicant who does not meet all of the admission standards. The cases that follow will be considered in the sequence of admission, termination, and limitation.

In *Don v. Okmulgee Memorial Hospital,*[53] an osteopathic doctor sought admission to the staff of a private hospital but did not meet all of the requirements for admission. His application was rejected without a formal judicial or quasi-judicial hearing. The court held that this did not violate due process of law.

The hospital bylaws provided for the admittance of osteopathic doctors, but required one year of internship and one year of residency. The plaintiff and his counsel met with the hospital board of trustees to discuss his application. The board waived the residency requirement and instead examined the plaintiff's professional experience in an effort to accommodate his application. Thereafter, the trustees rejected it.

The appellate court upheld the trial court's finding that the hospital had the discretionary authority to establish the residency requirement as an effort by the hospital staff and trustees to improve the standards of the hospital, and that it was not aimed at excluding the plaintiff. In fact, the hospital showed good faith in its consideration of the plaintiff's application by waiving that requirement for him.

Based on the examination of the plaintiff's experience, the court found that there was sufficient reason for the trustees to have excluded him. Among other facts, the plaintiff had been seeing "a daily excessive large number of patients" that raised the inference he was practicing osteopathy on a "mass production basis."

As to the due process requirement for a hearing the court said:

The law is not clear as to the type and extent of administrative hearing necessary to satisfy procedural due process where the matter before the board is admission to the staff. Where the proceedings seek suspension or expulsion from the staff, it has been held that an evidentiary hearing must be held at some point in the administrative process.[54]

The reason for this is that when a physician is being removed from the staff, he is being deprived of a right that has more or less, depending on the particular circumstances, vested into a "legitimate claim of entitlement."[55] However, when, as here, the physician is making an initial application and does not satisfy all the requirements, "the formal adversary hearing is less important." Nonetheless, "the applicant is though entitled to overall fairness and a good faith consideration of his qualifications and background."[56] (Citations omitted.)

The facts in the Don case indicate that his application was treated with fairness and in good faith. The reason for the hearing requirement is to afford the person with an opportunity to present his case. This was done at the trustee meeting. There was no need for a formal hearing because specific charges of misconduct were not being preferred against him, as might be the case in an action to dismiss him from the staff. The procedure required by due process is concerned with substance; if the particular steps taken vindicate the person's substantive rights, then due process will be satisfied.

The discretion of a hospital in dealing with the application of a physician for staff privileges that meets the established requirements is more limited. This was spelled out by the Supreme Court in *Goldsmith v. United States Board of Tax Appeals*,[57] where an individual had applied for admittance to the bar to practice before the board, and he met all the written requirements that were provided in the board's rules for admission. The rules also provided that the board could in its discretion deny admission to any applicant, or suspend or disbar any person after admission.

The board denied admission to Mr. Goldsmith under its discretionary power, without a prior hearing, and without giving him an explanation of the reasons for denial. He brought suit to compel admission. The court refused to order the board to admit him and disposed of the case on other grounds, but in its opinion it did state that the existence of the board's eligibility rules gave the plaintiff an interest and claim to practice before the board. It said that the board's discretionary power "must be construed to mean the exercise of a discretion to be exercised after fair investigation, with such notice, hearing, and opportunity to answer for the applicant as would constitute due process."[58]

The same rule should apply to hospital action on applications for staff privileges that meet the established criteria for eligibility.

In many large hospitals the determination of staff privileges will initially be made by a committee of staff physicians who will make a recommendation to the board of trustees who will, in turn, make the final decision. In such a case, and where the staff committee makes a decision adverse to the applicant, there is a hearing requirement before both bodies. Similarly, where the staff committee recommends admission of the applicant, and the trustees do not follow the recommendation, the applicant again would be entitled to a second hearing before the trustees, and before they take their action.[59]

In cases where existing privileges are to be limited, or where existing privileges are to be revoked, a full fact-finding hearing complete with counsel, the examination of witnesses, cross-examination of adverse witnesses, with the right of appeal, is mandated. The type of hearing that must precede the termination of privileges is best illustrated by comparing two cases—the first upheld the procedure that was employed, and the second remanded the case to the trial court with the order to grant an injunction to restrain the hospital from denying the physician his clinical privileges.

The opinion in the first case, *Woodbury v. McKinnon,*[60] is extremely well written. The concise explanation of the law, and of all the elements that must be satisfied, and what specific procedures will meet them make the opinion a valuable reference document for the purposes of planning a hospital credentialing program. It is, therefore, included as Exhibit 10-2.

The hospital in *Silver v. Castle Memorial Hospital*[61] provides a case study of how not to revoke a physician's clinical privileges. There the physician was granted probationary staff privileges for about one year, at the end of which time the hospital decided not to renew them. Although a hearing was granted the physician, it was a mere formality with no substance.

The physician was never provided with a list of specific charges against his professional conduct. In the Woodbury case the plaintiff was handed a written list of charges that contained the names of specific cases and hospital records in which he was alleged to have acted improperly. However, in the Silver case "he was merely read an indictment of general allegations at the hearing." This does not enable the physician to present his side of the case, which is the reason for holding a hearing. The hospital in the Woodbury case even offered the physician additional time to prepare his response to the charges made against him.

Compounding the problem in the *Silver* case, it appeared to the court from the record that the hospital board of trustees had reached its decision not to renew Dr. Silver's privileges prior to "the ineffective hearing granted appellant." It only bears stating that if the hearing is to have any meaning, the decisions that are to be based on the facts elicited in it must come after a full consideration by the board of the evidence presented at the hearing.

The court emphasized in the *Silver* case that it was not even approaching the question of whether there was sufficient evidence presented at the hearing to substantiate the board's action. Their attempt to rescind Dr. Silver's privileges was enjoined solely because they had not followed the proper procedure in considering the question. This could mean that where a hospital has abundant evidence to restrict or rescind a physician's privileges, its action to do so will be thwarted by court order if the proper procedure is not followed.

Where a hospital tries to limit, but not rescind entirely the privileges of a staff physician, the courts are more likely to indulge the hospital action so long as there is a valid purpose and a fair procedure. The Delaware Valley Hospital sought to upgrade the level of medical practice. Reading between the lines of the opinion, it becomes clear that the hospital was recovering from some problems in the recent past. It operated a surgical residency program up until three years before this case, when it lost the program following a review of the hospital by the American Osteopathic Association. Prior to this case, the chairman of the Department of Surgery was replaced, and the new chairman, after conducting a thorough review of surgical privileges in the hospital, reduced the privileges of all surgeons in an attempt to regain the residency program.

The case, *Citta v. Delaware Valley Hospital*,[62] arose when Dr. Citta's privileges were further restricted to allow him to perform gastrectomy procedures only when another surgeon was responsible for the case, and when the Chief of Surgery, Dr. Mogul, approved of the responsible surgeon. This action was taken summarily by Dr. Mogul after he observed the results of an earlier operation Dr. Citta had performed on a patient who subsequently died, presumably from complications of the operation.

Even after the restriction, the court stressed that Dr. Citta could still admit patients to the hospital and could even perform the procedure in question so long as another surgeon was responsible for it. Dr. Citta took an appeal, as allowed by the hospital bylaws, to the medical staff, the Corporate Staff of the hospital. Here, he had a hearing and was represented by counsel who examined and cross-examined witnesses. After the hearing, which lasted two complete evenings, a vote was taken, and only those physicians who had heard all of the evidence were allowed to vote. Again the vote upheld Dr. Mogul.

The plaintiff alleged in his suit that the hearing was not impartial because Dr. Mogul was the presiding officer. However, this was not enough to impugn the vote. The court said that this fact alone was not dispositive of plaintiff's claim. It noted that the standard that must be observed is "that the hearing must be meaningful." The plaintiff had "comprehensive safeguards" to protect him at the Corporate Staff hearing: a stenographic record was prepared; Dr. Citta was given timely written notice of the hearing and the charges; he personally appeared and testified along with counsel, who was allowed to participate; and a secret vote was taken with no proxy balloting permitted.

Referring to the initial summary action taken by Dr. Mogul to restrict Dr. Citta's privileges, the court explained that an administrative hearing is not always required before some action is taken, so long as a hearing is granted before final hospital action occurs. A competing interest of the hospital, and one that may allow for summary action as here is the "... overwhelming interest in maintaining the highest standards of medical care for its patients."[63]

On balance, after weighing the competing interest of the physician and the hospital, Dr. Citta comes up short. Only one of his surgical privileges was limited, and where a question is raised by his operating procedures that affect the quality of care his patients receive in a hospital, the hospital will suffer if a full administrative hearing process with appeals must be first allowed to run its course before disciplinary action can be taken. The result could be different if the action that is taken substantially reduces the physician's privileges or removes him completely from the hospital staff.[64]

State Licensing

As wide as the zone of permissible discretion is for hospitals, the state as the licensing authority has even greater latitude. Two cases serve as examples of this.

The New York State Medical Practice Act provided for suspension of a physician's license if he is convicted of a crime in any other jurisdiction. Dr. Barsky was so convicted; his license was suspended for six months, and he filed suit. The case was *Barsky v. Board of Regents of University of State of New York*.[65] He charged that the act, insofar as it allowed for the suspension of the license to practice because of the conviction in another jurisdiction of a criminal offense, was unconstitutional.

The court pointed to the serious responsibility states have to maintain the public health. It said: "the state's discretion in that field extends naturally to the regulation of all professions concerned with health."[66] It emphasized that "such practice is a privilege granted by the state under its substantially plenary power to fix the terms of admission."[67]

This state concern for health and the accompanying plenary power are not limited to just the initial licensing of practitioners, but rather, as the court noted "It is equally clear that a state's legitimate concern for maintaining high standards of professional conduct extends beyond initial licensing.

Without continuing supervision, initial examinations afford little protection."[68]

The second case that involves the licensing power was decided just last year in *Withrow v. Larkin*.[69] The Wisconsin Medical Practice Act authorized the Medical Examining Board to investigate, warn, and reprimand doctors who violate the licensing law, and to temporarily suspend the license of those physicians when it finds cause for such action. The board notified the doctor that it intended to conduct an investigation to determine whether he had engaged in certain proscribed conduct. Numerous witnesses testified at the hearing, and the doctor's counsel was present.

The board then notified the doctor that it intended to hold a "contested hearing" which would be an adjudicatory hearing open to the public to consider whether the doctor's license should be suspended on account of his professional conduct. At the hearing the board found probable cause to believe that the doctor had violated criminal provisions of the licensing law, and it filed a criminal complaint with the district attorney.

The district court found the Wisconsin law unconstitutional as a violation of the doctor's right to due process of law because it permitted the deprivation of his license to practice without the intervention of a neutral detached decision maker.

The lower court's order was reversed by the Supreme Court, which said that the combination of the investigatory and adjudicatory function in the same administrative body did not constitute a per se unconstitutional risk of the denial of due process of law. Courts are frequently called upon to reconsider their own decisions on motions for a retrial. Also, when a case is reversed and remanded for a new trial, that second hearing is usually before the same judge who conducted the first one.

To prevail on a charge that the decision maker is biased, the petitioner must show facts that would indicate that fairness is highly unlikely, as for example the adjudicator has a pecuniary interest in the outcome of the case, or where the judge has been the target of personal abuse/criticism from a party before the court. Claims of bias will not be lightly considered for "Without a showing to the contrary, state administrators are assumed to be men of conscience and intellectual discipline, capable of judging a particular controversy fairly on the basis of its own circumstances."[70] (Citations omitted.)

This case is cited as an example of the types of action a state licensing board can take within its authority to regulate a profession.

The range of credentialing options available to state licensing agencies is not appreciably restricted by the Supreme Court decision in the abortion case of *Doe v. Bolton*. At issue in the Doe case was the constitutionality of the Georgia state law that required a consultation by two additional state licensed physicians and the concurrence by them with the attending physician that an abortion was necessary. The court found that portion of the law to be unconstitutional because if "...a physician is licensed by the state, he is recognized by the state as capable of exercising acceptable clinical judgment."[71]

However, often overlooked is the court's reason for holding that such a statutory requirement "unduly infringes on the physician's right to practice." The court went on to say that such a consult requirement could not stand because "the required acquiescence by co-practitioners has no rational connection with a patient's needs...."[72] This decision is consistent with past decisions with regard to the regulation of medical practice. Such laws have always been required to demonstrate a rational connection with the purpose they serve. See *Roe v. Ingraham*.[73]

LEGAL PROTECTION
FOR CREDENTIALING PROGRAMS

Although specialty boards and hospitals have the clear legal authority to conduct credentialing programs, that does not mean they are immune from suit for such actions, as these cases attest to. No one, not even the President, is immune from suit. However, the boards and the hospitals have legal privileges to provide them with a personal defense should a physician seek to file a suit.[74]

A suit for damages against an individual physician or against the hospital whose medical staff committee of which he is a member would probably be based on a theory of defamation, libel, or slander. The complaint would be that in the process of considering the physician's application, the committee members made statements about the applicant that are untrue or critical.

The law recognizes both qualified and absolute privileges to a suit for defamation. The qualified privilege has four conditions that must be met for it to apply. They are as follows:

1. The communication that is complained of must be made in good faith without malice.

2. Reasonable care must be exercised to ascertain the truth of the matter communicated.

3. The information must be reported accurately and fairly.

4. The communication must be made only to others with a legitimate interest in the quality or economy of patient care.

This privilege could apply even if the statements that are made prove to be inaccurate, so long as they are made in good faith, and made after a reasonable effort has been made to determine the truthfulness of them. For example, if a latent error is made in the progress charts of a patient, medical staff committee members would probably not be liable for defamation. Whereas, if the error is patent, the privilege probably would not be availing.

The absolute privilege provides total protection even if there is malice, or if any of the other conditions are not met for a qualified privilege. This privilege is afforded participants in judicial and legislative proceedings, in administrative hearings, and in other quasi-judicial or quasi-legislative activities. Some state courts have held that hospital staff proceedings are quasi-judicial and, therefore, qualify for this absolute privilege.

What this privilege, either qualified or absolute, means to physicians is that should a suit be filed against them, they are entitled to a dismissal of the action or to a summary judgment in their behalf. Either of these judgments is granted without the need of a full trial; thus that expense and aggravation can be saved.

In addition to the common law privileges mentioned above, it is also possible for the state legislature to enact legislation to confer this protection to hospital staff committee members. The Report of the Secretary's Commission recommended that: "the committee members and the hospital should have qualified immunity from suit for their acts."[75]

In the absence of such a law, or until one is passed, many of the problems can be avoided by including in the statement that an applicant for privileges submits to the hospital a provision that authorizes the hospital, its committees and agents to consult with other hospitals where the applicant holds privileges, and with any other persons who "may have information bearing on my professional competence, character, and ethical qualifications." This consent would also provide a defense for any invasion of privacy action that might be filed.

To further ensure that there is no misunderstanding between the applicant and the hospital, it would be advisable to also include a release from liability for the hospital and its agents "for their acts performed in good faith and without malice in connection with evaluating my application and credentials and qualifications" as well as a release for all parties who may provide information to the hospital.[76]

Even after all of the above precautions have been taken, this does not provide total protection. A suit can still be filed. And for this possibility, the only option is insurance which would provide for legal representation sufficient to prepare the papers necessary to obtain a dismissal of the action based on privilege.

With a combination of thoughtful advance planning, good faith in carrying out the credentialing program, and insurance, a doctor should have no fear of legal repercussions from his participation in a program to improve the quality of medical care.

Exhibit 10-1: JCAH ACCREDITATION STANDARDS

STANDARD I

Each member of the medical staff shall be qualified for membership, and for the exercise of the clinical privileges granted to him.

STANDARD II

The medical staff shall be organized to accomplish its required functions; it shall provide for the election or appointment of its officers, executive committee, department heads and/or service chiefs.

STANDARD III

The medical staff organization shall strive to create and maintain an optimal level of professional performance of its members through the appointment procedure, the delineation of medical staff privileges and the continual review and evaluation of each member's clinical activities.

STANDARD IV

The medical staff shall participate in the maintenance of high professional standards by representation on committees concerned with patient care.

STANDARD V

There shall be regular medical staff and departmental meetings to review the clinical work of members and to complete medical staff administrative duties.

STANDARD VI

The medical staff shall provide a continuing program of professional education or give evidence of participation in such a program.

STANDARD VII

The medical staff shall develop and adopt bylaws, rules and regulations to establish a framework for self-government and a means of accountability to the governing body.

STANDARD VIII

The governing body shall delegate to the medical staff the authority to evaluate the professional competence of staff members and applicants for staff privileges; it shall hold the medical staff responsible for making recommendations to the governing body concerning initial staff appointments, reappointments and the assignment or curtailment of privileges.

STANDARD IX

The medical staff bylaws, rules and regulations shall be subject to governing body approval, which shall not be unreasonably withheld. These shall include an effective formal means for the medical staff to participate in the development of hospital policy relative to both hospital management and patient care.

STANDARD X

The governing body shall require that the medical staff establish controls that are designed to ensure the achievement and maintenance of high standards of professional ethical practices.

Exhibit 10-2: WOODBURY v. McKINNON

Philip S. WOODBURY, Plaintiff-Appellant,

v.

Neil McKINNON, Chairman, et al., Defendants-Appellees.
No. 30420.

United States Court of Appeals,
Fifth Circuit.
July 12, 1971.

Rehearing and Rehearing En Banc
Denied Sept. 24, 1971.

Before CLARK, Associate Justice,* and GEWIN and RONEY, Circuit Judges.

RONEY, Circuit Judge:

This case originated on the complaint of Dr. Philip S. Woodbury that he had been deprived of surgical privileges at Barbour County Hospital without due process of law in that no charges had been made against him and that no hearing had been held. After the complaint was filed, the medical staff of the hospital held a hearing to consider and act upon Dr. Woodbury's qualifications to handle surgery and conduct surgical procedures in the hospital. Amending their answers to allege that such hearing had taken place, defendants moved for a summary judgment.

Upon a complete review of a transcript of the hearing, affidavits and exhibits, the district court found that the hearing was in accord with the requirements of procedural due process and that the hospital authorities had not acted arbitrarily, capriciously or unreasonably in refusing to reappoint Dr. Woodbury to the surgical staff. Finding that there was no genuine issue as to any material fact on these matters, the district court held that no

---

* Honorable Tom C. Clark, Associate Justice United States Supreme Court (Ret.), sitting by designation.

substantive rights had been violated and granted summary judgment in favor of the hospital authorities. We affirm.

Plaintiff contends that he was denied procedural and substantive due process in both the administrative hearing and in the court below, and that there are issues of fact in this case which he is entitled to litigate.

It is argued that Dr. Woodbury's attorney was not allowed to question members of the medical staff of the hospital by deposition and written interrogatories and that he was not permitted to cross-examine or question them at the time of the administrative hearing. A determination of whether this violated due process depends entirely upon the purpose for which such interrogation was intended.

Appellant's brief states that this discovery would have shown that the cases, procedures and operations performed by the individual defendant members of the medical staff are no better and in some instances not as good as those of Dr. Woodbury, and that it would disclose that the rules and regulations which Dr. Woodbury is alleged to have violated are also violated by the very defendants who determine surgical privileges. He states that it is gravely material whether operations performed by other members of the medical staff are of a higher degree of skill, competence and ability than Dr. Woodbury.

The difficulty with the argument is simply that Dr. Woodbury has not brought that issue to court by any allegation of fact. Nor does the record support any such defense to the charges made against him in the administrative hearing. In any event, we think that the argument misses its mark as to Dr. Woodbury's rights in the posture of this case. It misconceives his substantive rights as balanced against the rights of the governing authority of the hospital.

[1] Once having become a member of the hospital surgical staff Dr. Woodbury had a right to reappointment until the governing authorities determined after a hearing conforming to the minimum requirements of procedural due process that he did not meet the reasonable standards of the hospital. The decision resulting from the hearing must be untainted by irrelevant considerations and supported by sufficient evidence to free it from arbitrariness, capriciousness or unreasonableness. This is the extent to which Dr. Woodbury is entitled to substantive due process under the United States Constitution. Foster v. Mobile County Hospital Board, 398 F.2d 227 (5th Cir. 1968).

[2] A doctor has no constitutional right to practice medicine in a public hospital. Hayman v. Galveston, 273 U.S. 414, 47 S.Ct. 363, 71 L.Ed. 714 (1927). However, there is no dispute that the operation of this hospital is state action and that it is required to meet the provisions of the Fourteenth Amendment in the admission of physicians to its staff. Foster v. Mobile

County Hospital Board, *supra;* Birnbaum v. Trussell, 371 F.2d 672 (2d Cir. 1966); Meredith v. Allen County War Memorial Hospital Comm., 397 F.2d 33 (6th Cir. 1968); see Annot. 37 A.L.R.3d 645 (1971).

[3] The Constitution, however, does not prevent the hospital from establishing standards for admission geared to the purpose of providing adequate hospital care. This court has recently spoken to the broad discretion that must be given to the governing board of a hospital in setting the standards and in admitting physicians to its staff. Sosa v. Board of Managers of Val Verde Memorial Hospital, 437 F.2d 173 (5th Cir. 1971). Judge Goldberg there placed in proper focus the restraint that must be exercised in judicial consideration of challenges to hospital administration.

"No court should substitute its evaluation of such matters for that of the Hospital Board. It is the Board, not the court, which is charged with the responsibility of providing a competent staff of doctors. The Board has chosen to rely on the advice of its Medical Staff, and the court cannot surrogate for the Staff in executing this responsibility. Human lives are at stake, and the governing board must be given discretion in its selection so that it can have confidence in the competence and moral commitment of its staff. The evaluation of professional proficiency of doctors is best left to the specialized expertise of their peers, subject only to limited judicial surveillance. The court is charged with the narrow responsibility of assuring that the qualifications imposed by the Board are reasonably related to the operation of the hospital and fairly administered. In short, so long as staff selections are administered with fairness, geared by a rationale compatible with hospital responsibility, and unencumbered with irrelevant considerations, a court should not interfere. Courts must not attempt to take on the escutcheon of Caduceus." *Id.* at 177.

It is within this setting that we consider Dr. Woodbury's appeal.

I. Procedural Due Process

The plaintiff contends that he was denied procedural due process in that (1) the notice of the charges was insufficient, (2) the right of cross-examination was denied, and (3) the medical staff was biased.

Considered in the light of opinions of the United States Supreme Court as to the requirements of due process, it is apparent that these arguments must fail.

" 'Due process' is an elusive concept. Its exact boundaries are undefinable, and its content varies according to specific factual contexts." Hannah v. Larche, 363 U.S. 420, 442, 80 S.Ct. 1502, 1514, 4 L.Ed.2d 1307 (1960).

"The very nature of due process negates any concept of inflexible procedures universally applicable to every imaginable situation." Cafeteria and Restaurant Workers Union, etc. v. McElroy, 367 U.S. 886, 81

S.Ct. 1743, 6 L.Ed.2d 1230 (1961); see also Bell v. Burson, 402 U.S. 535, 91 S.Ct. 1586, 29 L.Ed.2d 90 [1971].

"Expressing as it does in its ultimate analysis respect enforced by law for that feeling of just treatment which has been evolved through centuries of Anglo-American constitutional history and civilization, 'due process' cannot be imprisoned within the treacherous limits of any formula. Representing a profound attitude of fairness between man and man, and more particularly between the individual and government, 'due process' is compounded of history, reason, the past course of decisions, and stout confidence in the strength of the democratic faith which we profess." Joint Anti-Fascist Refuge Committee v. McGrath, 341 U.S. 123, 162-163, 71 S.Ct. 624, 643, 95 L.Ed. 817 (1951) (Mr. Justice Frankfurter's concurring opinion).

"Therefore, as a generalization, it can be said that due process embodies the differing rules of fair play, which through the years, have become associated with differing types of proceedings. Whether the Constitution requires that a particular right obtain in a specific proceeding depends upon a complexity of factors. The nature of the alleged right involved, the nature of the proceeding, and the possible burden on that proceeding, are all considerations which must be taken into account." Hannah v. Larche, *supra,* 363 U.S. at p. 442, 80 S.Ct. at p. 1515.

A. *Sufficiency of notice of charge.* Dr. Woodbury was charged in writing with lack of competence and judgment to perform surgery and surgical procedures. Four specifications were noted: (1) lack of surgical judgment, (2) lack of an assistant while performing surgery, (3) assisting another who had no surgery privileges, and (4) training and background. The first three specifications contained names of specific cases and the hospital records of those cases were furnished to the plaintiff. The plaintiff requested the exact nature of the fault in each case. The Medical Chief of Staff refused because he felt that any competent doctor could discover that from the records and further that the records must be read in context as a unit.

[4,5] We are concerned with whether sufficient notice was given to comply with minimum standards of due process and not whether the charges would survive the scrutiny applied to a criminal indictment. Bell v. Burson, *supra,* 402 U.S. at 540, 91 S.Ct. 1586. The notice was specific enough to permit the plaintiff to answer the charges against him. He was offered additional time to respond to the matters discussed at the hearing but the offer was declined. We conclude that Dr. Woodbury, as a professional person, was sufficiently notified of the basis upon which the medical staff was considering his competence for surgical privileges.

B. *Right to cross-examination.* It is plaintiff's position that inasmuch as his surgical judgment was being considered by members of the medical staff who practiced in the hospital, they must submit themselves to the test of their own surgical judgment. In effect, he would try the judges. We do not believe that this is a constitutional necessity. United States v. Morgan, 313 U.S. 409, 422, 61 S.Ct. 999, 85 L.Ed. 1429 (1941).

[6] The hearing was an informal discussion by the medical staff of the cases specified in the charges against the plaintiff. There were no witnesses presented at the hearing. Nor did any of the doctors testify in any sense of the word. The members of the medical staff, including plaintiff, were free to make comments or ask questions concerning each particular case as reflected in the hospital records. Under these circumstances, there was no one to cross-examine. The plaintiff's attorney, although present, was not permitted to question the other doctors present. However, the plaintiff was allowed to ask questions and exercised that privilege freely. Since the attorney and the plaintiff could confer at will, we see no due process violation in the refusal to permit the attorney to ask questions. Dr. Woodbury was in a familiar setting, with familiar people, discussing a familiar subject. His expertise and acquaintance with the facts of each case thoroughly qualified him to be effective in discussion with his fellow doctors.

[7] We have held that cross-examination need not be a part of every hearing in order to satisfy due process. Dixon v. Alabama State Board of Education, 294 F.2d 150 (5th Cir. 1951). Whether it is required depends upon the circumstances. Because of the nature of the charges (professional competence) and the nature of the hearing (informal discussion of medical records with no witnesses) cross-examination was not required in this case.

C. *Bias of medical staff.* The plaintiff contends that the medical staff was biased. This court has recognized that in a situation such as this, the tribunal should be impartial. Ferguson v. Thomas, 430 F.2d 852 (5th Cir. 1970). However, the record is bare of any indication that the medical staff was in fact biased by any matter not relevant to the proper consideration of Dr. Woodbury's qualifications. There were no allegations of bias in the complaint and there were no affidavits filed in opposition to the motion for summary judgment.

[8, 9] The only suggestion of bias contained in the record is in a letter from plaintiff's counsel to the Chief of the medical staff asking for an ad hoc committee to be appointed.[1] The effect to be given this letter as to these allegations is very limited. It is not within the material specified in Rule 56, F.R. Civ.P., to be considered on a motion for summary judgment. Even so, the allegations of bias are insufficient to raise a fact question even if contained in an affidavit. The consideration on a previous occasion of the plaintiff's qualifications would not demonstrate such bias as to constitute a denial of due process. United States v. Morgan, *supra,* 313 U.S. at p. 421, 61 S.Ct. 999; Goldberg v. Kelly, 397 U.S. 254, 271, 90 S.Ct. 1011, 25 L.Ed.2d

287 (1970); Richardson v. Perales, 402 U.S. 389, 91 S.Ct. 1420, 28 L.Ed.2d 842 [1971].

A reading of the transcript of the hearing fails to indicate any bias against the plaintiff by the medical staff. To the contrary, the hearing transcript reveals that the hearing was held in a decorous manner with a high degree of professionalism.

II.   Substantive Due Process

The questions here are whether the standards set by the hospital authority are reasonable and whether they have been applied without arbitrariness, capriciousness or unreasonableness.

The general standards investigated by the credentials committee of the medical staff, i.e., character, qualifications and community standing, are the same standards held reasonable in Sosa v. Board of Managers of Val Verde, supra. The language of that opinion is well-suited to this case:

"We think the stated factors used by the Credentials Committee of the Medical Staff to evaluate staff applicants are reasonable. This court has recently indicated that staff appointments may be constitutionally refused if the refusal is based upon 'any reasonable basis, such as the professional and ethical qualifications of the physicians or the common good of the public and the Hospital,' Foster v. Mobile County Hospital Board, supra, 398 F. 2d at 230. Admittedly, standards such as 'character qualifications and standing' are very general, but this court recognizes that in the area of personal fitness for medical staff privileges precise standards are difficult if not impossible to articulate. North Broward Hospital District v. Mizell, supra [Fla., 148 So.2D 1]. The subjectives of selection simply cannot be minutely codified. The governing board of a hospital must therefore be given great latitude in prescribing the necessary qualifications for potential applicants. Foster v. Mobile County Hospital Board, supra; North Broward Hospital District v. Mizell, supra; Sussman v. Overlook Hospital Association, supra [95 N.J.Super. 418, 231 A.2d 389]. Contra, Milford v. People's Community Hospital Authority, 1968, 380 Mich. 49, 155 N.W.2d 835." (p. 176 of 437 F.2d).

[10] The record of this case is devoid of any inference that considerations other than the medical competence of Dr. Woodbury were involved. There is

---

[1] "* * * In addition to the above, we call to your attention that you have set this hearing before the entire Medical Staff and we point out that on January 12, 1970, at a Medical Staff meeting, the Medical Staff voted to withhold the privileges of Dr. Woodbury based upon the vague and general allegations set forth in the Credential Committee minutes of January 7, 1970.

In view of the bias and prejudice generally shown by the Medical Staff, we request that an ad hoc committee of disinterested doctors, not affiliated with Barbour County Hospital, be selected for the purpose of conducting this hearing * *."

not the slightest suggestion shown by the facts that the hospital action was for any reason other than the concern of the authorities for the standard of medical practice and the welfare of the hospital patients.

[11] The claim that Dr. Woodbury may be getting uneven treatment because other members of the medical staff are no better than he gives little support to his constitutional argument. Where there is no intentional or purposeful discrimination, and a standard reasonable on its face is applied in good faith, the one who fails to meet the standard has not been denied constitutional equal protection just because others have not likewise been held accountable. Snowden v. Hughes, 321 U.S. 1, 64 S.Ct. 397, 88 L.Ed. 497 (1944); Oyler v. Boles, 368 U.S. 448, 82 S.Ct. 501, 7 L.Ed.2d 446 (1962); Moss v. Hornig, 314 F.2d 89 (2d Cir. 1963); Stanturf v. Sipes, 335 F.2d 224 (8th Cir. 1964); Delia v. Court of Common Pleas of Cuyahoga Co., 418 F.2d 205 (6th Cir. 1969); Davis v. Georgia State Board of Education, 408 F.2d 1014 (5th Cir. 1969); Zayre of Ga. v. Marietta, 416 F.2d 251 (5th Cir. 1969).

III. Summary Judgment

[12] The plaintiff argues that the district court should have conducted "a full scale trial" with full discovery. Again he would try the medical staff in the district court. This misconceives the limited scope of judicial review in cases of this kind. Sosa v. Board of Managers of Val Verde, *supra*. As stated in Ferguson v. Thomas, *supra,* in an analogous school employment case:

"Federal Court hearings in cases of this type should be limited in the first instance to the question of whether or not federal rights have been violated in the procedures followed by the academic agency in processing the plaintiff's grievance. If a procedural deficit appears, the matter should, at that point, be remanded to the institution for its compliance with minimum federal or supplementary academically created standards. This should be done so that the matter can first be made ripe for court adjudication by the school authorities themselves. Stevenson v. Board of Education of Wheeler County, supra [5 Cir., 426 F.2d 1154]. See also, French v. Bashful, 425 F.2d 182 (5th Cir. 1970). If no federal right has been violated in the procedures followed, then the court should next look to the record as developed before the academic agency to determine whether there was substantial evidence before the agency to support the action taken, with due care taken to judge the constitutionality of the school's action on the basis of the facts that were before the agency, and on the logic applied by it. Johnson v. Branch, supra [4 Cir., 364 F.2d 177]. If the procedures followed were correct and substantial evidence appears to support the Board's action, that ordinarily ends the matter." 430 F.2d at 858.

Although when originally filed the complaint would have required a remand to the hospital authorities for compliance with the minimum standards for procedural due process, those requirements were met before final disposition of the case.

The defendants had a duty to provide the patients of Barbour County Hospital with competent professional medical services. The practice of major surgery is a highly specialized field and is recognized as a delicate art. The citizens of Barbour County are entitled to have the defendants, who have been charged with that responsibility, make the sensitive and critical judgments as to the medical competence of the hospital staff. Once having determined that the judgment was supported by substantial evidence and was made using proper criteria, after a satisfactory hearing, on a rational basis, and without irrelevant, discriminatory and arbitrary influences, the work of the court came to an end. There was nothing further to try and the entry of summary judgment was entirely proper.

Affirmed.

ON PETITION FOR REHEARING AND
PETITION FOR REHEARING EN BANC

PER CURIAM:

The Petition for Rehearing is denied and no member of this panel nor Judge in regular active service on the Court having requested that the Court be polled on rehearing en banc, (Rule 35 Federal Rules of Appellate Procedure; Local Fifth Circuit Rule 12) the Petition for Rehearing En Banc is denied.

NOTES

1. U.S. Department of Health Education and Welfare, Report of the Secretary's Commission on Medical Malpractice 57 (1973).

2. *Id.* at 57.

3. 33 Ill.2d 326, 211 N.E.2d 253 (1965), *cert. denied,* 383 U.S. 946 (1966).

4. 229 Ga. 140, 189 S.E.2d 412, 51 ALR3d 976 (1972). See, discussion and cases at 51 ALR3d 981 on the issue of the hospital's liability for negligence in the selection and appointment of staff physicians and surgeons.

5. 189 S.E.2d at 414. In *Gonzales v. Nork,* No. 225866, Sup. Ct. Cal. Sacramento Co. November 19, 1973, Judge B. Abbott Goldberg summarized earlier court opinions, and articulated the following legal duty for hospitals:

> The hospital has a duty to protect its patients from malpractice by members of its medical staff when it knows or should have known that malpractice was likely to be committed upon them. Mercy Hospital had no actual knowledge of Dr. Nork's propensity to commit malpractice, but it was negligent in not knowing...because it did not have a system for acquiring the knowledge; it did not use the knowledge available to it properly; it failed to investigate the Freer case (a previous malpractice charge against Dr. Nork) .... Every hospital governing board is responsible for the conduct of their medical staff.

6. 498 P.2d 136 (Mont. 1972). But see, G. Annas, The Rights of Hospital Patients (1975). The decision in *Nork*, "is probably the beginning of a trend to hold hospitals accountable for failure to monitor the performance of the physicians it permits to practice within its walls." at 32.

7. Report of the Secretary's Commission, *supra* note 1, at 55.

8. *Id*, at 55.

9. *Id*, at 55.

10. *Id*, at 53. The above findings and recommendations of the Secretary's Commission do not make these credentialing proposals reasonable per se. But, they are persuasive evidence, coming after a study of the medical malpractice situation in the United States. These proposals should not be considered lightly. This is the type of evidence that a court will look for when credentialing programs are challenged for lacking a purpose.

11. Assembly Bill No. 1. The law amends numerous sections of the California Code.

12. Cal Bus. & Prof. Code §2123 *et seq.*

13. *Id*, §2101.6 *et seq.*

14. Florida, Indiana, and Nevada.

15. 42 U.S.C. §300k *et seq.*

16. Pub. L. 93-641 §2(a)(3)(B), 42 U.S.C. §300k(a)(3)(B).

17. Pub. L. 93-641 §3, which added section 1502 to the Public Health Service Act. 42 U.S.C. §300k-2. This section contains the national health priorities.

18. §1502(1), 42 U.S.C. §300k-2(1).

19. See, for example, Wallis, "Will Tomorrow's Health Care Be Controlled by Lawyers?" *Resident and Staff Physician* (August, 1975); Ingelfinger, "Legal Hegemony in Medicine," 293 *New England Journal of Medicine* 825 (October 16, 1975).

20. 15 U.S.C. §1.

21. 44 L. Ed. 2d 572 (1975).

22. 44 L. Ed. 2d at 584.

23. 44 L. Ed. 2d at 585.

24. 44 L. Ed. 2d at 585.

25. 44 L. Ed. 2d at 585.

26. *New York Times,* September 23, 1975, at 22, col 4.

27. Thomas E. Kauper, Assistant Attorney General, Antitrust Division, U.S. Department of Justice, is quoted in PSRO Letter, November 1, 1975 pp. 1-2 as saying:
    Let me state that we regard the demise of the learned profession exemption as complete. Professional organizations that do not conform their conduct to the dictates of the *Goldfarb* decision run a substantial risk of antitrust prosecution.

28. This provision does not impose an absolute prohibition on state action to deprive a person of life liberty or property. Rather, it requires the state to follow the due process of law before it does deprive. To satisfy this balancing test the state must meet a burden of proof, *e.g.*, rational basis, or compelling state interest being the two most frequently employed. State action of the type contemplated by this chapter must meet the former standard.

29. 408 U.S. 564 (1972).

30. 408 U.S. at 577.

31. 408 U.S. at 572.

32. 408 U.S. at 573.

33. 408 U.S. at 571-72.

34. 42 U.S.C. §291 *et seq.*

35. *Don v. Okmulgee Memorial Hospital,* 443 F.2d 234, 235 (10th Cir. 1971). However, other courts have held that the receipt of Hill-Burton funds is not enough to give the state action characterization to the acts of a private hospital. *See, Greco v. Orange Memorial Hospital Corporation,* 513 F.2d 873 (5th Cir. 1975), *cert. denied,* 44 U.S.L.W. 3328 (Dec. 2, 1975); *Doe v. Bellin Memorial Hospital,* 479 F.2d 756 (7th Cir. 1973).

36. 40 N.J. 389, 192 A.2d 817 (1963).

37. In another case involving a private hospital which had received Hill-Burton funds, the public function theory provided an alternative basis for finding state action in the medical staff selection process. *Ascherman v. Saint Francis Memorial Hospital,* 45 Cal. App. 3d 509, 119 Cal. Rptr. 507 (1975). A doctor sought admission to the medical staff, but was summarily rejected because he did not have the requisite three letters of recommendation from active staff members. The Fourteenth Amendment protection of due process applied to him:

> "...because of the fiduciary responsibilities arising out of 'public service' functions membership decisions of professional associations, like those of the hospital staffs... must be rendered pursuant to minimal requisites of fair procedures required by established common law principles." 119 Cal. Rptr. at 509.

The opinion is clear that the phrase "fair procedures" is the same as due process. In commenting on the property right that is involved here, the court stated that it is not necessary for a physician to make a showing of "economic necessity" that he be admitted to the medical staff. Rather the proper test is whether denial would effectively impair the doctor's right to fully practice his profession. Here Dr. Ascherman held staff privileges at other hospitals in the area, but wanted privileges at this hospital because it would be more convenient for some of his patients and for himself as well.

38. 273 U.S. 414 (1927).

39. 273 U.S. at 416-17.

40. 273 U.S. at 417.

41. 18 Ill. App. 2d 263, 152 N.E.2d 205 (1958).

42. As a practical matter, anyone challenging hospital action because it was an abuse of discretion would have to successfully maintain that there is no conceivable valid purpose to be served by the decision made. This is a much higher standard of proof than the "beyond a reasonable doubt" standard required in criminal prosecutions. However, courts will still examine the hospital conduct, the reasons and the policies behind the conduct, and will reject it if it is arbitrary or unreasonable.

43. 495 P.2d 605 (Nev. 1972).

44. 437 F.2d 173 (5th Cir. 1971).

45. The three paper qualifications that the physician met were: graduation from an approved medical school, license to practice in the state, and practice within a reasonable distance of the hospital. In addition to these the medical staff considered in this case: the applicant's character, his professional qualifications and his standing in the community. The court held the latter three to be reasonably related to the purpose of the operation of the hospital, and therefore, not objectionable.

46. 392 F. Supp. 393 (E.D. La. 1975).

47. 72 Ariz. 58, 230 P.2d 526, 24 ALR2d 841 (1951).

48. In *Meredith v. Allen County War Memorial Hospital Commission,* 397 F.2d 33 (6th Cir. 1968), the plaintiff-physician was denied reappointment to the staff based on the letters written

to the Commission by five other staff members. In the letters the physicians complained that the plaintiff was generally uncooperative, that he refused to handle emergency room cases, and that he had been dismissed from several medical associations. The court noted that these letters did not challenge the plaintiff's professional competence, and therefore, that the accusations were just too vague to allow the plaintiff to answer.

49. 398 F.2d 227 (5th Cir. 1968).

50. 398 F.2d at 230.

51. 398 F.2d at 230.

52. 398 F.2d at 230. Other courts have reached this same result in cases that have considered the same type of bylaws provisions. *Ware v. Benedikt,* 225 Ark. 185, 280 S.W.2d 234 (1955). *Hamilton County Hospital v. Andrews,* 227 Ind. 217, 84 N.E.2d 469, 85 N.E.2d 365 (1949).

Also held unreasonable was the requirement that members of the hospital staff maintain an office within the county where the hospital was located. *Sams v. Ohio Valley General Hospital Association,* 413 F.2d 826 (4th Cir. 1969). It was pointed out that where the county boundary was formed by a street running through the middle of a town, half of the town would be "off limits" for a doctor's office.

53. 443 F.2d 234 (10th Cir. 1971).

54. 443 F.2d at 238.

55. *Board of Regents of State Colleges v. Roth,* 408 U.S. at 577.

56. 443 F.2d at 238.

57. 270 U.S. 117 (1926).

58. 270 U.S. at 123.

59. In *Shaw v. Hospital Authority of Cobb County,* 507 F.2d 625, (5th Cir. 1975), the hospital medical staff and the hospital corporation both had bylaws that contained admission requirements for staff privileges. The court held that in situations such as this, an applicant for staff privileges is entitled to a hearing before each body, the medical staff and the hospital trustees, before either can take adverse action on an application.

60. 447 F.2d 839 (5th Cir. 1971).

61. 497 P.2d 564 (Hawaii 1972).

62. 313 F. Supp. 301 (E.D. Pa. 1970).

63. 313 F. Supp. at 309.

64. Report of the Secretary's Commission, *supra* note 1 at 53 expressed concern over the serious problems caused by delays in attempts to remove clinical privileges of physicians who have had malpractice judgments returned against them, and still continue to practice medicine, possibly causing more harm to their patients.

65. 347 U.S. 442 (1952).

66. 347 U.S. at 449.

67. 347 U.S. at 450.

68. 347 U.S. at 451.

69. 95 S. Ct. 1456 (1975).

70. 95 S. Ct. at 1468.

71. 410 U.S. 179 (1973).

72. 410 U.S. at 199.

73. 480 F.2d 102 (2d Cir. 1973). This case concerned a constitutional challenge to a New York statute which required that when certain controlled drugs were prescribed, a copy of the

prescription form be sent to a state-maintained computer file to detect persons who obtained prescriptions for the same drug from several physicians, and those who received more than a 30-day supply of the drug within a month. The law was later held unconstitutional as an invasion of privacy of the doctor-patient relationship by the U.S. District Court for the Southern District of New York sitting as a three-judge court, 73 Civ. 1303 (August 13, 1975).

In this latter opinion the court said:

" ... we read ... *Doe v. Bolton* ... as holding explicitly that the doctor-patient relationship is one of the zones of privacy accorded constitutional protection." slip at 12.

It seems clear that a credentialing program will be upheld under *Bolton* and its progeny so long as it doesn't intrude on the privacy of the doctor-patient relationship as by requiring the disclosure of the identity of a particular patient and the details of the treatment that has been rendered.

Reliance on the *Bolton* line of cases to attack regulation of the practice of medicine without this intrusion is misplaced. See, *e.g.,* 293 *New England Journal of Medicine* 828 (October 16, 1975) an article criticizing Senate Bill No. 1948 in the Massachusetts State Senate which would establish a patient's bill of rights as an invasion of doctor-patient right of privacy.

74. An excellent analysis of the law in this area is, C. Jacobs and S. Weagly, "The Liability Myth Exposed: Hospital Review Activities Pose No Risk" (JCAH 1975). This paper, written by two staff attorneys at the JCAH, contains numerous references to the state statutes that grant a privilege to hospital credentialing communications.

75. Report of the Secretary's Commission, *supra* note 1, at 57.

76. "The Liability Myth Exposed," *supra* note 74, at 6. This language is taken from JCAH Guidelines for the Formulation of Medical Staff Bylaws, Rules and Regulations.

Chapter 11
Alternative Legislative Strategies
for Licensure: Licensure and Health

Rick J. Carlson

INTRODUCTION

There are two very different formulations of this topic. The first is what legislative alternatives are available to control the entry and practice of manpower resources in the medical care system? The second, on the assumption that medical care resources are intended to produce health in the population, is what alternative strategies are available to optimize that objective? While some of the same ground may be traversed in each formulation, the resulting discussions nevertheless may be very different. I feel strongly that the first question is barren without consideration of the second. Yet, exclusive concentration on the second might result in abstraction. Hence, in a time-honored sense of compromise, I will wrestle with both, but in the reverse order.

MEDICAL CARE RESOURCES AND HEALTH

In no single study have the nature, type, and qualifications of health care personnel been definitively correlated with the health of the population. The same can be said of the health care institutions. But let's be clear about this. There are studies which show that certain kinds of personnel and specific types of institutions are associated with such things as income, infection rates, and "satisfactory performance," whatever that is.[1] To the extent that these are proxies for quality, the argument can be made that some correlations may exist. But if the test is the outcome to the patient, then any correlations which have been found are weak.[2] But more pointedly, if the health of the population is the measure, then no correlations have been shown to exist.

Perhaps this is too dramatic. After all, questions about licensure have been framed for so long in terms of the quality of care that we have forgotten that we don't know the relationship (except in a few limited instances) between the quality of care and the health of the population. Given the baldness of the point then, what I am saying should be put into a broader context.

Medicine and Health

The major improvements in health over roughly the last 200 years, up until the 1930s, have been principally due to public health measures. The introduction of sanitary services, coupled with greatly improved nutrition, were chief among them. Then as health levels stabilized early in this century, some major and decisive medical care technologies were deployed, principally surgery and drug therapy. These measures, in turn, contributed to improved health and longevity. Since that time the provision of medical care, rather than public health, has been the tool society has chosen to achieve health.

But today health levels are no longer rising; in some population groups they may even be deteriorating.* The reasons for this are complex. The lack of new public health measures geared to the health problems of today is among them. But undeniably the limitations of medical care to enhance health is also a reason. Medical care today, with its emphasis on the disabilities and diseases of individuals, is correspondingly limited in its capacity to further improve the health of the population. Moreover, since so much disease is self-limiting—and as a corollary, health, a function of individual responsibility—medicine's power and mystique have eroded the will of many individuals to assume responsibility for themselves. The result is that the bulk of the health problems of today are beyond the reach of medical care.

The public health measures of the 1800s were designed to deal with the health problems of an industrial era: waste matter, unpotable water, poor diet, harsh labor practices, and unsanitary and debilitating living conditions. Almost all of these conditions were either eliminated or significantly ameliorated through public health programs. Then, building upon this base—the base of fundamentally healthy living conditions—medicine turned its technologies to focus on the specific disorders of individuals which were unamenable to public health interventions. But today, although many conditions remain which require curative medical care (and many traumas occur which require acute treatment), health and longevity can no longer be improved without the development of new technologies designed to treat the unhealthly conditions of post-industrial society.

---

* In recent months, overall longevity has slightly increased, but the increases are so small as to be statistically insignificant.

The health problems of the industrial era lay largely in the physical environment—water quality, sewage and waste, coldness and dampness, and poor food. Today, these conditions have largely succumbed to public health and medical care interventions; new disabling conditions have arisen. They include stress, smoking, air quality, congestion, overly refined diets, over-indulgence in drink and rich foods, ignorance about the body and bodily functions, and the lack of physical activity. Most of these problems simply cannot be treated by physicians. Medical care is still required for all those diseases and traumas for which the application of modern medical technology is demonstrably effective. But, if improvement in the health of the population is the objective, new approaches must be developed. And these measures will have to be largely social and cultural in nature, unlike the public health measures of nearly two centuries ago.

Now it is fair to ask, "Where is the evidence for this claptrap?" There is evidence, but rather than take up the time to go through it all, I'll just quote Thomas McKeown extensively, from a recent paper, "The Determinants of Human Health: Behavior, Environment, and Therapy."[3]

Between 1900 and 1935, medical measures undoubtedly contributed in some diseases: antitoxin in the treatment of diphtheria; surgery in the treatment of appendicitis, peritonitis, ear infections, etc.; salversan in the treatment of syphillis; intravenous therapy in the treatment of diarrhoeal diseases; passive immunization against tetanus; and improved obstetric care resulting in the prevention of puerperal fever. But even if these measures were responsible for the whole of the decline in mortality from these conditions after 1900—which clearly they were not—they would account for only a small part in the decrease in deaths which occurred before 1935.

I must now summarize the reasons for the decline in mortality which was responsible for the modern improvement in health and growth of the population. It was due initially to a large increase in food supplies, which changed the relationship between micro-organisms and man, against the parasite and in favor of the host. In the second half of the 19th century this advance was supported powerfully by the reduction of exposure to infection, which resulted indirectly from the falling preva-lence to disease, and directly from improved hygiene affecting, in the first instance, the quality of water and food. With the exception of vaccination against smallpox, the effect of immunization and treatment and disease was restricted to the 20th century, mainly since 1935, and although now significant, over the whole period since the 18th century they have been less important than the other influences.

I have concluded that the influences responsible for the modern improvements in health were mainly behavioral ... and environmental (comprising two changes, an improvement in food supplies and removal of hazards from the physical environment). The contribution of immunization and therapy has been recent, and, over the whole period, relatively small .... However, the conclusion that behavior is still predominant rests in the significance of another class of influences, personal behavior in relation to smoking, diet, exercise, etc. ... Smoking consumption of refined foods, and sedentary living are all profound departures from the conditions under which man evolved. ... [The result is that] in developed countries the individual's health is largely in his own hands, for if he is fortunate enough to be born free of congenital disease or disability, and to have an income which meets the cost of essentials, by controlling his behavior he can do more to preserve his health and extend his life than can be achieved by specific preventive or therapeutic medicine.

After having made these points, McKeown then comes to the rather obvious conclusions that "It is essential that the public should come to understand ... and to realize that the health of the individual is determined essentially by the pattern of life which he adopts."

All of this is obvious and yet very hot to handle. In a wonderfully understated way, McKeown draws out his own policy implications:

The medical services of today are the result of more than a century (three centuries in the case of hospitals) of unplanned development which reflects both the predominant interest in the diagnosis and prevention of acute illness and the relative lack of concern for population measures and the provision of care.

And, using the example of cancer, he goes on:

We should ask ourselves which approach offers the better prospect of a solution of the problems presented by the common forms of cancer: extension of the traditional lines of laboratory and clinical investigations; or cessation of cigarette smoking (or second best, removal of the carcinogenic constituents of the smokes) and consumption of high residue foods; and the identification of those features of reproductive practice which are responsible for the high incidence of breast cancer.

To me the implications can be put much more heavy-handedly: if it is the health of the population which is our objective, then continued reliance on the provision of medical care as it is now practiced represents a massive misallocation of resources.

Speaking of tempests and teapots, then, what about licensure? It's a little like this: picture a bar graph which represents health,*

---

* I am aware that the use of the schematics in this section is subject to criticism for the lack of adequate representation of coordinates, and the due degree of sophistication one associates with the use of schematics in papers of this sort. Nevertheless, I am trying to sketch the ideas visually and graphically, leaving questions of statistical nicety to those who wish to ask them.

```
┌─────────────────────────────────────────────────┐
│                    (Health)                     │
└─────────────────────────────────────────────────┘
```

and picture above it five major clusters of variables which influence health:

| Genetics | Medical Care | Environment | Society | Lifestyle |

```
┌─────────────────────────────────────────────────┐
│                                                 │
└─────────────────────────────────────────────────┘
```

Then plot the influence of these sets of variables on the dimension "health," given the current state of the art (which is admittedly poor):

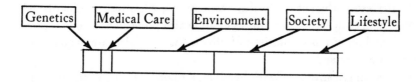

If medical care makes the contributions suggested above, what part of that contribution is owed to licensure? If we are generous and say 25 percent, then what we are saying is that a small amount of health is conceivably due to licensure controls:

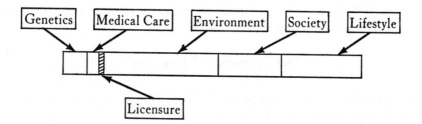

Having said this, then we know what we're talking about. This doesn't mean that licensure isn't worth talking about. It only means that we shouldn't trade in over-inflated assumptions about the significance of the subject.

LICENSURE TODAY

Legislative Alternatives

There have been few, if any, significant changes in licensure practices in recent years. In 1970 I authored a paper[4] in which I laid out six major alternative approaches to licensure. They included:

1. maintenance of the status quo;

2. expanding the licensure scheme to (a) expand or contract the functions defined by existing licensure laws, and (b) legally recognize new health professions;

3. the certification of paramedicals, which, among other things, would accomplish some degree of legal control over health auxiliaries subject to the delegation of authority by physicians;

4. enactment of specific and general delegatory statutes to make more precise the responsibility for the performance of services by various health professionals subject to the delegation of the physician;

5. the establishment of health manpower committees or boards which would subject licensure procedures of all health professionals to one common board, including representatives of all the major health professions and lay representatives; and

6. investing institutions with licensing authority in lieu of the licensing of individual practitioners.

In the five intervening years, no major innovations have been introduced on any scale—the status quo has largely been maintained. There has been some further sharpening of delegatory authority; a few states have launched modest experiments with health manpower boards;[5] and finally, a few lay representatives have been allowed to invade licensure boards in a few states.[6] Essentially, the changes have been cosmetic.

The Impacts of Licensure[7]

Despite the absence of significant statutory change, some recent studies have illustrated some of the impacts of licensure on the practice of medicine.

None of these impacts can be directly translated into definitive statements about the quality of medical care or, more importantly, about the effectiveness of medical care in producing health for the population. The research, however, occasionally and indirectly bears on the questions.

Derbyshire's[8] comprehensive review of licensure in the United States is the most complete examination of licensure practices available. Among the more provocative of his findings are those relating to disciplinary actions. Derbyshire found evidence of 938 disciplinary actions by state physician licensure boards in the five-year period from 1963 to 1967. The most common penalty was probation, followed in frequency by revocation of license. Almost one-half of disciplinary actions were occasioned by violations of narcotics laws, followed by medical incompetence as the second most common cause.

Derbyshire also supplied information about other aspects of the licensure of physicians. Two of his other findings are that the composite licensure board member was "a caucasian man a little over 58 years of age; most likely a general practitioner; if not, a general surgeon or an internist." Another finding of interest was that the National Board of Medical Examiners substantially improved the tests which were utilized in medical licensure.

In 1974 Derbyshire updated his original findings, and again found a very low rate of disciplinary actions by state licensure boards.[9] During the period 1968 to 1972 only 1,034 disciplinary actions were undertaken, which, when combined with his earlier findings, show that for the 10-year period of 1963 to 1972 only 1,972 actions were taken against physicians by state licensure boards. This means that about one in 1,500 physicians had been disciplined by state licensure boards in each of the years studied.

The most important point, however, is not evident from the data. Since the grounds for action against a physician under licensure statutes only rarely, if ever, go to the question of the performance by that physician in the duties for which he or she was trained, the actions taken by licensure boards against physicians are related to quality only in the most indirect sense.

Another question which has been examined in studies of licensure is the effect of licensure on interstate mobility among health professionals. Since problems of distribution and access have always plagued the medical care system, this has been a question meriting attention. Shimberg, Esser, and Kruger[10] examined a series of occupations, including three in the health area—practical nurses, dental hygienists, and opthalmic dispensers. On the criterion of mobility, practical nurses were the most mobile, and ophthalmic dispensers the least, with dental hygienists falling somewhere in between. In 1962, Holen undertook a study to determine the effects personnel licensure had on interstate mobility of various professions.[11] In the case of medicine, she found that personnel licensure created few barriers to mobility because of the high degree of reciprocity which exists between the states, and partially because of increasing use of the National Board of Examination. Dentistry exemplified the least degree of reciprocity in licensing between the states and hence erected a substantial barrier to interstate mobility. Although interstate mobility for dentists seems to have been proven, Holen's conclusions about the medical profession are inconclusive.

Schaffner and Butter initiated several studies to investigate the geographic location and mobility of Foreign Medical Graduates (FMGs).[12] Despite the fact that barriers did exist to the interstate migration of FMGs, nevertheless they were able to find their way into practice settings in most states. Hence, whatever the barriers may be, they are certainly not absolute.

On a question which is arguably more closely related to quality, Lewis and Hassanein look at the effectiveness of continuing medical education activities at the University of Kansas Medical School.[13] They were unable to demonstrate any relationship between gross measures of the outcomes of medical care and continuing education programs. There were, however, two other significant findings. The first was that there was a strong positive relationship between participation in continuing education and recent graduation from medical school, which, of course, is a rather perverse result, since the intent of continuing education is to re-educate physicians who have been around for a while. A second finding was that 43 percent of the physicians in active practice in Kansas refused to participate in any post-graduate continuing education activities. Either physicians in Kansas believe their skills to be impervious to the ravages of time, or the programs were poor, or both.

There are a number of articles and papers which examine the legal aspects of health manpower licensure. The argument made in almost all of them is that activities which could be undertaken by allied health personnel, especially physician assistants, are unduly limited by existing state licensure legislation. However, there has been some modulation in many state licensure laws in recent years to permit a greater range of activities by health professionals other than the physician.

Legal analysis has also contributed the argument that there is a gradual movement towards increased institutional responsibility for medical care and towards the establishment of national, or at least regional, standards for the practice of medicine. This suggests that schemes for institutional licensure may make more sense in the future.

Overall, the amount of research focused on licensure has not been substantial. And among those studies which have been undertaken, few, if any, of the findings demonstrate particularly useful policy implications for the quality of care. Almost all of the studies have focused on licensure as essentially a process measure, and few, if any, have attempted to examine the relationship between licensure and the outcome to the patient, much less the relationship to the health of the population as a whole. Thus, while licensure does seem to have an impact on manpower utilization patterns, the mobility of practitioners, and to some extent the involvement of health professionals in continuing education programs, there is little evidence which can be used to demonstrate the relationship of licensure to quality of medical care.

LICENSURE AND THE CRISIS IN CONTEMPORARY MEDICAL CARE

The "crisis" in medical care is customarily put in terms of cost, distribution, access, and quality. Arguably, the failure of medicine to deliver care of impeccable quality wherever it is needed at an acceptable cost has led to the demand for some type of national health insurance program. Cost, distribution, access, and quality are useful analytical containers, but to me they still do not reach the roots of the crisis. The real crisis in medicine today is one of "fit," not one of cost, distribution, etc. Simply stated, today's medicine is not calibrated with fundamental social needs. This doesn't mean that medicine doesn't meet some needs, nor contribute to the well-being of many patients.[14] But it does mean that medicine is failing to meet the health and well-being needs of society, and that as time passes, unless it is transformed, medicine will more demonstrably fail to meet those needs. The manifestations of this lack of "fit" are many, but key among them are:

• the almost sudden aggravation of the medical malpractice problem;
• the uneasiness in the Congress about national health insurance;
• the general disaffection consumers share about doctors and hospitals;
• the slowly mounting evidence about the "limits" of medical care to produce health in the population; and
• the renewel of interest among consumers in alternative therapies and healing practices.

These conditions can be translated into three specific policy-salient issues: the doctor-patient relationship; the limits of medical care; and the role of government in the production of health. These to me are the fundamental crises in medical care; accordingly, the viability of licensure depends on the degree to which these questions are reflected in its design.

The Physician-Patient Relationship

When I was 14, I had a fairly bad case of osteomyelitis. Our family physician came to the house, chided me, joked with my parents, and endured a cup of my mother's eight-day-old swamp-brown Swedish coffee. Today, I am 20 years older, and in that time either I have forgotten how to develop that sort of relationship with a physician, or there are only a few doctors around who are willing to treat patients in that way. Only 20 years have passed; yet we all know that in that time the style of medical practice has been radically altered.

The relationship of physicians to patients has always been somewhat schizoid. Historically, physicians functioned not only as healers, but also as counselors, confidants, and friends—roles which displayed the anthropological side of medicine. But with the advent of new and more sophisticated medical hardware, and the specialization that characterizes today's medicine, the technical aspects of the physician's practice are now emphasized. Many physicians still dispense "homey" wisdom and act as friends and counselors to patients. But, specialization and assembly-line processing of patients has become inevitable. The patient can no longer be treated as a whole person because few physicians are equipped to do so.

The relative importance of the technical and anthropological aspects of care has been controversial in medicine. But the proponents of technical medicine have had the better of the argument and, as a result, have dramatically influenced the evolution, nature, and style of the medical care system. However, the argument is far from over; neither is it an either/or question. Proponents of anthropologic practice do not argue that medical technology has not contributed (and cannot contribute) to the quality of care. What they emphasize is the profound importance of the texture of the relationship between physician and patient.

Although the issue is not yet resolved, all sides to the debate agree that change, and particularly change in the relationship between healer and patient, is possible only if both the role and the function of the physician is transformed. Michael G. Michaelson, a critic of the medical care enterprise, suggests a direction for change:

> It is impossible to understand the pathology of American medical education and care without first understanding the essential obsolescence of the American physician. And it is only on the basis of this understanding that the fundamental restructuring of American medicine... can amount to anything more than the "patchwork approach."[15]

The problem with Michaelson's analysis, and for that matter a lot of the critiques of today's practitioner, is that the alternatives aren't spelled out. Is the implication of Michaelson's characterization of the physician as obsolete that the physician must become an even more highly trained technician, or more of a humanist? My argument is that essential technologies must be retained, and that technicians must be available to implement the machines. But the physician—the one who deals with the patient face to face—must once again become the healer and friend and counselor. I know this is just pop sociology, but I strongly feel that patients just don't trust the doctor anywhere near the extent to which they did in the past, and that this is a major failing of medicine.

Still, even this is too easy. The physician is not entirely to blame. We as patients have allowed ourselves to be used as cannonfodder, *and* to be convinced that we know little or nothing about ourselves, *and* as a concomitant that the responsibility for health lies with the physician. The only occupation we expect more from is the police—and they don't deliver either. Our failure as consumers is that we do not gauge our expectations with the real capabilities of medicine. And, because we have failed to do so, medicine continues its mad march toward more growth and more control over diverse human behaviors in its effort to be effective. Irving Zola, a sociologist at Brandeis, in his paper "Medicine as an Institution of Social Control," points to medicine's insatiable thirst for human behaviors to medicalize. Obesity, sexuality, disability, smoking, and drinking are just a few of the pockets of human behavior which the physician seeks to invade, and by doing so, to cure. The fat shall become thin, the impotent tumescent, the lame vigorous, and the sinful virtuous. As Zola says,

> The list of daily activities to which health can be related is ever growing and with the current operating perspective of medicine seems infinitely expandable.[16]

This march, seemingly unstoppable because of the tractability of consumers, may, as Peter Sedgwick suggests, lead to "a future [which] will belong to illness."[17]

Yet, in the final analysis, part of the problem still lies in the nature of the physician. True, we as patients have demanded technicians, and that is what we have gotten. But medical schools have been positively hell-bent to produce expertise to the exclusion of the experientially wise. Of course, there are humane, caring physicians, but they are outnumbered by the technocrats, and further, they are forced to practice in a medical care system which squeezes out individuality and refuses to reimburse caring. Licensure simply buys the product—warts and all. Licensure as an input measure is little more than a rubber stamp for whatever medical schools push into the water. And if this is true, as an input control, licensure has contributed to the disintegration of the physician-patient relationship—a relationship which is salient to the phenomenon of healing.

The Limits of Medical Care

Despite the evidence that medicine, as it is now practiced, may have reached technological limits to the production of health for the population, most of us continue to demand more of it. Nowhere is the sound more strident than in the United States, where the Congress is about to endorse decades of ineffectiveness by the passage of national health insurance legislation. The prescription for the legislation has been written by the physicians; the only arguments have been about the extent of coverage, not whether there will be universal coverage. The lessons of other countries are being ignored. It is clear that the National Health Service in England hasn't achieved a millenium in health for the English population. And it is also clear that Canadians are no healthier as a result of massive expenditures for medical care. This is forthrightly acknowledged in *A New Perspective on the Health of Canadians*.[18] This quotation from the introduction make my points better than I can:

> The health care system, however, is only one of many ways of maintaining and improving health. Of equal or greater importance in increasing the number of illness-free days in the lives of Canadians have been the raising of the general standard of living, important sanitary measures for protecting public health, and advances in medical science.
>
> At the same time as improvements have been made in health care, in the general standard of living, in public health protection and in medical science, ominous counter-forces have been at work to undo progress in raising the health status of Canadians. These counter-forces constitute the dark side of economic progress. They include environmental pollution, city living, habits of indolence, the abuse of alcohol, tobacco and drugs, and eating patterns which put the pleasing of the senses above the needs of the human body.
>
> For these environmental and behavioral threats to health, the organized health care system can do little more than serve as a catchment net for the victims. Physicians, surgeons, nurses, and hospitals together spend much of their time in treating ills caused by adverse environmental factors and behavioral risks.
>
> It is evident now that the further improvements in the environment, reductions in self-imposed risks, and a greater knowledge of human biology are necessary if more Canadians are to live a full, happy, long, and illness-free life.

This is really very obvious. Yet we still thrash around tinkering with the medical care system. I suppose that there's nothing wrong with some tinkering. It is probably true that if we tore down the gates of licensure, a host of crazies would rush in, and possibly harm some patients in their attempts to treat, heal, and make some money along the way. So licensure has a role, but it must be reconceived if, once again, the purpose of medicine is to make the population and most people healthy.* Today's physician knows a lot—a wealth of detailed information has been programmed into each product of medical education. But what kind of information? Today, the physician knows how to repair and replace parts in what he perceives as a machine. Since all machines are essentially alike, the physician chooses to use the same treatment modalities for each machine manifesting the same symptoms. In short, the physician is a highly trained technician who possesses special skills—skills which are finely calibrated with our prevailing perceptions of health and disease in the advanced Western world. But the limits of this vision, and these skills, are now becoming clear. If—and to me the "if" is very real—as a culture we choose to live differently and think differently about health, new healing professions will be needed. What will these professions be like?

First, and perhaps most important, what we will need is health counselors. Some physicians function this way now, but they are rare. The health counselor is not a technician; in fact, he will function largely as "triage"—less for the purpose of channeling for medicine than for providing basic information about health. The health counselor must be trained in the workings of the body-mind combination and its interaction with its environment. The fundamental objective of the counselor is to educate individuals to take care of themselves and each other. When specialized help is needed, it should be made available. Expertise must be retained, but it should not be allowed to drive the system to technological sophistication. Rather, it must be harnessed to allow the individual to draw upon it, with the help of a health counselor.

Second, since so much of our emerging understanding of health and well-being is dependent on understanding the dynamics of the interaction of the individual with the environment, persons must be trained to formulate an "ecology" of health. This is properly the transformed role of the public health practitioner. Relieved of the duty to monitor alleys full of garbage, the new health ecologist, while doing that as well, will focus on more subtle interactions between humans and their environment.

The role of the health educator, long neglected in the United States as well as elsewhere, needs enhancement. The health counselor can supply information to those who seek it, but given the costs of care, some—even with expanded insurance coverage—will not travel traditional corridors. Hence, health information must be provided by means more acceptable and acces-

---

* This need not be the sole purpose for medicine. If medicine is simply to treat what it can, with proven efficacy, then tight licensure controls designed to permit only the practice of highly skilled technicians may be perfectly appropriate.

sible to those who need it. The school and the hospital are the most likely candidates. Health education in the school must far transcend the art of brushing one's teeth, and hospitals must be compelled to furnish space to community health education programs featuring film, workshops, written materials, symposia, etc.

Health "ombudsmen" will also be needed. It is unlikely that the medical care system of the future will be much less complex than today's. Since patients will only slowly grow in wisdom about themselves, health ombudsmen will be needed to guide them through the system. But there is a more important role for the ombudsman to play. Many of the assaults on our health today are not made by germs, but by the combined actions of large institutions and manufacturers. We are continuously assaulted by disease-producing agents released into our environments by producers of goods and services. For example, it is generally known that carcinogens lurk everywhere, but there have been few systematic attempts (except for the limited attempts of the Food and Drug Administration in the United States) to abate pollutants. In addition, then, to the advocacy of individuals in a byzantine medical care system, health ombudsmen should foment abatement actions in the public interest.

Finally, ancillary personnel now rapidly filling jobs available in the medical care system must be given more recognition and more status. Nurses and various other helpers in the profession of medicine should be encouraged to overcome their inferiorities and work directly with patients as counselors. In addition, home visits must once again be instituted since the evidence shows that restoration of health in the home, with some exceptions, is more effective.

We will never be without the physician. That role has been played throughout history, but by different people with different orientations. Today a class of technicians occupies the role and dictates the shape and evolution of the medical care system. But plainly, health is far more than the application of purified technology. So, if we succeed in a reconceptualization of health (in the face of great odds), a concomitant reconceptualization of the health professional must follow. In the future, if it is health we are to have, we will need professions of the healing arts that are to serve the individual—not the reverse. And, if this is to happen, we must first find and then train people differently; then we must adjust licensure controls to allow the entry of the "new" physician.

The Role of Government

This is a very hard issue. It is clear that there are still some unmet needs in the United States for threshold medical care—medical care that works, including emergency services, ambulatory practice, and acute care. This is naturally one of the premises for the passage of a national health insurance program. But, if national health insurance is only to pay for what works, it need not be the ambitious, bloated program which is promised.*

National health insurance was a major issue in the 1972 presidential election, and the debate has continued in Congress since then. Thus, the assault proposed against inequitable access to care in this country is being made with dollars rather than with structural reform. The solution being advanced, despite differences in details, is to increase consumer purchasing power to a level that presumably would be relatively uniform throughout the population. But those with expanded purchasing power will be buying more of the same. This indictment applies to all of the major national health insurance proposals, including the polar approaches espoused by U.S. Senator Ted Kennedy and the American Medical Association. To be sure, there are differences of real substance in the pending proposals. But, when measured against the arguments made here, the plans are all of a piece. The current debate is proceeding along a narrow track. Rarely is discussion of the issues raised in this chapter heard. And failure to engage these issues will have two profound and irreversible consequences.

The first is that major expansion in the financing system will lock in the current system for delivery of care for the indefinite future. This is the pitfall of the otherwise salutary means being taken to assault inequities in medical care through an expansion of purchasing power. The issue must be so stated as to make it possible for those who wish to limit the scope of the existing system to fix on that goal and not be deflected by the benefits that comprehensive health insurance will ostensibly provide. This does not mean that opposition to national health insurance is in order. But it does mean that the form it takes must meet real threshold needs for medical care and leave enough resources to begin to attack the social, environmental, and behavioral conditions which compromise not only the efficacy of medical care, but all our efforts to be healthy as well.

The second is that underwriting the costs of medical care through a comprehensive health insurance plan will inevitably result in even steeper escalations in the cost of care and more disproportionate consumption of the gross national product (GNP) by medical care. Enoch Powell, based on his years of experience in administering England's health service, has marveled

---

* Naturally, any attempt to truncate the medical care system today would be followed by a significant level of trauma among patients whose dependency on medical care has developed to such an extent that their assumption of responsibility for themselves is exceedingly ifficult if not impossible. Hence, there is a "turnaround time" problem.

at the capacity of patients to consume large doses of care. The passage of a national health insurance plan will dissolve the last consumption constraint—the lack of uniform purchasing power. As a nation we will have then decided to further feed an already bloated system and, in so doing, divert monies that could otherwise be spent to ameliorate social and environmental conditions that have a demonstrably greater impact on health, such as poor housing and malnutrition.   And, most tragically, we will deepen the dependency of consumers on services and providers.

Because we are on the verge of putting public monies to the task that private money and health care professionals have not accomplished, the prospects for a new medicine are dim. Thus, passage of a national health insurance plan poses a real and poignant conflict to those who wish to devise and implement a system of medical care that will deal with causes, not cures, and with health rather than disease. The failure to promote a new medicine according to Peter Sedgewick, means that,

> [W]e are just going to get more and more diseases, since our expectations of health are going to become more expansive and sophisticated. Maybe one day there will be a backlash, perhaps at the point where everybody has become so luxuriantly ill ... [B]ut for the moment, it seems that illness is going to be "in;" a rising tide of really chronic illness.[19]

It is this latter problem that casts the largest shadow. If individual responsibility for health is as important as it is, as Lester Breslow and his associates found in their study in Alameda County,[20] how can this be achieved when more and more professional resources are pumped into the system—resources which inevitably further diminish the role of the individual? The answer here is related to points previously made. First, fewer practitioners should be allowed to practice who refuse to entrust their patients with substantial responsibility for themselves. Second, new practitioners must be trained—like those identified earlier—to counsel and encourage patients to assume the responsibility for themselves to the practical limits of self-care.[21] This again requires a retreading of licensure law and practice.

WHAT CAN BE DONE WITH LICENSURE?

I will separate the possibilities into short-term and long-term strategies, short-term being within the next one to five years and long-term being anything from five years on.

Short-Run Possibilities

The resistance to change in licensure laws and practice is legendary. Health care professionals, particularly physicians, have always strenuously opposed change in licensing practices because licensure has been easily manipulated to control the number and type of practitioners. And physicians have been granted control because to argue for relaxed licensure standards is, they say, to argue in favor of exploitation and charlatanism. Yet, some relaxation is exactly what I have in mind, along with a few other measures.

In the short run, the following proposals are worth looking at.

* the relaxation of some licensure standards;
* the establishment of licensing boards with jurisdiction over a wide range of health professions;
* lay control of licensure boards; and finally
* a shift to institutional licensure whenever feasible.

The arguments for and against each of these proposals can be briefly stated.

Relaxation of Licensure Standards

The rationale here is simple. The skill of healing and/or providing health-related services is not confined to licensed practitioners. Moreover, the failure of most physicians to deal humanely with their patients might also be partially overcome by the legitimation of practice by humane practitioners of other origins and disciplines. Nevertheless, despite the easy appeal of this proposal, the objections to this scheme are easily anticipated.

The major objection arises from a concern that quackery is sure to result if the system is deprofessionalized. There are some dangers, but nevertheless, since many other reforms will founder unless professionalism is eroded, it is necessary to do so. There will be some quackery; it is unavoidable where money is to be made out of human suffering. But there are two serious arguments. First, as I have said, we do not know much about what heals and what does not. As conventional research is conducted, we discover what conventionally works. But we also know that there are less conventional factors at work—factors that are unlikely to be assessed, or in some cases allowed into the healing equation in the first place. Some of these are the scale of the facility in which care is rendered; the nature and behavior of health personnel; the setting for the care—home, outpatient, hospital; the powers of healing of those who claim to be healers; and the roles of the family and the patient. Unless the barriers to practice are lowered to allow the interplay of new mixtures of personnel and facilities and interpersonal interactions, these factors are unlikely to be fully assessed.

The second argument is closely related to the first. The theories and practices on which contemporary medicine is premised are not the only ones.

There are other theories and other medical practices. And there is evidence, some of which has been discussed, that these systems of medicine are effective. The rigorous professionalization of modern medicine has succeeded in barring, or at least constraining, practitioners employing alternative therapies and techniques, such as acupuncture and chiropractic. The opportunity to learn from alternative practices should not be lost, but it will be if the prevailing barriers to practice remain. One example: Sister Justa Smith, a biochemist, has isolated a factor that may be associated with healing. Since her hypothesis is that enzyme activity is related to the healing process, she examined persons who claimed to be healers to determine whether they could accelerate enzyme activity. Her research thus far is confirmatory. Some of those who claim to be healers and appear to have had success in healing can dramatically elevate enzyme activity in controlled experiments.[22] If this is so, although much more research needs to be done, why should the natural healer be a hunted species?

The argument against alternative therapies is always that the quality of care would be compromised. It is said that these alternatives haven't been shown to be "effective." They are said to be fraudulent; to fail to use accepted tools and techniques—in short, to be unscientific. The result is that the battle between modern medicine and other healing therapies is joined on the wrong question. The question of the impact on the patient is not raised—but it is the crucial question. One of the reasons that the question is not asked is that the answer is potentially embarrassing. Few procedures and processes used in modern medicine can be correlated with a beneficial outcome to the patient.[23] To repeat, patients can be cured by contemporary allopathic medicine and by practices like psychic surgery, but there is little more hard evidence that the technologies used in contemporary medicine have anything more to do with the outcome to the patient than those utilized in psychic surgery. This is not to say that fraud is widespread in today's medicine, but rather to say that the question of fraud is irrelevant, if a healthy outcome to a patient is the concern.

Quackery will occur, but it can be dealt with in two ways. First, as information becomes available linking the processes of care with patient outcomes, information will be available to aid people in making choices about healers. Second, that same information will make it possible to bar some practitioners from practice when it is clear that harm is being done to patients.

Licensing Boards and Lay Control

The idea here is that as long as physicians control the licensure process, they will continue to do what they have always done—control the supply by number to ensure adequate compensation levels, and by type of qualifications to preserve that same monopoly. Hence, by empowering one board to license, not only should more rational patterns of manpower utilization result, but physicians will lose their stranglehold. Then, by coupling this reform with lay control, consumers will gain authority over the passkey to the system. This simply will give consumers that authority necessary to calibrate the entry of resources into the system with their needs and wants. While most consumers may not exercise this authority any differently than physicians, and in fact may initially choose to tighten entry into the system as opposed to relaxing it, eventually they may choose to relax entry standards. Many consumers are far more elective when they seek cures than is commonly assumed. They may sample chiropractors, allopathic medicine, and the community "kahuna" all for the same problem. But, even if they don't force an immediate change in licensure practices, at least one of the barriers between physicians and patients will have been breached.

Institutional Licensure

As the scale of the medical care system increases, impersonality appears to be a concomitant. Yet, whether good or bad, the scale of the system is increasing, and one result is that more and more health professionals are becoming parts of larger organizations. And, as they do, it makes more sense to license organizations rather the many individuals who populate them. One of the advantages of this scheme is that it would be free to employ and deploy whomever it pleases, and hence relax entry standards. Moreover, institutional licensure schemes would ease the malpractice crisis.

Yet there are some disadvantages. Some of the questions that can logically be raised are these:

1. How would the scheme affect utilization of institution-based personnel by independent physicians who presumably would bear no responsibility for their employment and utilization;

2. The scheme presents a solution for institutions, but does it offer any solutions to extra-institutional utilization of personnel, such as physician practices, except in those instances in which a physician group practice may have achieved institutional status;

3. Although purporting to offer a solution to the rigidities of licensure, doesn't the scheme reintroduce inflexibility at a different level—i.e., to the extent to which job descriptions for health professionals become fixed, the functional scope written into the job description becomes limiting, and thus becomes another form of licensure, and hence a constraint to optimal utilization; and finally,

4. Is description developed in one institution readily transferable to another?

None of these disadvantages is insurmountable, but they do suggest that the implementation of institutional licensure will not be easy.

The reason for all of these proposals is that the system needs to be loosened up. What have we got to lose? Medicine as it is now practiced is not significantly improving the health of the population. Perhaps medicine has reached technological limits which, without new biomedical breakthroughs, will fundamentally constrain its further development. Hence, if we are to have a medical care system, which of course we will have, then some modest experimentation seems warranted. None of the proposals urged thus far is much more than modest. They may sound radical, but given the compromises which will necessarily attend their implementation, they won't tear the system apart.

Long-Range Proposals

Licensure can never be radically transformed unless medicine itself is first transformed. Licensure simply is not an unattached issue. Hence, in order to effectively use the licensure process to engage the crises in medicine I have identified, most of our perceptions about health and medicine must be altered. This is no place to argue all these points. Most of them are raised in my book, *The End of Medicine*.[24] Nevertheless, a few points can be made.

First, there is no sense in talking about long-range proposals for the reform of licensure without considering the changes which are first necessary in medical education. The key to the new practitioner—one who can relate to patients in a technologically limited medical care system—is a new system of medical education. Medicine, like other highly developed systems, is reaching its technological limits. This is not to say that biomedical breakthroughs will not occur; they probably will. But it is to say that we may not be able to afford them. What we may need in the future is a medical care system that does what it does well for everyone, and does not grow by leaps and bounds at the cost of the health of the population as well as the cost of an appreciable part of our GNP. Medicine must necessarily utilize advanced technology and rely on expertise. But it must trust the patient as an ally in the process, and in most cases as the boss. This shift is profoundly dependent on a thorough-going reconceptualization of the purposes of medical education.

Second, a great deal more work must be done to fully conceptualize our emerging understanding of health. For so long now we have thought only of disease and the medicine needed to treat it. There simply is far more to it, but we don't have a cogent framework within which to work. There are, however, some promising leads. To take just one, Howard Brody in "The

Figure 11-1: Hierarchy of Natural Systems Constituting Man*

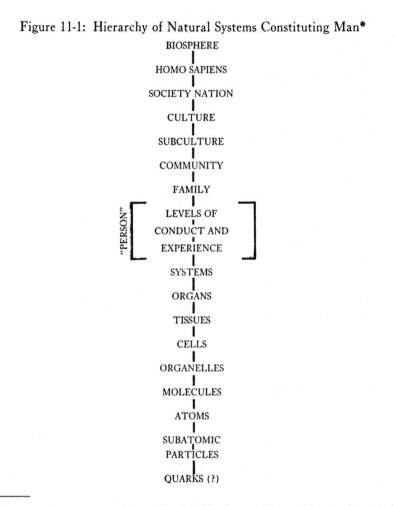

Systems View of Man: Implications for Medicine, Science and Ethics"[25] characterizes health as " ... the harmonious interaction of all hierarchical components, while 'disease' is the result of a force which perturbs or disrupts hierarchical structure." He illustrates his argument with the schematic in Figure 11-1.

There are a few critical points about the figure. First, the steps in the schematic are not discontinuous—they flow into one another and naturally interact through feedback loops. Second, disease in this schema isn't an

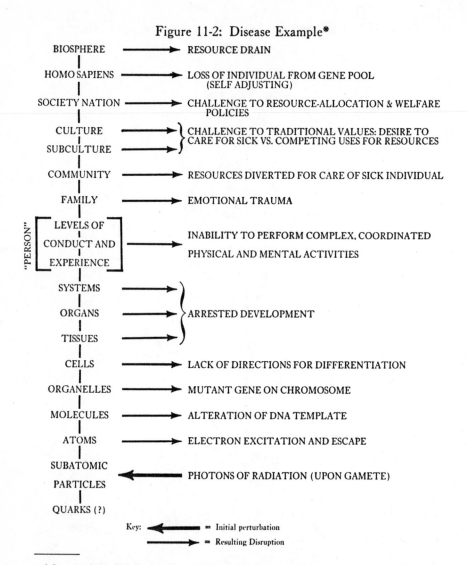

Figure 11-2: Disease Example*

BIOSPHERE	RESOURCE DRAIN
HOMO SAPIENS	LOSS OF INDIVIDUAL FROM GENE POOL (SELF ADJUSTING)
SOCIETY NATION	CHALLENGE TO RESOURCE-ALLOCATION & WELFARE POLICIES
CULTURE / SUBCULTURE	CHALLENGE TO TRADITIONAL VALUES: DESIRE TO CARE FOR SICK VS. COMPETING USES FOR RESOURCES
COMMUNITY	RESOURCES DIVERTED FOR CARE OF SICK INDIVIDUAL
FAMILY	EMOTIONAL TRAUMA
"PERSON" [LEVELS OF CONDUCT AND EXPERIENCE]	INABILITY TO PERFORM COMPLEX, COORDINATED PHYSICAL AND MENTAL ACTIVITIES
SYSTEMS / ORGANS / TISSUES	ARRESTED DEVELOPMENT
CELLS	LACK OF DIRECTIONS FOR DIFFERENTIATION
ORGANELLES	MUTANT GENE ON CHROMOSOME
MOLECULES	ALTERATION OF DNA TEMPLATE
ATOMS	ELECTRON EXCITATION AND ESCAPE
SUBATOMIC PARTICLES	PHOTONS OF RADIATION (UPON GAMETE)
QUARKS (?)	

Key: ◄——— = Initial perturbation
———► = Resulting Disruption

* Severe physical and mental retardation caused by a readiation-induced mutation in the gamete: example of spread of disruption upward through the hierarchy.

*Reprinted by permission. Howard Brody, "The Systems View of Man: Implications for Medicine, Science and Ethics," *Perspectives in Biology and Medicine* (Autumn 1973). ©1973 by the University of Chicago. All rights reserved.

entity, but a perturbation which, when introduced, disturbs the equilibrium state. Brody includes the Figure 11-2 to illustrate how the perturbation causes disruptions.

Figure 11-3: Disease Example*

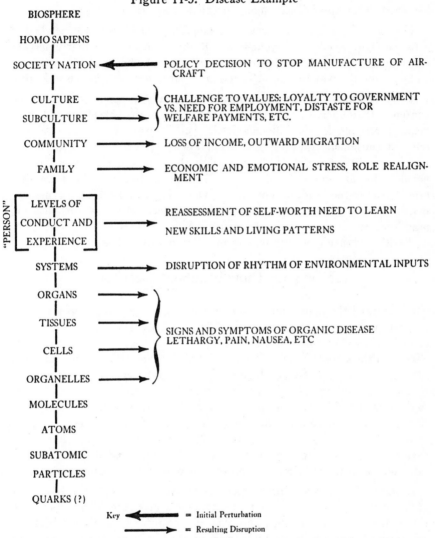

* Stress-related psychosomatic illness in an unemployed aerospace engineer: example of spread of disruption downward through the hierarchy.

*Reprinted by permission. Howard Brody, "The Systems View of Man: Implications for Medicine, Science and Ethics," *Perspectives in Biology and Medicine* (Autumn 1973). ©1973 by the University of Chicago. All rights reserved.

Then, to illustrate how a social or political decision perturbs the system, he introduces Figure 11-3.

The strength of the systems approach is that it overcomes the reductionist bias in the prevailing disease model implicit in medicine.

The point here is not to argue for adoption of a systems view, whether articulated by Brody or anyone else. Rather, the point is that emergent conceptual work holds the promise of clarifying our understanding of health and pointing the way to a reconstruction of our society's approach to health.

Third, as I have implied, a new medicine depends far more upon a changed consumer than upon a converted provider. If all of the physicians and other health professionals who influence health policy were replaced by randomly selected consumers, the decisions about allocation of resources for health which would be made would be essentially the same—or if anything, would be more in favor of medical care. Thus, no matter how hard we beat providers over the head, or how persuasive we are with health policymakers, it still is the consumer who makes the ultimate decision. What this means in practical terms is that unless consumers gain a new, more holistic perspective on health and medicine, any long-term solution will be frustrated.

A Few Last Thoughts about Licensure

I have used the opportunity afforded me to harangue about issues which interest me—which are perhaps only tangentially related to licensure. But I can't help it. For too long now, in my opinion, we have spent too much energy on the wrong issues. There's a lot of skill and talent at a conference like this, as there is at many high-level health conferences. If just some of that skill and talent could be diverted from the recycling of old information to the task of building a new approach to health—one which will incorporate the capacities and contributions of modern medical practice—our progress toward that goal might be accelerated. Nevertheless, I still feel that I have construed the broad topic to my own ends. Consequently, I will offer one last salvo on just plain old licensure in order to sum up the possibilities.

Licensure today is a captive process—captive to forces that have decided and continue to decide how we will spend our health care dollar. As long as this is the case, the modifications that can be introduced to the licensure process are likely to be modest. At the most, the following alternatives should be considered for the reasons given.

• some relaxation of entry standards in order to facilitate the wider practice of qualified practitioners of alternative systems of healing;

• a shift to comprehensive licensure boards, charged with the responsibility to license all health professionals;

• lay determination of such boards; and

• institutional licensure in lieu of individual licensure wherever feasible.

Beyond this, licensure is simply not a tool that can be used to turn the system around. The transformation of public education does not depend on changing the number of years that teachers must languish in schools of education before their certification. The same is true in medicine. If licensure is ever to be transformed in order to alter the nature and type of resources we as a society choose to entrust with our health money, other transformations must occur first. When and if that happens, we can talk about licensure again.

NOTES

1. See Paul Elwood *et al., Assuring the Quality of Health Care* (Minneapolis: InterStudy, 1973) for a review of the major studies.

2. *Ibid.,* pp. 29-30.

3. Thomas McKeown, "The Determinants of Human Health: Behavior, Environment and Therapy," unpublished paper, 1975.

4. Rick J. Carlson, "Health Manpower Licensing and Emerging Institutional Responsibility for the Quality of Care," *Law and Contemporary Problems* (Autumn 1970), p. 849.

5. See, for example, recent legislation in Minnesota.

6. See recent legislation in California.

7. This section draws heavily on Carl Slater *et al., Personnel Licensure* (Denver, Col.: Policy Center, Inc., 1975).

8. Robert C. Derbyshire, *Medical Licensure and Discipline in the United States* (Baltimore: Johns Hopkins Press, 1969).

9. Robert C. Derbyshire, "Medical Ethics and Discipline," *JAMA,* 228 (April 1, 1974), 59-62.

10. Benjamin Shimberg *et al., Occupational Licensing: Practices and Policies* (Washington, D.C.: Public Affairs Press, 1973).

11. Arlene S. Holen, "Effect of State Licensing Arrangements in Five Professions on Interstate Labor Mobility and Resource Allocation," M.A. Thesis, Columbia University, New York, 1962.

12. R. Schaffner and I. Butter, "Geographic Mobility of Foreign Medical Graduates and the Doctor Shortage: A Longitudinal Analysis," *Inquiry,* 9 (March 1972), 24-33.

13. Charles E. Lewis and Ruth S. Hassanein, "Continuing Medical Education—An Epidemiologic Evaluation," *New England Journal of Medicine,* 282 (January 29, 1970), 254-259.

14. Rashi Fein makes the point quite forcefully that whatever the effect of medicine on health, consumers still want more and more medical care. He points out that:

"In the case of health and medical care, we are dealing with a sector in which, because of customs and folkways, image may be even more important than reality. Because some (even if relatively little) medical care deals with matters of life and death, because of fear, because of infatutation with science and technology—as well as because medicine oftentimes does help some individuals and, therefore, each individual can hope that it will help him—persons have come to believe that medical care services and intervention by the physician make significant contributions to health. This view is not likely to change."

Rashi Fein, "On Achieving Access and Equity in Health Care," *Milbank Memorial Fund Quarterly,* 50 (October, 1972), 158-159.

15. Michael G. Michaelson, "The Failure of American Medicine," *The American Scholar,* 39 (Autumn, 1970), 702.

16. Irving K. Zola, "Medicine as an Institution of Social Control," a paper presented at the Medical Sociology Conference, British Sociological Conference, Nov. 5-7, 1971.

17. Peter Sedgwick, "Illness—Mental and Otherwise," *Hastings Center Studies,* 3 (1973), 37. Even "disability" is now defined as "deviance." See Eliot Freidson, "Disability as Social Deviance," in M. Sussman, ed., *Sociology and Rehabilitation* (American Sociological Association, 1965).

18. Marc Lalonde, *A New Perspective on the Health of Canadians,* a publication of the Government of Canada, 1974.

19. Sedgewick, *op. cit.*

20. The research was reviewed in *The Los Angeles Times,* November 14, 1973.

21. There is, unfortunately, very little hard research work on the possibilities and limits of self-care. There is an unpublished paper by Lowell Levin at Yale Medical School and a modestly annotated bibliography put together by Levin and his associates.

22. See Sister Justa Smith, Ph.D., "Paranormal Effects on Enzyme Activity," *Human Dimensions,* 1 (Spring 1972).

23. See A.L. Cochrane, *Effectiveness and Efficiency* (London: The Nuffield Provincial Hospitals Trust, 1972).

24. Rick J. Carlson, *The End of Medicine* (New York: John Wiley and Sons, 1975).

25. Howard Brody, "The Systems View of Man: Implications for Medicine, Science and Ethics," *Perspectives in Biology and Medicine* (Autumn 1973), pp. 71-92.

Part V

Financing Mechanisms and Costs in Quality Assurance Activities

Chapter 12
The Private Role of Financing of Quality Assurance Systems

Daniel W. Pettengill

In the manufacture of goods, it is common to have both quality controls and cost controls. Indeed, it is almost axiomatic that there be some standard of quality for the product in order for the cost control program to operate and have validity. Furthermore, the expense of operating these control programs is normally included in the price of the final product.

Quality is more difficult to measure with respect to a service than to a manufactured good. The provider of the service may think the quality excellent, while the recipient may think it most unsatisfactory. This is especially true of health care services. In manufacturing, if one controls the input and the process, one is virtually assured of a quality output. In health care, however, the physician generally has to start with an imperfect input—namely, a diseased or injured patient. The physician may use the highest quality process—i.e., treatment, and yet come out with a most unsatisfactory result from the patient's point of view—namely, death or permanent disability. Accordingly, in the field of health care, one generally talks about quality assurance (QA) rather than quality control. Furthermore, the term "assurance" is normally used in the sense of inspiring confidence rather than guaranteeing results.

When one discusses the financing of QA systems, it is essential to indicate which, or what combination, of the three phases of QA is to be financed—the input, the process, or the outcome.

To date, the emphasis has been on the process because it is the least difficult to define and measure. Furthermore, one needs to realize that if QA is to be more than empty words, considerable expense may be involved, and someone has to be willing to pay for the expense, or else the QA system will not long be viable. With health care services themselves so expensive today, most QA activities will, and should, be measured in terms of their cost/benefit effectiveness.

There will also be pressure to combine the QA program with a cost control program and to place major emphasis on the latter. Certainly, the original Medicare requirement that each participating hospital have a utilization review (UR) committee was such a combination, and the new Professional Standards Review Organization (PSRO) program may be much the same.

The demand for QA programs comes essentially from three sources: management (medical staffs, administrators, or boards of trustees); regulators; and purchasers. Some of the programs now required of hospitals in order to be licensed by a state or certified by the Joint Commission on Accreditation of Hospitals (JCAH) were originally instituted voluntarily by hospitals in order to satisfy management that the services rendered were of top quality. Tissue committees are a case in point.

The expense of QA programs instituted by management is almost always merged with other hospital expenses and is paid for by the patient or his insurer. Thus, if the patient is self-insured or has private insurance, this type of QA is paid for by the private sector. To the extent that the patient's bills are paid for by government as charged, the expense becomes funded by tax revenues. Where a government program, such as Medicare, pays on the basis of allowable costs, this type of QA program is financed by tax revenues to the extent, and only to the extent, the government recognizes the costs of the program as an allowable expense.

The hospital's license to operate is a rudimentary form of QA program. In general, QA programs required by law or regulation for all patients are financed the same as programs voluntarily instituted by the hospital's management.

METHODS OF QUALITY ASSURANCE

Private insurers have seldom required actual QA programs designed solely for their own insureds. One reason for this has been their lack of negotiating power with hospitals. However, insurers have attempted to give their insureds some rough assurance of quality by the following means.

One method used primarily by insurance companies is to include in the insurance policy a strict noncontracting of what constitutes a hospital for purposes of that insurance policy and to refuse to pay benefits unless the insured was confined in a hospital meeting that definition. Although this method is still in use today, its effectiveness has been reduced in some states by the enactment of laws requiring insurance policies to pay benefits to any institution that the state licenses as a hospital.

A second method, used primarily by hospital service plans and prepaid group practice plans, is to make contracts only with certain hospitals and to decline to pay any benefits to hospitals with whom no contract had been made. This method has likewise been rendered less effective by the enactment in most states of legislation requiring these plans to pay some benefit for confinements in noncontracting hospitals. It is interesting to note that Medicare originally intended to use a combination of these two methods, but ended up with such a lenient administration of its definition of a hospital that it made contracts with most hospitals and does pay for emergency care in those hospitals with which it has no contract.

A third method, used by all insurers, is to encourage the hospital's medical staff to review the practices of its members by studying their use of diagnostic tests, modes of treatment, lengths of stay, and plans for treatment following discharge, and to bring about any needed changes by intensive continuing education rather than punishment.

Regrettably, this third method has not yet inspired much confidence on the part of the public because, to date, the progress toward improved quality has been so slow. Accordingly, Medicare tried to speed up progress by denying its benefits to any hospital whenever the UR committee found an instance of unnecessary care involving a Medicare beneficiary. Combining cost control with QA in this manner has saved some money for the Medicare program itself, but the resulting unreimbursed expenses have become either a burden on the Medicare patient himself or on non-Medicare patients whose charges have been increased to cover the hospital's loss.

It would seem wiser and more effective had Medicare paid such claims and put the hospital on probation. If the hospital had then repeatedly failed to reduce its improper utilization of services, its contract should have been canceled and no Medicare benefits paid at all thereafter.

Be that as it may, Congress instead decreed in the fall of 1972 that UR should, to the maximum extent possible, be done on a concurrent rather than a retrospective basis, and that it be done on the basis of professional standards with oversight by an organization independent of the hospital. Congress called this new program "Professional Standards Review" and agreed to pay its cost in the form of either direct charges by the PSRO or as part of the reimbursable costs of the hospital. This new government program is Part B of Title 11 of the Social Security Act and applies only to health care services payable under that act. This PSRO program will be discussed in greater detail in other chapters. It is mentioned here because it raises most of the issues with which this monograph is concerned.

MAJOR ISSUES

First, will all QA programs be tied to cost control programs in the future? Second, is the PSRO concept a sound combination of QA and cost control, how much will it cost to operate, and will it be reasonably cost/benefit effective?

Third, if the PSRO concept is sound, then should it not be applied to all patients rather than just those covered under Titles 5, 18, and 19 of the Social Security Act?

Fourth, if the PSRO concept is sound but is not applied to all patients, will two standards of care emerge? (For those who believe two standards already exist, the question is whether the disparity in those standards will increase.)

Fifth, how will the detailed patient record information, needed to establish and keep current the professional standards, be developed and managed, and who will have access to this data base so that essential needs of all parties concerned are promptly served with due regard for the patient's right of privacy?

Sixth, how will the new Health Systems Agencies, which are charged with health planning, fit in?

Seventh, how will the agencies responsible for prospective rate review fit in and be satisfied that the costs of the program are proper to be included in the hospital's regular charges?

Eighth, if the PSRO concept is not sound, what type of cost control quality assurance program would be?

Ninth, how should whatever QA system is used be financed?

Rome was not built in a day, and neither will the multitudinous problems of the health care delivery system be solved in one lifetime. However, the willingness of private insurers and, more particularly, their insureds to pay their fair share of the cost of experiments to improve the system is going to be governed in large measure by the degree to which such experiments effectively serve all people and give appropriate representation or voice to each of the major interests involved.

It is important to realize that much private health insurance is provided through the employee benefit plans of very large employers. Insurance companies do endeavor to persuade such clients to participate in worthwhile experiments but cannot force them to do so. If a carrier attempted to require an employer to participate against his will, the employer could transfer his group plan to another carrier or even self-insure it. This is why voluntary experiments have to be fair for all if they are to have broad-based financial support.

Subject to the above caveat, the insurance business supports the development and implementation of programs of peer evaluation of quality health care, provided such programs:

1. Are carried out by the medical profession working in cooperation with hospital administration and other health professionals as appropriate;

2. Are carried out as a permanent community-wide monitoring and

evaluation system assuring the public that the care rendered meets professional standards of quality and is delivered on an economical cost basis;

3. Identify and correct through the process of continuing education and, when necessary, disciplinary action, practices which result in care that does not meet professional standards of quality;

4. Identify and eliminate wasteful and unreasonable practices and correct deficiencies in the system which unnecessarily inflate costs; and

5. Inform the public of the objectives of the program and its potential effect on the cost and quality of health care in order to secure the public's understanding, cooperation, and support.

Although the insurance business wants such programs to encompass all types of care, it realizes that their establishment must proceed on a gradual basis. Accordingly, it urges that the initial effort be made with respect to care in hospitals.

ESTABLISHING A PROGRAM

A first step in the establishment of such a program would be the definition of professional standards and the development of statistical norms and other criteria needed to facilitate the review process. This step needs to be performed by the medical profession in the area concerned, with special input from the medical staffs of the hospitals involved. The norms and other criteria should permit economical review, for the more common diagnoses, of the appropriateness of the admission, the duration, and the services rendered or omitted. Less common diagnoses will have to be evaluated on a judgmental basis until adequate data can be accumulated to permit the establishment of specific norms and criteria.

To keep the cost of the program reasonable, the screening norms should be set so that, for a quality institution, somewhere between 85 percent and 95 percent of the cases will meet the norms, and only the balance will have to be individually reviewed by physicians. The screening process itself should be handled by computer where the volume warrants, otherwise by carefully trained personnel other than physicians. Furthermore, there should be periodic evaluation on a sample basis of the cases found acceptable by the screening process to assure the continued validity of the norms. This sampling would normally be done by reviewing all or a significant portion of the cases involving a given diagnosis for which the norms or other criteria are to be checked.

A second step would be for the PSRO, by whatever name called, to consult with representatives of the hospitals and the carriers with respect to how the program should be operated and the role of each. The carriers should monitor and provide input for the policymaking decisions of the PSRO. Ultimately, written memoranda of understanding should be reached with each hospital and lists of participating hospitals made public.

A third step, which should be carried on in conjunction with the second step and which should also involve the Health Systems Agency or Agencies in the area to be served by the program, would be the development of a community-wide health care data system that will provide the data needs of not only peer evaluation but also health care financing and health care planning. The system must safeguard the confidentiality of the patient's record while permitting essential access thereto by the organizations concerned with the delivery, evaluation, financing, and planning of health care. All such organizations should be involved in policy decisions with regard to the nature of the input, output, and control of the data system. Furthermore, in order to avoid conflicts of interest and minimize possible misuse by any one such organization, the computer system used to store all the patient records and to print out the necessary data should be that of an entity which is independent of all of them. In short, no one vested interest, even an insurance company or a service plan, should have all the data within its own computer.

A fourth step would be the determination of the means of financing the various components of the program. Inasmuch as most such programs will commence on a voluntary basis for patients insured by private carriers, it would be desirable, if not essential, that all the costs of operating a given peer evaluation of the quality health care program be allocated equitably to the participating hospitals and made an integral part of their respective charges. This would assure that all patients and their carriers participate in the financing of the program. Admittedly, this approach would require the approval of any existing state hospital rate review agency. Such approval should be virtually automatic if the program is performing properly. If the cost of the portions of the program that are performed by other than hospital personnel were to be financed by direct charges of the PSRO to participating carriers, then some carriers or some of their large group policyholders might refuse to participate, with the consequent danger of either underfunding the program or saddling it with a high, unattractive cost per hospital admission.

A final step would be to establish mutually acceptable criteria for evaluating the cost/benefit effectiveness of the program at periodic intervals, with special attention to its effect on the quality of health care.

Regardless of their form, there need to be specific professional standards, and they need to be kept up to date. Likewise, regardless of the organizational structure, there does need to be an entity of professionals that will give the public reasonable assurance of both the necessity and the quality of the treatment rendered. The medical profession and hospitals are faced with just two ways of responding to this increasing pressure for assurance that the quality of care rendered meets professional standards. One way is defensive compliance with the specifications laid down under the PSRO law. If this occurs, the program carried out as a function of the medical profession will probably be of short duration, as it will exert little impact on the quality of care, and the cost of the reviews can be expected rapidly to exceed the savings generated under the program.

The other way, which the author recommends but for which he sees relatively little evidence of broad-based cooperation and support, is a recognition on the part of the medical profession and hospitals that taking the initiative now to establish an economical but effective quality of care monitoring and evaluation system for all patients is the best approach for both the public and the health care providers. While the program must address at least the same elements as are contemplated by the law mandating PSROs and should discourage overuse of hospital facilities and the delivery of poor care, it should, simultaneously, be organized to correct underuse and to raise the quality of care for all patients by retrospective evaluation of the care rendered. Corrective action should take the form of more intensive continuing education and, in rare instances, disciplinary action where required.

The present activities which have been established, generally in anticipation of the PSRO law, are geared largely to the required review of government programs. The likely result could be not only to deny private patients of the benefits of the program, both from the standpoint of dollar savings and the quality of care, but also to cause the resulting loss of revenue to the institution under the government program to be made up by increasing the cost of care to the private patient. This would then be another illustration of how the application of fragmented government controls works against the interest of the private patient, since he inadvertently becomes the buffer to protect the institution's financial position.

The insurance business is seeking the cooperation and support of the medical profession and hospitals to establish and operate a quality of care and evaluation system for all patients, and is prepared to underwrite its share of the cost involved. It urges the help of all interested parties in persuading the medical profession and hospitals that both the public's and their own interests will be better served by such a system which leaves great flexibility with the attending physician in managing the care of the patient, but requires him to be ultimately accountable to his peers for the judgments applied.

Chapter 13
Implementation vs. Experimentation:
The Federal Financing Question in PSRO

*William A. Knaus**

This chapter will summarize the current role of the federal government in financing the Professional Standards Review Organization (PSRO) in relationship to the possible costs of this activity and the policy implications of various sources of fiscal support. It will assume basic familiarity with the PSRO program, its design, and current operation.

COST**

Total cost predictions for the PSRO program have ranged from modest estimates of $150 million to over one billion dollars. The program is currently undertaking an in-depth cost study, but precise data is not presently available. Therefore, in order to arrive at rough cost estimates for this chapter, the actual experience of existing conditional PSROs was examined. For this analysis certain assumptions have been made:
(1) only the costs of review in short term care general hospitals conducted on Medicare and Medicaid admissions are included;
(2) the cost for PSRO review will be the same as the cost of utilization review (UR), excluding administrative costs;
(3) start-up costs are not included;
(4) physician reimbursement will be made for all but policy functions, the reimbursement rate will be $35 dollars an hour, and approximately 20 percent of admissions will require review; and
(5) the 11 million yearly Medicare and Medicaid admissions will remain constant.

With these definitions in mind, the conditional PSRO's costs were divided

---

* The opinions, conclusions and proposals in the text are those of the author and do not necessarily represent the views of the Department of Health, Education, and Welfare.

** This portion of the chapter relies heavily on work completed in the Office of Controller, DHEW, by Gregory Lear.

into review and administrative segments. Table 13-1 displays this information.

Table 13-2 summarizes this data on a per admission cost basis. Based upon this information, review costs can be estimated to range from $8 to $22 per admission, and administrative costs could range from $2.50 to $14.50. Thus, the total per admission costs of a PSRO could be from $10.50 to $36.50.

Utilizing these estimates the annual cost of a fully implemented national PSRO can be seen to vary from $136 to $422 million (Table 13-3).

There are a number of limitations in this type of analysis that also have policy implications. The estimates assume cost controls and limitations on physician reimbursement. Reimbursement without controls might significantly increase costs. In addition, the estimates do not consider the expansion of PSRO into the long-term and ambulatory care areas. They do not completely account for quality or medical care evaluation studies, mandated by PSRO, in their totals. Finally, of great importance, they do not include the cost implications of establishing a national data system under the aegis of PSRO.

Therefore, even this crude analysis, which does not include many desirable elements of PSRO, demonstrates that it will be an expensive federal program with the prospect of increasing costs as it expands into new areas of responsibility. How much of the cost of peer review the government should assume, and how it should monitor PSRO's financial and regulatory growth have been the topic of numerous and at times heated discussions.

Since its inception, PSRO represented a departure from the model of UR which it was designed to replace. URs costs were borne solely as part of the Medicare program and effectively hidden from definitive analysis. PSRO, on the other hand, has been a line item in the Public Health Service (PHS) budget and has had to compete with other PHS programs for health funds and with other service programs for Congressional appropriations. The overall budgeted amount, however, has included monies from both trust funds and general revenues. This is shown below.

	In Millions				
	FY 74	FY 75	FY 76	FY 77 (est.)	
Total........................	32	37	50	100 (high)	70 (low)
Amount from Trust Funds*...................	16	27	20	55	40

---

* As an interim financing approach, the costs of PSRO review delegated to hospitals are now reimbursed through the traditional Medicare and Medicaid mechanisms—i.e., Medicare benefit trust funds and Medicaid program on a 100 percent financing basis.

Table 13-1: Available Cost Data from Conditional PSROs

Conditional PSRO	(1) Amount Awarded	(2) Period	(3) Annualized Amount	(4)[a] Review Amount	(5)[a] Administration Amount	(6) Admissions Reviewed 1975	(7)[b] Total Admission In PSRO Area	(8)[c] Review Cost Per Admission	(9)[d] Administrative Cost Per Total Admission in Area
Colorado	$2,700,000	6/28/74—12/28/75	$1,800,000	864,000	936,000	119,000	117,000	$ 7.26	$ 8.00
Utah	951,495	6/18/74—12/18/75	634,330	310,822	323,508	28,000	42,000	11.10	7.70
Wyoming	604,502	6/28/74— 6/28/75	604,502	386,881	217,621	16,000	15,000	24.18	14.51
Multnomah	662,848	6/28/74—12/28/75	441,899	185,597	256,301	8,000	30,000	23.20	8.54
Minnesota	886,000	6/28/74—12/28/75	590,667	324,867	265,800	0	100,000	—	2.66
Prince Georges	212,458	6/29/74—12/29/75	141,639	50,990	90,649	0	12,000	—	7.55
Mississippi	1,227,954	6/28/74—12/28/75	818,336	515,552	302,895	0	124,000	—	2.44
Tennessee	1,626,305	6/29/74—12/29/75	1,084,203	444,523	639,680	0	109,000	—	5.87
Average			764,477	385,404	379,056	68,625		$16.44	$7.16
Weighted Average[e]								10.21	5.52

[a] Based upon estimates from the program. Medicare and Medicaid admissions only.

[b] From "Professional Standards Review Organization Study (Draft)" by Office of Associate Administrator for Planning, Evaluation, and Legislation, HSA, April 30, 1974. Medicare and Medicaid only.

[c] Column 4 + Column 6

[d] Column 5 + Column 7

[e] Weighted by number of admission.

Table 13-2: Per Admission Costs of Conditional PSROs

	Review Cost Per Admission	Administrative Cost Per Admission
DATA FROM CONDITIONAL PSROS		
Low	$ 7.26	$ 2.44
High	24.18	14.51
Average	16.44	7.16
Weighted Average	10.21	5.52
HSA STUDY [a]		
Low	9.00	NA
High	31.30	NA
OPSR STUDY [b]		
Low	16.63 [c]	—
High	26.99	—
Average	17.49	
PROGRAM ESTIMATES		
Average	12.00	4.55 [d]

[a] From "Professional Standards Review Organization Study (Draft)" by OPEL, HSA, April 30, 1974.

[b] From "Cost and Benefits of the PSRO Program (Draft)," OPSR, October 10, 1974.

[c] Figure reflects total cost per hospital review.

[d] Based upon administrative costs of $250,000 per PSRO with the average PSRO having 55,000 annual admissions.

Distribution of the amounts between review and administrative costs are based upon information supplied by the program. The number of admissions in FY 1975 are estimates based upon anticipated reviews the PSRO plans to conduct.

How and why the original decision was made to fund PSRO in this manner is difficult to trace historically, but there is no difficulty in defining the current objections to this financing structure. Prior to that discussion, however, it is worthwhile to record that Section 1168 of the Social Security Act, Title XI, that defines the structure of PSRO financing:

Expenses incurred in the administration of this part (Title XI, Part B) shall be payable from—
(a) funds in the Federal Hospital Insurance Trust Fund;
(b) funds in the Federal Supplementary Medical Insurance Trust Fund; and
(c) funds appropriated to carry out the health care provisions of

Table 13-3: Cost of a Fully Implemented PSRO System

		LOW	HIGH
1.	Total Annual Medicare and Medicaid Admissions..	11,000,000	11,000,000
2.	Review Costs = Annual Admissions × Review Cost per Admission [a]	88,000,000	242,000,000
3.	PSRO Administrative Costs = Annual Admissions × Administrative Cost per Admission [b]..	27,500,000	159,500,000
4.	Salaries and Expenses and Overhead, BQA	10,000,000	10,000,000
5.	Contracts (Criteria Development, etc.)	5,900,000	5,900,000
6.	Evaluation..	1,000,000	1,000,000
7.	State Councils [c]	3,600,000	3,600,000
	TOTAL..	$136,000,000	$422,000,000
	Less Reimbursement through Medicare and Medicaid for Delegated Review (50 percent of review delegated)	44,000,000	121,000,000
	Budget Amount for PSRO...........................	$92,000,000	$301,000,000

[a] Based upon a low estimate of $8.00 per admission and a high estimate of $22.00 per admission.

[b] Based upon a low estimate of $2.50 per admission and a high estimate of $14.50 per admission.

[c] Based upon 18 state councils at $200,000 each.

the several titles of the Act; in such amounts from each of the sources of funds as the Secretary shall deem to be fair and equitable after taking into consideration the costs attributable to the administration of this part with respect to each of such plans and programs.

Persons who wish to remove control of PSRO financing from the Congress cite Section 1168 as giving the Secretary of DHEW responsibility for assigning funds from the Social Security Act. This interpretation has been supported by the Assistant General Counsel for Public Health.

The desire for a change to DHEW-controlled financing is supported by the following arguments:

1. The current financing approach slows the progress of PSRO, while UR remains intact. By returning control over appropriations to DHEW, more rapid development through increased monetary support would be possible.

2. The current mechanism encourages local PSROs to delegate review.

Table 13-4: Financing Alternatives

Left-margin labels (upward arrows): Greater Visibility of Total Program Costs; Greater Control over Cost; Encouragement of Delegated Review

1. Utilize the annual appropriation mechanism for all PSRO costs.

2. Continue the existing system.

3. Utilize the appropriation approach for all PSRO costs except review costs in both delegated and non-delegated hospitals which would be paid through Medicare and Medicaid funds through the existing hospital reimbursement mechanism.

4. Use the Secretary's authority to transfer Medicare and Medicaid funds to a PSRO account for support of all aspects of the program except administrative costs which would be obtained through annual appropriations.

5. Establish a special PSRO account from Medicare and Medicaid funds for support of the entire program.

Right-margin labels (downward arrows): Faster Implementation; Less Individual Recognition of PSRO; Less Congressional More DHEW Control

Because delegated review does not draw on the local PSRO's budget, this type of review is preferable regardless of the quality of the actual review process. Proponents of this change feel the decision to delegate review should be removed from financial considerations.

3. The current approach fails to fully recognize PSRO as a regulatory component of Titles 18 and 19 and, therefore, as an integral part of these programs.

In view of these criticisms, a number of alternatives have been proposed. They are listed in Table 13-4, along with the directions in which they change overall policy (indicated by labeled arrows).

DISCUSSION

Rather than present each of the individual alternatives with specific arguments, it is helpful to emphasize the policy directions that their adoption or rejection imply.

Greater Visibility of PSRO's Total Costs

Despite our inability to precisely predict costs, there can be little argument that PSRO will be an expensive program. Furthermore, given the established annual trend of all major federal health programs to substantially increase costs, one's immediate reaction is to maintain maximum visibility over total costs. This is especially true since the future financial benefits of PSRO are unknown.

Despite optimistic admissions, that peer review will significantly decrease expenditures through decreased length of stay and reduction of inappropriate admissions, there are disturbing limitations. One limitation is the possibility that following an initial decline in length of stay new norms will be established that will limit any ongoing savings. In addition, there is the growing fear that through adoption of rigid norms and standards by local PSROs, additional laboratory and diagnostic support will be encouraged, actually *adding* to total costs. The final answers to these questions are not yet available.

On the other hand, high visibility of the program's costs may expose the program to the vicissitudes of Congressional funding and in a time of economic depression could result in premature destruction before real benefits could be appreciated. Within the federal bureaucracy line item identification also makes a program susceptible to easy reductions. Indeed, one of the arguments used by PSRO administrators is that progress has already been severely hampered by poor funding support within the administration.

Direct Control over Costs

This policy direction is, quite naturally, tied to the visibility of the program's total expenditures. The cost of UR, PSRO's predecessor, is impossible to precisely define—indeed the FY 1975 Social Security Administration budget does not even indicate a level of funding for the administrative cost of UR. Therefore, it is difficult even in retrospect to say how much this activity costs the federal government. For a similar situation to develop in respect to PSRO is, at best, undesirable.

Furthermore, as more information does become available from new PSROs, it is important that any benefits be compared to the cost outlay.

Of course, the beneficial effects of increased quality of care are immeasurable in dollars. This argument, however, does not reduce the need to control federal spending for PSRO.

Delegated Review

Under the present system, each PSRO can maximize its allocated funds by delegating review to hospitals within its area. Only the costs for non-delegated review draw on the local budget. Given this strong incentive, it is feared review will be delegated regardless of individual adequacy and that local PSROs' oversight function will be weakened. In addition, as occurred with UR, costs could significantly increase at the hospital level without a corresponding increase in results or efficiency.

On the other hand, the concept of delegated review was to maintain maximum individual flexibility and to allow for experimentation on the local level. Since the precise manner in which review should be conducted is far from clear, this type of diversity on the part of individual hospitals and physician groups might prove extremely beneficial.

Increased Recognition of PSRO as Part of Titles 18 and 19: Time for Implementation

The argument to incorporate PSRO into these two federal programs is an obvious attempt to reduce some of the resistance still operating against implementation. There is little disagreement that PSROs have been viewed as a separate and very controversial federal program by some American physicians. Although intended by Congress to replace UR, the law does have much broader consequences. The argument that there needs to be a direct relationship between the financing of care and the financing of review makes little historical sense. Separate identification will certainly make future evaluation easier, and, vice versa, incorporation will make it more difficult.

Those persons who wish to return financial control over PSRO to DHEW wish to do so in order to more rapidly complete implementation. They point out that budget projections for FY 76 will not allow them to fund all the new planning PSROs and, in addition, will not allow them to convert existing plannings to conditionals. Within a given PSRO area budget, restrictions will make uniform implementation of review difficult. Therefore, in their viewpoint, unequal application of the law will occur; in addition, selection of which conditional PSROs to fund with limited resources is a difficult procedural problem.

On the other side are those persons who feel that the federal effort should move with more caution. They emphasize the lack of operational data upon which to calculate benefits.

From the private sector has come recent criticism that in the haste of attempting to implement and run the program, DHEW has given too little support to private initiative for individual experimentation. This, it is argued, reduces the potential of PSRO to be maximally effective.[1]

Finally, the rush toward implementation has resulted in neglect of a potentially beneficial aspect of the PSRO program. One of the most frequently heard complaints from the public is the multiplicity of required federal forms.

A data collection system, designed with the PSRO program as its impetus, could go far to address and possibly correct this problem. Although initial studies have been completed, little attention has continues, paid to them as emphasis is placed on expansion. If this continues, PSRO will be open to criticism that it is attempting to solve health problems through random inputs without overall total organization.

Congressional vs. Bureaucratic Control

Thus, discussion over the cost of financing structure for PSRO provides a classic example of legislative, governmental, and public interaction.

Combined with disagreements over how much to spend, where the money should come from, and exactly how much say the public should have in designing the program is the usual emphasis on economics. Within this emphasis on costs and potential cost savings, however, other policy goals are implied.

By maintaining Congressional control, financial resources will probably remain limited and, provided support does continue at a reasonable level, nationwide implementation could await more definitive operational and cost benefit analysis. This would require a coincident decision by the operating agency (the Bureau of Quality Assurance) to provide maximum support for operational PSROs and limit further expansion. At the least, this would permit the public and government more time, if not resources, for experimentation.

This option accepts the risk that Congress, dissatisfied with preliminary results, might permaturely dissolve the program. It also assumes that the information and experience gained by operational PSROs would be incorporated into policy.

The alternative to this approach—namely the return of all or part of the funding support to the bureaucracy—will hasten complete implementation. It will closer associate PSRO with Titles 18 and 19 and will decrease the possibility of a precipitous withdrawal of funds. It would certainly allow for the more equitable support of developing PSROs nationwide.

The government presently finds itself in the uncomfortable position of denying funds to physician groups who have organized in response to a federal mandate. Measured in terms of numbers of planning and conditional PSRO, the program is behind schedule.

In terms of federal health policy the PSRO program is perceived as a significant undertaking, but one whose total cost remains largely unknown. Although substantial optimism exists for eventual cost savings and quality influences, current medical and economic evidence can be used to support either a policy of rapid implementation or cautious experimentation.

Policy in Action—Current Update

Since this chapter was written, Public Law 94-182 was passed by the Congress, and on December 31, 1975 it was signed into law. This amendment to the Social Security Act changed the federal financing structure of PSRO. In effect, it adopted financing alternative number three in Table 13-4.

The amendment allows a local PSRO to bill each individual hospital within its area for all review costs. In turn, the hospital will obtain reimbursement from the Medicare and Medicaid programs. Prior to this amendment only delegated review costs were handled in this manner.

As outlined in Table 13-4, this statutory change will permit more rapid implementation of the PSRO program. Projections for FY 1977 now have 120 PSROs in the conditional category, with the remaining 83 to be in planning phases by the end of 1978. Before passage of 94-182, it was unknown whether the level of appropriations would be high enough to support this effort. Now that all hospital review costs are removed from the appropriations process, financial support is assured.

Another effect of this change will be a reduction in the recognition of PSRO's total costs. Since only administrative costs and review costs outside of the hospital will be obtained via appropriations, the level allocated will decrease while the total costs continue to increase.

For example, the FY 1977 budget level for PSRO is $89 million. However, it is estimated that, under the new amendment, $62 million of that total will be obtained from the Medicare trust funds and the Medicaid program. Thus, only $27 million need be appropriated by Congress.

Naturally this change also decreases Congressional control over PSRO and transfers major financial responsibility to the administration (third policy arrow on Table 14-4 leading to administration). Decisions as to what limits are applied to the total costs and how expenditures are recorded are now within control of the federal bureaucracy. It is expected, given the experience with UR, that attempts will be made to closely monitor PSRO's total costs.

Therefore, this most recent amendment to PSRO provides for more rapid implementation with less time for experimentation, decreased Congressional supervision, and, depending on future policy decisions, somewhat decreased control over total costs. Whether the future will see further movement toward a more autonomous role for PSRO merits close observation.

NOTE

1. P. J. Sanazaro, "Private Initiative in PSRO." *N. Engl. J. Med.*, 293 (1975), 1023-1028.

Chapter 14
Benefit/Cost Analysis of
Quality Assurance Programs*

*Charles E. Phelps***

INTRODUCTION

The costs of medical care, and the resulting benefits in terms of improved health, have become topics of increasing concern in the United States and in other countries around the world. Third parties (private insurance and government) have become more and more involved in the financing of medical care, and have come to a position where stronger interest in the outcomes of the medical care market seems desirable. Thus, the government (in particular) and private markets (doctors, hospitals, and private insurance companies) have started down a path of evaluating the outcomes of medical care and of controlling, through regulation or law, the ways in which medical care can be undertaken.

The evidence used to justify these various regulations of quality has been, to be generous, sparse. The primary justification for many of these programs is that the present state of affairs is scandalous, so that change must lead to improvement. While not necessarily quarreling with the premise, the conclusion is unwarranted. It, therefore, seems appropriate to begin to evaluate the evaluators, to develop a framework with which one could assess the gains to society from undertaking a quality assurance (QA) program of one type or another. The purpose of this chapter is to set forth a general framework for conducting such an analysis, to provide where possible some

* Support for this research was provided through General Research Support Funds from the DHEW Health Insurance Study, Grant Number 016B-7401-P2021. The opinions and conclusions expressed herein are solely those of the author and should not be construed as representing the opinions or policies of any agency of the United States government.

** The author would like to thank Will Manning and Joseph P. Newhouse for helpful comments on a previous draft of this chapter.

examples of how the analysis might be undertaken in specific cases, and to indicate some likely pitfalls in which the QA analyst might be entrapped.

The methodology adopted for this analysis is a basic benefit/cost calculation. The value of this approach has been well proven over a variety of fields, even though proponents and opponents of a given project may calculate immensely different benefit/cost ratios for the same project. The reason such discrepancies can occur is because methods of assessing benefits and accounting of costs are sometimes ambiguous. The value, nevertheless, is that the framework forces the attention of decision makers onto many, if not all, of the relevant considerations.

Much of the effort of this chapter will be devoted to the propositions that casual benefit/cost analysis, particularly as demonstrated in current literature, will likely *overstate* benefits and *understate* costs of QA programs. The resultant benefit/cost calculation, of course, would overly encourage the undertaking of the QA programs which had been so misassessed. The methodology can be applied to find those programs which will provide the greatest improvement in public welfare for the least cost. The essence of benefit/cost analysis is simple and pure; one computes the aggregate benefits and the aggregate costs for a QA program and then takes their ratio. The wise decision maker selects first those QA programs with the highest benefit/cost ratio and proceeds down the available list until either, (1) the benefit/cost ratio falls below 1.0; or (2) available funds for QA programs are expended.

Unfortunately, the actual computation of benefits and costs for any large program is difficult, frustrating, and often ambiguous. Thus, while the essence of this method appears simple, the actual analysis needed to complete it is likely to be quite complex. This chapter will investigate some of these complexities.

Discounting Future Benefits and Costs

QA programs generally have benefits and costs that extend over many years, rather than being concentrated in a specific short time interval. Indeed, while the costs are incurred early in a project, benefits may not be realized for some years in the future. Thus, it is necessary when assessing the benefit/cost ratio of QA programs to account properly for the temporal pattern of benefits and costs. The usual method for undertaking this is to use *discounting*. Discounting is based upon the notion that a benefit received (or a cost expended) next year is of less value than one received (or expended) today. If the discount rate is specified as "r," then any stream of benefits can be "discounted" back to its "present value" by the following formula:

$$(1) \qquad \begin{array}{c} \text{Present Value} \\ \text{of Benefits} \end{array} = \text{PVB} = \sum_{i=1}^{n} \frac{B_i}{(1+r)^i}$$

where B_i is the benefit received in the ith year. Similarly, the stream of costs undertaken for a project can be discounted to its present value by:

$$(2) \qquad \begin{array}{c} \text{Present Value} \\ \text{of Costs} \end{array} = \text{PVC} = \sum_{i=1}^{n} \frac{C_i}{(1+r)^i}$$

where C_i is the cost incurred in the ith year. Clearly, if the pattern of benefits or costs is identical in each year, then the discounting is irrelevant because B_i or C_i would be factored out of the summations. However, if the pattern changes over time, then discounting is essential to reach the correct conclusion about the value to society of undertaking a project. Thus, for a project which has a multi-year lifespan, the correct calculation for benefit/cost analysis is the ratio of PVB to PVC.

It is also of obvious importance to select the proper discount rate. This choice has been a subject of debate among economists for years, and the issue is still far from resolved. At one extreme, some persons argue that the appropriate discount rate is a weighted average of the private interest rate on commercial securities (bonds), on the grounds that any investment (either government or private) could (as an alternative) be moved into private industry, where the private rate would apply. Others suggest that a lower rate should apply to government projects, because the private rate includes payments for risk that are not applicable to government projects, and because the government can, by its size, more easily bear risk than can private individuals and firms. Still others argue for an artificially low government discount rate on the grounds that future generations' preferences are not expressed well in present day markets, and that society owes future generations some sort of protection which a low discount rate will provide. Finally, some argue for project-specific rates which reflect the risk of each project on the grounds that there is identifiable separate risk on each project undertaken. My reading of this literature is that a single rate should be applied, and that risk should be accounted for in the benefit and cost streams (i.e., by making B_i and C_i random variables), rather than by introducing risk into the discount rate. A rate at or very near the private market interest rate should be applied to assessing governmentally undertaken projects, primarily on the opportunity cost argument. Current operationalization of this concept in such agencies as the Office of Management and Budget (OMB) suggests using a rate of 10 percent.

Dealing with Inflation in Cost/Benefit Studies

Two important aspects arise when dealing with inflation in benefit/cost analysis. First and foremost, in periods of inflation, it is clear that even if costs and benefit streams are identical in terms of resources used to undertake a project, inflation would give a different indication. Thus, aside from the problem of discounting, it is necessary to put all benefit and cost measures and the discount rate into the same unit of measurement. To do this, one must assume a path of inflation or deflation that will occur throughout the life of a project, and make adjustments from nominal to real dollars accordingly. A valuable discussion of discounting and inflation adjustment is included in Hanke, Carver, and Bugg[1] for persons interested in more detail on this subject. In general, if project costs and benefits C^i and B^i are measured in nominal terms (i.e., in dollars that become inflated over time), then the joint solution of discounting and adjustment to constant dollars involves calculating the present value in real dollars of costs (PVRDC) as:

$$(3) \quad \text{PVRDC} = \sum_{i=1}^{n} \frac{C_i}{(1+r)^i (i+p)^i}$$

where r is the discount rate and p the annual rate of inflation. If a known pattern of inflation is to be substituted, rather than assuming some constant rate of inflation, then the appropriate divisor for PVC is $\pi_{j=1}^{i} (1+p_j)$, where p_j is the inflation rate in year j. A similar formula, of course, is applied to calculate the present value of real-dollar benefits, PVRDB. In practice, since future inflation is difficult to predict, one commonly assumes a constant rate of inflation and uses the method shown in (3).

Justifications for Public Production of Quality Assurance

Two basic premises behind governmental mandated or regulated intervention in the medical market along quality of care dimensions are that there is insufficient information being *produced* or *used* privately. These two dimensions are quite different in their implications for appropriate action in general. If the production of information is not optimal, this may be because: (1) there are persistent economies of scale in production of information (as, for example, there are in national defense, telephone, and water systems, etc.); or (2) because there are artificial restrictions on the amount of information in the medical sector (as, for example, from suppression of advertising). Even these two cases lead to different actions, and the costs and benefits of QA programs will depend quite heavily on whether appropriate action is taken.

If the first reason for insufficient supply of information is correct, then appropriate action is either a direct subsidy to production of information (i.e., government subsidy of QA programs carried out in the private market) or direct government production of QA programs. Alternatively, if the second reason holds, then removal of the interfering mechanisms should suffice. Naturally, both reasons could simultaneously cause an underproduction of information on quality, in which case the appropriate response includes activities on both fronts.

The other widely espoused reason for governmental QA programs is that there is insufficient use of information by patients (in the economist's jargon, insufficient demand), the reason usually being given that the subject is so complex and difficult that the patient cannot understand what is happening, and thus capitulates to the suggestions of his physician.

From a personal viewpoint, I find this argument rather paternalistic, and not convincing. As is discussed later, a parallel argument could be made concerning the citizen-consumer's inability to understand the processes involved in such things as televisions, automobiles, high fidelity systems, restaurant meals, or even professional athletic events. Yet, the market has responded with mechanisms that allow the consumer to evaluate these areas if he so chooses, including advertising by firms, warranties on quality, specialized magazines providing consumer information, and even restaurant rating services. To accept that medical care is so radically different from these areas seems incorrect to me, at least as a general proposition. Thus, the case for government intervention in the QA field rests on questions relating to the adequacy of supply, and upon possible economies of scale in the production of QA information. This chapter supplies a method of evaluating specific QA programs, whether they are undertaken publicly or privately.

A FRAMEWORK FOR ASSESSING BENEFITS OF QUALITY ASSURANCE

In order to characterize adequately the benefit/cost ratio of QA programs, a basic starting point must be to understand what benefits are being derived from the program. This basic model is that the consumer derives utility from being healthy, and that he produces health by combining inputs of medical care with his own time, efforts, and knowledge. This production process may be likened to those undertaken by any business or firm, and subject roughly to the same rules of efficiency. In either case, the problem is to select the best amount of output (health to the individual, widgets to the firm), and to produce that at the lowest possible cost. More formally, the problem can be described as follows: The consumer sets about to maximize a utility function, $U(x,H)$, where x is his consumption of other goods (defined in units such that the price $= 1$), and H is his consumable level of health. The consumer is faced with a budget constraint, $I = x + pM = wT + NWY$, where I is his income, w the wage rate (value of time), T his total productive time available, and NWY his income from other than wage sources (non-wage income). He buys medical care, M, and produces health, H, by combining that care with his own time. Thus, there is a production function for health described by $H = f(M,t)$, which describes the process by which health is produced.

From this general framework, one can derive a theoretical relationship between the amount of medical care a person would purchase (for any given set of conditions) as a function of the price of that care. This relationship is that characterized generally as a demand function, and it is normally thought of as a downward-sloping line when the quantity of medical care is plotted against the price of care. This relationship between quantities demanded and the price of each item is derivable from simple maximization of a utility function coupled with a constraining budget.

General demand theory has been applied more directly to medical care with particular modifications by several persons (Grossman,[2] Phelps,[3] Phelps and Newhouse,[4] Acton,[5]) to show in particular how such things as insurance, nonprice restrictions on care availability, and random illness affect the demand curve. The important things established from this work are: (1) demand for medical care is derived from a more basic demand for health itself; (2) demand for medical care (as for other goods and services) shows an inverse relationship between quantities demanded and price. Put differently, demand curves for medical care are downward sloping; (3) more serious illnesses shift demand curves outward, so that holding constant everything else, *including the price of care,* sick people will demand more medical care than healthy people. A set of demand curves showing this relationship appears in Figure 14-1 for illnesses ℓ_0, ℓ_1, and ℓ_2, each more serious than the preceding illness; (4) the price of care facing the individual at the time care is sought is the relevant price variable for medical demand. Thus, if a person is insured, the out-of-pocket price is relevant, not the list price; (5) time can act as a rationing device, just as can medical prices. Thus, holding constant such things as income, insurance, and medical prices, an inverse relationship is established between the amount of care people demand and the amount of time (or distance traveled) necessary to obtain care.

Figure 14-1: Demand Curves for Medical Care at Different Illness Levels

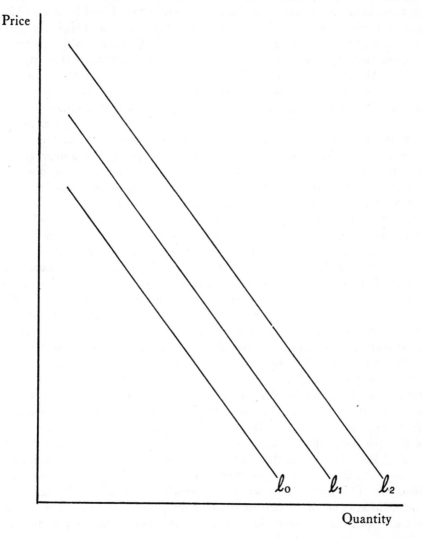

To this structure it is necessary to add two complications which show the essence of the QA problem, and which will lead to useful and estimable functions showing the value of QA in the medical market.

The first complication is really a well-known phenomenon—health is not a certain event, but is in fact highly random. It is indeed this random component of health which leads consumers to purchase insurance against medical cost variability (Phelps,[3]).   Thus, we can better describe the problem facing the consumer as choosing a final level of health after he has faced a drawing from a random illness distribution. That is, if H_0 is the level of health at the beginning of the period, and if ℓ is the health loss from sickness, then the final level of health the consumer can enjoy is $H = H_0 - \ell + g(M,t)$. The *distribution* of illness is thus an important part of the problem facing the consumer—it tells him how much insurance to buy, and it tells the insurance company what to charge him for that insurance.   But, buying medical care is a separate problem—the consumer receives a drawing from this random distribution, and he must then decide how much medical care to buy, so that (coupled with his own time inputs) he can improve his health. Thus, Figure 14-1 can be interpreted as showing various demand curves *conditional* on the actual illness facing a person—i.e., what behavior would be for any random ℓ_1 actually drawn from the $f(\ell)$.

An important part of QA in medical care is simply assuring that unbiased estimates of the severity of ℓ are given to the patient by his doctor, so that he can act rationally thereafter. Patients normally do not have direct observations of the size of   (the severity of their disease), but rather they must seek expert advice and opinion as to how sick they really are. Thus, physicians are able to induce consumers to spend more on medical care than is optimal. This line of argument formalizes one way in which physicians might be able to increase demand for their own services beyond the appropriate amount. (For another interpretation of this phenomenon, see Monsma[6] and Pauly.[7]

The second problem to add to this structure is one relating to the production function of health—$g(M,t)$. This function has standard characteristics of all production functions, namely that more of either input will increase output (i.e., that the first derivatives g_M and g_t are positive), but at a decreasing rate (g_{MM} and g_{tt}, the second derivates, are negative). Thus, (g_{MM} and g_{tt}, the the production function is concave, as shown generally in Figure 14-2. A key parameter in the consumer's decision about seeking medical care is the marginal productivity of medical care, g_M, which is the slope of the function. This parameter describes how much more health will result from the addition of one more unit of M, other things held constant. The second key complication of this model is that the marginal productivity of medical care is random—i.e.,

$$g_M = f(M,t) + u$$

where u is a random variable unknown to the patient when he seeks care. Thus, with an unfavorable drawing from the distribution of u, the marginal productivity of medical care may fall, and may even become negative. When this occurs, the patient is said to have contracted an iatrogenic disease. The structure of this random component of the marginal productivity of medical care is of keen interest. Several factors combine to determine u: the competence of the physician performing the medical service, the nature of the patient and his disease; the state of medical knowledge; and blind luck. I allege here, and will discuss further below, that a major and important function for QA programs can be to identify knowable components of the distribution of u, and to pass that knowledge along to consumers.

It is helpful to think of the various components that make up the random variable u. Some are doctor-specific; I assume that a distribution exists describing the average error component attributable to doctors in the community. A more common way of stating this is that some doctors are better than others, and that the distribution of their skills may be observed. It is of major importance to note that most existing QA mechanisms in practice today or proposed for tomorrow operate on exactly this problem—they attempt to identify, and hence to correct or remove those doctors who form the lower tail of this quality distribution. The stated purpose of licensure examinations is exactly this—to eliminate "bad" doctors. Bad doctors are those whose marginal productivity is much lower than community standards. Licensure would nominally cut off the lower tail of the skill distribution. Similarly, the apparent operational intent of the Professional Standards Review Organization (PSRO) will be to identify bad doctors and make them change, or to remove them from the distribution, although it has been forcefully argued (White,[8]) that a more promising approach would be to attempt to modify the distribution as a whole.

Malpractice suits as a quality control device present a slightly different picture. If there is a further element making up the random variable u that is outside of the control of the doctor and is uncorrelated with physician behavior, then unfortunate outcomes can occur even if a "good" doctor undertakes care on a given patient. Malpractice suits nominally attempt to isolate which component (doctor-specific or doctor-independent) is responsible for a maloccurrence, and reward the patient when it is a doctor-specific component. To the extent that these awards could be correctly made, and to the extent that malpractice insurance premiums accurately reflected doctor-specific components of quality, then malpractice activity in the courts would serve as a powerful way of screening out low-quality doctors from medical practice. Current insurance practices, however, seldom incorporate physician-specific characteristics in determination of malpractice insurance premiums; rather, group rating is used.

Other QA mechanisms attempt to determine, by force of law or regulation, that only certain production processes are undertaken to achieve cures in the medical market. These laws specify types and amounts of various types of medical care that must be used in certain circumstances, and prohibit the use of alternative processes. Perhaps the most prominent forms of such laws at a governmental level are the Food and Drug Administration (FDA) drug

Figure 14-2: Health Production Functions for Two Time Inputs ($t_2 > t_1$)

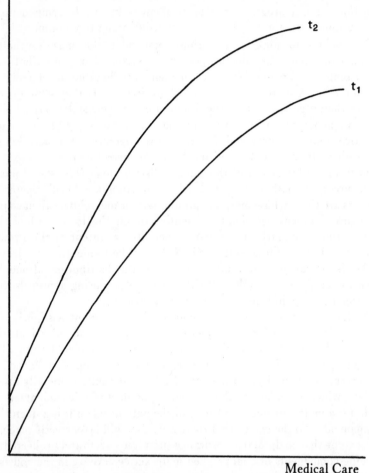

regulations, prohibition of non-M.D. practitioners undertaking certain activities (e.g., injections, acupuncture), required nurse-staffing levels, etc. At the institutional level, many hospitals specify certain procedures to always be done in certain circumstances (e.g., type and cross-match blood samples before surgery) and place absolute prohibitions on other procedures (e.g., the use of cyclopropane and other explosive anesthetic agents). The implicit assumptions necessary to make such regulations useful is that they must either raise the average marginal productivity of medical care in the community explicitly, or they must eliminate the lower tail of the outcome distribution. These two objectives may conflict. While removing the lower tail of outcome distribution, it may be also necessary to reduce the average outcome, at least in the long run.

THE VALUE OF EXACT INFORMATION ON THE SEVERITY OF ILLNESS

I have characterized the consumer as optimizing a utility function with respect to three decision variables: his own time allocation; his consumption of other goods; and his health. These in turn imply an optimal amount of medical care for a given disease. I have shown elsewhere (Phelps,[3] Phelps and Newhouse,[4]) that these conditions in general lead to a set of demand curves for medical care, each one shifting to the right for more severe illnesses. I have drawn them in Figure 14-3 in typical fashion, so that the less care is purchased, all other things held equal, the higher the price of care. I show demands for medical care for two illnesses, ℓ_1 and ℓ_2, the latter being more severe. Suppose the event ℓ_1 has actually befallen the consumer. Then his optimal amount of medical care would be q_1, the point where his demand curve is intersected by the price of care, p. Suppose now a doctor deceives the patient, and convinces him that he really has a disease of severity, ℓ_2, and the consumer then purchases what he believes to be the optimal amount of care, q_2 (similarly determined). How much value has he lost?

As a general proposition, a demand curve shows the marginal valuation for each succeeding unit of care, so that the area under the demand curve describes the value placed by the consumer on the total amount of care he has received. For that value, he gives up the rectangle described by $Opaq_1$, the quantity q_1, times the price p. This is the expenditure for care we observe with survey data, for example. The additional value to the consumer, the triangle pac, is often described as "consumer surplus," and can be estimated from demand curves. A similar technique can be used to measure the loss to the consumer from having false information given to him about the severity index . Suppose he thinks he has a disease of severity ℓ_2, and buys the quantity of care q_2 (which would be optimal if ℓ_2 were the correct severity). His total expenditure for care is now q_2 times p, or the rectangle Oq_2bp. The total value he places is the area under the demand curve labeled ℓ_1, in the sense that optimal levels of health would then be obtained. Thus, the loss to the consumer is the triangle abc—the area above demand curve ℓ_1 but under the price line.

Note that this is less than the additional expenditure $(q_2 - q_1) \times p$ that we might observe. Although the consumer has "too much" care, he still places some (but diminishing) value upon it. To simply count the additional medical expenditure arising from false information as waste is incorrect.* Put differently, to count total expenditure savings as a benefit to QA programs would overstate the benefits from such programs. The correct measure would be to use triangles similar to abc in Figure 14-3, summing them for all possible diseases for all persons. The extent of overstatement depends upon the elasticities of demand for each illness, and upon the degree of misinformation supplied.**

Towards an Operational Measure of the Value of Quality Assurance Regarding Illness Severity

The correct measure of benefits of QA can be derived by assessing state-specific demand curves for care under two states of the world: (1) existing consumer information about the value of treatment; and (2) optimal consumer information about the value of treatment. The latter state of the world is difficult to observe. Several comparisons are possible; however, each contains some potential biases. First, the argument has been made that the amount of care delivered in prepaid practice plans is optimal in the sense that the marginal revenue to the provider is zero for any particular service delivered to a particular patient. This argument would suggest that the standard of comparision would be prepayment practice levels vs. comparable fee-for-service levels. Some difficulties arising from this comparision are:

1. Prepayment groups generally have zero monetary price for services, particularly for inpatient care, whereas the fee-for-service market, even with insurance, normally contains some copayment feature which will reduce observed utilization in the fee-for-service market. Thus, comparisons would have to be made holding constant the copayment status of patients, or adjusting for coverage. Without adjustment for copayment, the comparison will understate the true differences in demand between informed and

---

* An example of this error in logic appears in Wallace and Donnelly.[9]

** Note that this argument is conceptually similar to statements about the welfare loss from "excess" health insurance.[10,11,12] In those models, the subsidy from health insurance induces persons to acquire additional medical care by lowering the effective price. The "welfare loss" is described as the triangle above the demand curve and below the price line bounded by the quantities that would be purchased at market prices and at the insured subsidy price. In general, I view this as a mistaken argument. What is really being measured there is not the welfare loss from excess health insurance, but a lower bound on the transactions costs of administering perfectly an insurance plan that paid an indemnity amount to consumers dependent upon the actual illness that had occurred. For this study, however, the presence or absence of insurance (and its effect on demand) are irrelevant except for estimation problems. Any additional demand induced by false information can be treated identically in concept.

Figure 14-3: Demand Curves Showing the Welfare Loss (Cost) of Medical Misinformation

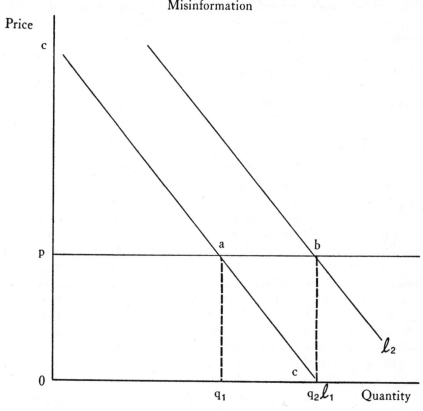

uninformed consumers, and will hence understate the value of QA programs.*

2. The relative prices of inpatient and outpatient care are different in the fee-for-service market and the prepayment market, because of differences in insurance coverage. Thus, there would likely be relatively more hospital care in the fee-for-service sector, all other things being equal, than in the prepayment sector.

3. The prepayment plan has an incentive, all other things being equal, not to deliver care, because marginal costs are positive for each service delivered, and marginal revenues are zero. Thus, using prepayment plan data as a comparison base may overstate the differences between informed and unin-

---

* If nonprice rationing (waiting, queues) deter medical use in a prepaid group more than copayments do in the fee-for-service sector, the bias would be reversed.

formed demand, other things being equal.

4. Patients in prepayment plans are self-selected, and may thus have basically different underlying characteristics from those in fee-for-service markets.

The optimal comparison would be between a fee-for-service group of persons who had full coverage for all services and a prepayment plan group with full coverage. This would eliminate the first two problems, except for differences in time-price and other nonprice rationing systems that would alter observed demand. The fourth problem could be eliminated by randomization of persons into and out of prepayment plans in an experimental setting.* The remaining (third) problem listed provides a boundary condition. Comparisons of such controlled groups could provide an upper boundary on the value of perfect information about the level of severity and/or the efficacy of care.

It is important to note that there is a substantial private market currently actively providing information about the true severity of illness—the market for second opinions. In a sense, the demand curve for second opinions is a close approximation to the theoretical demand curve for information along dimensions of true illness severity. Thus, while no such study has been undertaken along these lines, it would be conceptually possible to use (for example) survey data on purchases of medical care to assess how much information (e.g., second opinions) people sought at various prices, and from that assess the demand for the service provided by QA programs. It also provides a conceptual test of the efficacy of a QA program. If the program is successful, the demand for second opinions should fall.

Finally, the point should be made clearly that the value of perfect information (i.e., the benefits from QA of this type) depends upon the level of copayment for care, and upon the price elasticities of demand for care. Figure 14-4 shows why this is true. Even if the medical care demand curves (with and without QA programs) are parallel, the areas of consumer surplus to be gained by QA may differ at different levels of copayment, if the demand for care is ever "sated." At the smaller coinsurance rate (C_2) shown in Figure 14-4, the lower part of the welfare loss triangle B drops off. If the informed and uninformed demand curves are not parallel, the welfare loss areas can be either larger or smaller at full coverage than at no coverage.

It may also be possible to assess the benefits of specific QA programs directly by conducting medical care demand analysis in certain sites before and after a program is undertaken. To do this, one would essentially require

---

* The Health Insurance Study at the Rand Corporation, in cooperation with Group Health, Inc. in Seattle, Washington, is undertaking such a study.

Figure 14-4: Welfare Loss from Misinformation Varies by
Coinsurance Level

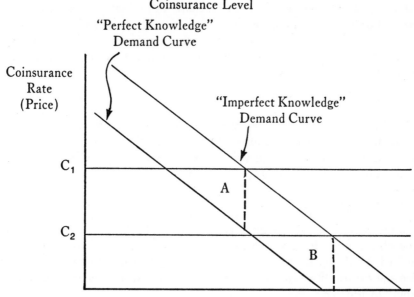

data on quantities, prices, insurance coverage, and other important variables before and after a QA mechanism were established in the community. From such a before/after study, a direct assessment of the welfare gains from the QA program could be derived.

A simpler way to make this type of comparison would be to assume that a functional form for the relevant demand equation existed. It would then be necessary to assume that the QA program caused parallel shift in the demand curve (presumably to the left), which could be measured by the change in observed utilization before and after the QA program were instituted. The correct area under the demand curves could then be calculated, given the assumptions about functional form, the way in which QA affected demand, and the fact that no other relevant variables had changed. These are strong assumptions, indeed, but they allow one to proceed with cost-benefit analysis of this dimension of QA programs at low cost. An example of such a calculation follows:

Suppose the estimated demand equation is of the form

(4) $y = a_0 + a_1 \times$ (Income) $+ a_2 \times$ (Health Status) $+ a_3$
$\times$ (Coinsurance $\times$ Price)
$+ a_4 \times$ (Wait Time $\times$ Value of Time)

The quantity demanded at various insurance levels can be derived by assuming other relevant variables (income, health status, time costs, and medical prices) have not changed in the period before and after installation of the QA program. Average demand in the community can be summarized by inserting average values for income, health status, time value, etc., leading to a new equation specifying

(5) $y = a_0' + a_1' \times \text{Price}$

where a_0' embodies all other variables' effects (which have been held constant). If demand shifts after QA is installed in the community, that is taken as a shift in a_0, which will also be a shift in a_0'. Call the shift in demand b. Then the post-QA demand curve is

(6) $y = a_0' + a_1' \times \text{Price} - b$

and the welfare gain is the integral of the area above the QA demand curve (possibly limited by zero), below the price line for the community and limited by the quantities demanded at the prevailing price for the two demand curves. For parallel linear demand curves, the welfare gain (WG) from QA programs is*

(7) $WG = \dfrac{\frac{1}{2} b^2}{a_1}$

A common and mistaken method of assessing the benefits from a QA program such as this would be to value the entire reduction in demand, b, at the market price, P, so that benefits would be stated for the QA program as bP. In general, this cannot be true, except if demand curves were perfectly price inelastic, which is not the case. In fact, this method of assessing benefits must overstate the benefits by at least a factor of two. To show this, I first note that the price P must be at least b/a_1 (comparable to the height CD in Figure 14-5), if the welfare gain measure is to include the entire triangle of relevance (the triangle ABC in Figure 14-5). Thus, $P > b/a_1$, and therefore $Pb > b^2 a_1$. Thus, the naive method of assessing benefits from this type of QA program overstate the true benefits (compare with Equation (7)).

The sole counterexample would be if demand curves were completely inelastic, as is shown in Figure 14-6. In that case, the QA program would simply shift the demand curve backward to the left, and the welfare gain

---

* The computation is made as follows: The welfare gain is a triangle with a base of b (the change in demand from the QA program), and a height which reflects the necessary price change to induce an "informed" consumer to purchase an amount $y = a_0 - a_1 P$. That price differential is exactly b/a_1, where a_1 is the slope of the demand curve. Thus, the welfare gain is $\frac{1}{2} b \times b/a_1 = \frac{1}{2} b^2 / a_1$.

would be the entire area Pb. Literature on demand for medical care shows, however, that this case is irrelevant.

The Case of the FDA Proof-of-Efficacy Requirements

Probably the most widespread QA program in current operation in the United States is the FDA's evaluation of new chemical entities (NCEs). One of the few examples of an actual benefit/cost analysis of a QA program involves the 1962 amendments to the Food, Drug, and Cosmetic Act of 1938. These amendments specified that, in addition to previously required proofs that the NCEs were not harmful, the chemical combination would have to be proved to be efficacious before it could be marketed in the United States. An analysis of the effects of these amendments on consumer well-being has been published by Peltzman[13], with subsequent criticism[14] and rebuttal.[15] adopted a methodology similar to that proposed in this chapter. The drug-efficacy laws are designed to prevent pharmaceutical companies from selling drugs which were not efficacious, but which were convincable as efficacious to doctors through massive advertising. Peltzman estimated demand curves for various types of drugs at various time intervals after their introduction. He argued that for those drugs which were not truly efficacious, use should fall off over time as physicians became aware of the incorrect claims made for the drug in advertising. In effect, he was estimating *uninformed* and *informed* demand curves by viewing using information on market shares over time. The major cost of the drug-efficacy laws, he argued, was that a substantial delay was imposed in the introduction of new drugs, so that even those with high efficacy were not available for consumption for a period of time while efficacy trials were underway.

This loss in value (measured by area under demand curves observed when the drugs were eventually permitted on the market) was aggregated over the time during which the drug was not available, but would have been available in the absence of the proof-of-efficacy requirement. In summary, Peltzman estimated (1) reduced waste of purchases of ineffective new drugs, producing a benefit of under $100 million; (2) missed benefits (a cost) of $300 to $400 million from the reduced flow of new drugs; and (3) higher prices for existing drugs because of reduced competition from new drugs, producing a loss of $50 million. Thus, he concludes that "These measurable effects add up to a net loss of $250 to $350 million, or about 6 percent of total drug sales.... Consumer losses from purchases of ineffective drugs or hastily marketed unsafe drugs appear to have been trivial compared to gains from innovation." Criticism of the work raises some questions about the methodology employed,[14] but the residual evidence seems to imply that the costs imposed by the 1962 amendments were greater than the benefits.[15] The

Figure 14-5: Method of Assessing Benefits

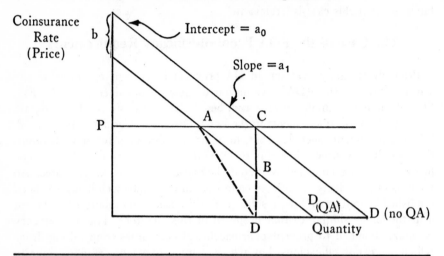

Figure 14-6:   Assessing Benefits with Inelastic Demand Curve

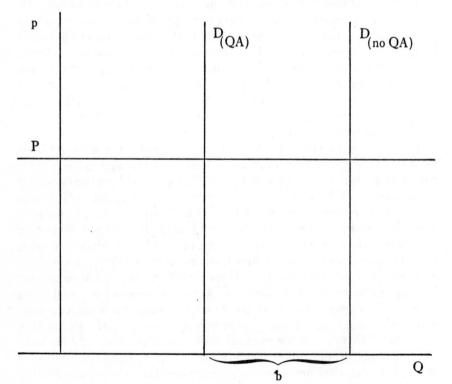

purpose here is not to adjudicate the debate on the value of Peltzman's estimates, but rather to commend them to the reader as an excellent example of the value of searching beyond simple program administration costs to assess the true benefit/cost ratio of a QA program that has substantial impact upon the American people today.

Some General Considerations

A 'model of demand for medical care has been set forth which explicitly introduced the concept that medical outcomes were uncertain (i.e., that the marginal productivity of medical care may vary considerably during an attempted cure). Similar uncertainty pervades our lives in other areas as well. A meal bought in a restaurant may turn out to be substandard; an apple purchased from a roadside vendor may already have been partly consumed by a resident worm; a television set, with an accuracy bespeaking an internal timing device, may self-destruct the moment the warranty expires. These and a multiplicity of similar uncertainties are a common characteristic of our world. Each case is essentially similar to the problems facing a medical consumer. One learns to avoid restaurants with systematically bad food or surly waiters; the roadside worm vendor will likely be driven from business by higher quality competitors; and such things as brand identification of television sets, coupled with more extended warranty lives, will allow the choice of a set which will more reliably keep us aware of the unfortunate events in the world around us on the evening news. The case of television sets (or any other major appliances) is particularly interesting as an analog to medical care, because the consumer is placed in roughly the same position in the purchase of both commodities: a purchase is made only infrequently; it is a substantial amount of money when the purchase is actually made; and the consumer is purchasing something involving a complex technology that is almost certainly far beyond his own ability to analyze or even remotely grasp.

To extend the analogy, there are known differences between different television brands, reflected in both quality, characteristics, and price. Furthermore, within any given brand or even for any given model, some television sets will turn out to be more reliable than others. Thus, the total variance in quality outcomes can be decomposed into firm-specific and firm-independent components. In both markets, some types of information assist the consumer/patient in identifying some of the inter-firm differences. Advertising and brand identification, for all of the supposed evils associated with them, turn out to be a remarkably valuable piece of information to the consumer selecting a television set, because he has seen similar sets in homes of his friends, can purchase ratings from consumer and electronics magazines that will describe the different brands and models in high detail, and can go and view the different sets in a store. Doctors also have means of identifying their own quality, although laws and ethical proscriptions vastly limit such information relative to other markets. Nevertheless, the doctor can show where he received his medical training, the extent of his specialization, and membership in societies and clubs which convey, rightly or wrongly, that the doctor has higher-than-average quality.

For manufactured products, there is also a warranty—a description of explicit conditions and duration of time under which the manufacturer is strictly liable for defects in the operation of the television set. The warranty is the consumer's insurance against an unfortunate drawing from the distribution of luck. It guarantees him the outcome based on continuing performance of his television set, no matter whether it was something common to all sets made by a particular manufacturer, or whether only one set ever had such a defect. There is nothing analogous to this in medical care whatsoever. (In malpractice cases, the doctor must be proved negligent before liability is assigned, although recent analysis suggests that court decisions are moving more in a direction towards strict liability for physicians as well as manufacturers.) Thus, in medical care, the patient is left facing a considerable risk concerning the outcomes of a medical care process for which there seems to be little opportunity to reduce the underlying uncertainty.

QA programs could be directed against both of these basic types of quality variation—doctor specific and luck. My observation is that the primary emphasis of most QA programs—licensure, hospital privilege committees, Experimental Medical Care Review Organizations (EMCROs) and Professional Standards Review Organizations (PSROs), to name but a few—is to attempt to identify doctor-specific components of this variance (i.e., to find bad doctors and to reduce or eliminate their bad activity). Graphically portrayed in Figure 14-7, these programs appear to be an attempt to identify and eliminate the behavior causing the outcomes shown in the shaded (left-tail) area of the distribution of doctor quality.

Other QA programs appear to modify, or at least to attempt to modify, the variance of doctor-independent variations in outcomes. These, for example, specify certain ways in which certain procedures must be carried out. Thus, patients with certain symptons and/or diagnoses are always treated in a particular fashion. This has the effect of reducing the variance of luck, as diagrammed in Figure 14-8. While it will likely remove the most unfortunate outcomes, it may also prevent some of the potentially most favorable outcomes from ever occurring, because such standardization removes certain treatment methods from the available list of therapies. The disallowance of cyclopropane as an anesthetic agent, for example, reduces danger of explosion, but it also deprives some patients of the unique high-oxygen administration that is feasible with that agent.

It is important to note the difference in philosophy between these two types of regulation and control of quality. One attempts, in effect, to remove producers with low average quality (i.e., those with systematically low marginal productivity), while the other attempts to reduce essentially the variance of doctor-unrelated incidents. One reason why these are essentially different problems is that, if left to their own devices, consumers and the marketplace would likely come up with radically different solutions to these problems. This suggests that nonmarket QA control should do likewise. Again, let me consider television sets as an example. The problem of firm-specific variations in quality is dealt with primarily through brand identification, advertising, and strong association of particular producers with particular levels of quality. (Note also that varying levels of quality remain on the market. Some persons are willing to pay more for higher quality; others prefer a less expensive television set for less money. In general, the ratio of prices of television sets to their marginal productivity—producing entertainment—would roughly be equal.) For the remaining problem (unspecific random error or luck), the market solution has been a form of insurance, either direct consumer-purchased insurance or a product warranty making the manufacturer liable if *anything* untoward occurs. Assignment of liability in a case such as this (e.g., having the consumer or the manufacturer liable) is normally thought of as a problem of minimizing transactions costs and minimizing probabilities that treatable defects will indeed be treated.[16,17,18,19]

The medical market seems characterized by only the barest minimum of product-brand type identification, along dimensions outlined above. I would propose here that a major increment in quality of care might be forthcoming if doctors (and other practitioners) were allowed to advertise both their qualities and their prices. If kept in check by general laws and regulations pertaining to fraud and deceit, a clear gain would occur with more information supplied to the patient-consumer.* The argument is primarily that, like any other goods, information is costly to acquire, and that the higher the acquisition cost, the less will be sought. Current barriers to the provision (or collection and dissemination) of information in the medical market can simply be thought of as raising the price of information. Unless a convincing case can be made that the information would have negative value to the consumer (a premise with which a majority of economists, at least,

---

* Since this paper was presented at the Boston University Conference in November 1975, the Federal Trade Commission (FTC) has entered a restraint-of-trade suit against the American Medical Association on the basis of advertising restrictions. Similar FTC suits have also been lodged against other professional organizations, including lawyers.

Figure 14-7: Truncating Lower End of Distribution of
Physician Marginal Productivity

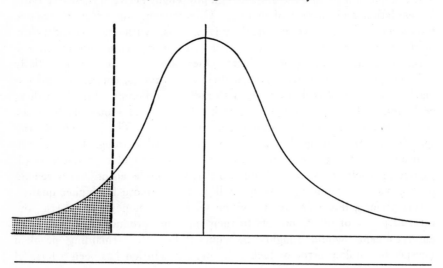

Figure 14-8: Reducing Variance in Physician Productivity

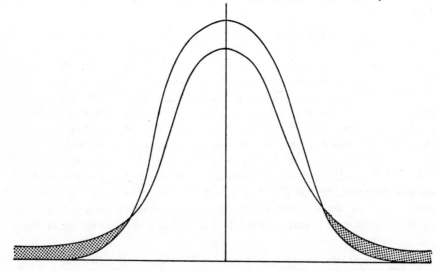

Left shaded area represents reduction of bad practice. Right shaded area
represents reduction of unusually good (innovative?) practice.

would disagree), the restrictions on advertising and information flow would seem to have a significant effect both in reducing quality and raising prices. (For a study of the latter effect in the eyeglass industry, see Benham.[20])

An Operational Benefit Measurement for Variance Reduction QA Programs

If a QA program is successful in reducing that variance, the demand for medical care should rise on net. To be more specific, the demand curve for medical care would shift outward, so that more care would be demanded at each price. Thus, I would argue that before-and-after QA program demand curves could give some evidence on how much value had been obtained by consumers by having the variance of outcomes reduced.

The argument that demand would shift outward can be made quite complicated, but its essence is that people dislike risky events, be they financial, medical, or whatever, and that something is more preferable if it is less risky. This is true even if one holds constant the average outcome. Thus, other things held equal, more medical care would be demanded if the outcome distribution were made tighter (less risk).

The situation in general is shown in Figure 14-9. There are (as before) two demand curves—one with high variance, and the other with low variance in outcomes. Again, as before, I have drawn them as straight and parallel lines. At the prevailing market price of P, consumers would demand q_0 in the high-variance case, and q_1 in the low-variance case. There is some equivalent tax T which would make the consumer in the low-variance case demand only q_0 rather than q_1, as I have indicated in Figure 14-9. (This tax is the implicit cost to the consumer imposed by the variance.) Consumer surplus, the measure of welfare I have adopted for this chapter, is again the area under a demand curve but above the price line. Consumer surplus without the QA program is the triangle abc, and after the QA program is undertaken (and variance in outcomes thereby reduced) the consumer surplus measure is the triangle ade. The gain, and thus the benefit from the QA program, is in this simple case the difference between the triangle ade and the triangle abc, which is the trapezoid cbde. Its area can be calculated by observing demand curves for care before and after a QA program designed to reduce variance in outcomes.

Unfortunately, this simple case is not even likely to hold. If the QA program is undertaken in a fashion such that the price of medical care rises, then even though the demand curve shifts, the quantities demanded may not shift by as much, because of the price increase. This is shown in Figure 14-10, where a price of P_0 exists in the high-variance case, and a price of P_1 in the low-variance case. The welfare gain is now the difference between the triangle abc and the triangle fhe.

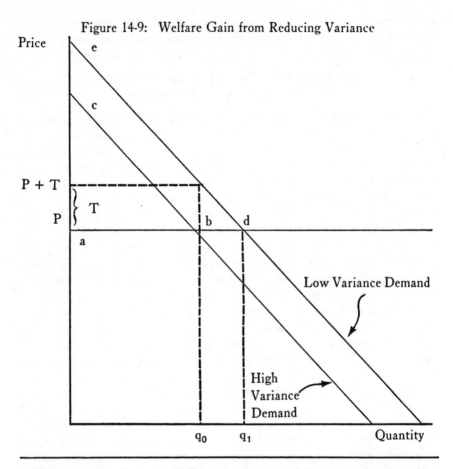

Figure 14-9: Welfare Gain from Reducing Variance

Thus, because of the possibility of variance reduction causing P to rise, there is no simple and useful formula relating the change in quantity demanded to the welfare gain, as was the case for the other type of QA program.

COST MEASUREMENT FOR QA PROGRAMS

The basic premise of this section will be that most benefit/cost studies undertaken in quality of care or QA areas will most likely understate the costs involved, because there will be a tendency to look over a far too narrow area in which costs might be incurred. While measurement of costs is relatively straightforward in most cases, identification of the true realm of costs often requires imagination and perseverance that proponents of a particular project may be loathe to undertake. I shall enumerate several

Figure 14-10:   Welfare Gain from Variance Reduction

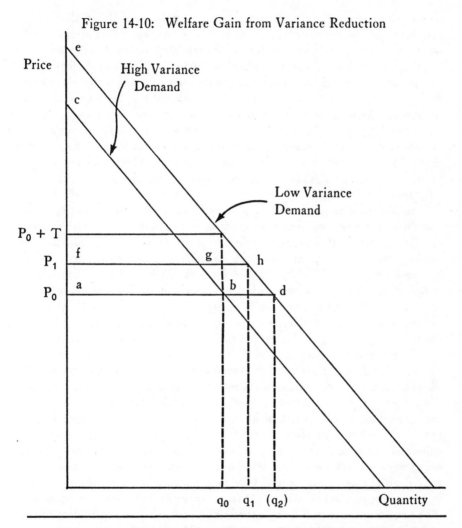

categories where search for costs will generally be fruitful when analyzing regulation of any broad sort, and provide, wherever possible, examples drawn from existing regulation in the health field and in other areas of the economy.

Direct Costs

The first category discussed is direct cost measurement. The recipe for cost/benefit analysis suggests that the appropriate costs to include are additional costs to society that are added if the project is undertaken. As simple a prescription as this may seem, existing studies of benefit/cost analysis tend to make two serious types of errors in assessing costs. First, they often overstate costs by including costs that are fixed (i.e., costs that are incurred whether or not the new project is undertaken) or by inappropriately spreading joint costs over several projects. Fixed costs are forever fixed, and should not enter marginal decisions about whether or not to undertake a new project. Thus, for example, in a hospital, costs such as heating, janitorial service, and general administration should not be spread to a new project when deciding its worth. Those costs will be incurred whether or not a new project (e.g., a tissue committee) is undertaken. Allocation of fixed costs should forever be taboo when they will be incurred whether or not a new project is undertaken. They should not alter decisions about the value of the new project.

Similarly, some projects produce joint products, and these present unusual and difficult accounting problems when assessing costs. The reader interested in pursuing this matter further is probably well-off to consult the existing literature on joint costs in economics and accounting; serviceable accounts are given in Alchian[21] and Allen and in Henderson and Quandt.[22]

A further mistake is often made in cost benefit analysis by not valuing resources used at their true cost to society. Indeed, one of the virtues of competitive markets so widely admired by economists is that prices at which goods and services are sold are exactly equal to the costs (in resources) necessary to produce more of the product. However, this equality is often not met in medical care sectors, and the careful analyst of benefit/cost ratios will likely have to use care and imagination to assess resource use at its true value. Two widespread examples come to mind: The first would be to place the cost of medical care delivered at its cost to the patient. This is generally in error because health insurance (private and public) reduces the price paid by consumers to some fraction of actual costs. A person with a major medical policy pays only 20¢ for each $1.00 of resources expended on his behalf at the time decisions are made to consume medical care. Thus, to use patient payments for medical care in a cost framework would be highly misleading. The correct measure would value the resources at the cost of providing them.

A similar error emerged in a recent study of a QA program within a specific hospital.[11] Much of the work was undertaken in that QA program by staff physicians whose time was donated in return for access to the hospital facilities. The computation of costs for that program allowed nothing for the time of the physicians on the grounds that the hospital had to pay nothing to them for their time. While this procedure may have been accurate on literal accounting grounds, it is an unfortunate error from the point of view of society—the physicians involved in that study could have been undertaking other activities which saved lives, stamped out disease or relieved itching, and it is the value of that time which is the opportunity cost of having them perform QA program work for free. The opportunity cost of the resource is of primary importance in assessing costs of projects.

The variety of cases in which nominal or measured costs do not actually match actual costs in health care is indeed wide. It remains for the analyst to assess properly the correct costs in each study undertaken.

Indirect Costs of QA Programs

This section relates several general areas in which indirect costs of QA mechanisms are likely to be generated, and some specific examples of these types of costs are given. My view is that the indirect costs of QA programs are likely to be large, difficult to detect, and probably the subject of considerable debate as to their magnitude. The types of costs discussed fall generally into three categories, as follows:

1. Those types of QA programs which have substantial effects on the economic incentives facing providers or patients, or which alter the market power of one or the other of these parties. Licensure and hospital privilege committees are explicit examples.

2. Those types of QA programs that are applied in inappropriate situations or to inappropriate populations, so that the very nature of the QA program engenders hidden costs. Some types of compulsory mass screening may be examples of this.

3. Those types of QA programs which, for whatever reason, employ inappropriate decision rules, thereby generating costs beyond those which would be found if appropriate decision rules were used. Any classification scheme which uses inappropriate decision rules falls into this category; interpretation of simple hospital laboratory tests is a mundane example. Classification of a hospital length of stay as excessive or not excessive is a particular example involved in implementation of the PSRO law.

Examples of each of these types of problems are discussed further in this section.

Regulation That Alters Market Power—The Case of Licensure

Quality control has been a favorite argument used by persons seeking to have legal or regulatory authority to limit entry into their profession or business. A common argument is raised that it is necessary to have some public control of entry to protect the public from entry by unscrupulous operators, frauds, cheats, or incompetents. Indeed, this is the primary and widely espoused logic for medical licensure, as well as control of the civil aviation industry, the interstate transportation, the pharmaceutical market, the taxicab industry (in many cities), trades such as plumbing, barbering, and beauticians, and others too numerous to account here. Few would deny that at least some of these licensure programs achieve their stated objective—to reduce the amount of incompetent or fraudulent practitioners, and to increase safety in the specified areas. This is not my point, which is rather that these gains are achieved at costs that may far exceed the actual costs of the licensure operations themselves.

In medical circles, it has long been argued by Kessel and others[23,24,25] that because entry into the medical profession has been heavily restricted by licensure, there has been created an economic return to those in the profession heavily exceeding returns to education of similar length and difficulty. This excess economic return is primarily reflected in higher prices to the profession members, the argument goes, that is achieved by restricting output in the fashion of a monopolist. In medical care, the argument is based upon restrictions to the supply of a particular input in a medical practice (the physician), rather than on the argument that each physician has colluded with all others to achieve a cartel-like monopoly. Thus, each physician can indeed act as a pure competitor (in his operation of his physician-firm) and still achieve the excess "rent" on his scarce input (physician time). The actual cost in value terms to society is best measured by reference to a demand curve. As is discussed above, a demand curve for any product reflects the additional (marginal) value which people place upon various quantities of the product they receive, and the area under a demand curve reflects the total valuation that describes how well off they are. In Figure 14-11, the output and pricing decisions of a monopolist and a perfectly competitive industry are shown when they face identical demand and supply conditions. The monopolist produces q_0, and charges a price $0a$ for each unit. The competitive industry result leads to production of q_1, which is sold at a price $0d$. The welfare loss to the consumer because of the monopoly is the area bounded by $abcd$. Note this is *more* than just the additional expenditure necessary because of the higher price (that is the area of the rectangle $abed$), but also includes a loss because of the restriction of output—output which would have a value to the consumers higher than the costs necessary to provide it. A monopoly in medicine, if it exists, will induce similar losses.*

The ability of producers to marshall legal assistance in maintaining a monopoly should not be dismissed as trivial, even if the arguments for the legal action correctly point out that some quality increases may be obtained (e.g., through licensure) for those units of production actually reaching the market. (Note that the quality of those suppressed units—$q_1 - q_0$ in Figure

---

* Note that the subsidy of health insurance leads to overconsumption of medical care, while a monopoly market would lead to underconsumption. The two may cancel each other to some extent.[27]

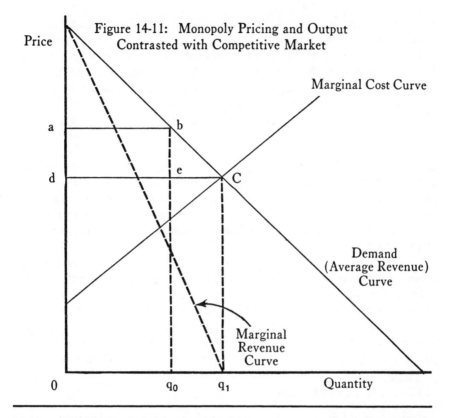

Figure 14-11: Monopoly Pricing and Output
Contrasted with Competitive Market

14-11—should be included in the calculation at zero quality to be perfectly complete in the quality calculation.) Recent theory and empirical work[26] suggest that this legal advantage is most likely to be sought and obtained in circumstances where legal forces are necessary to bind together a cartel. (For natural monopolies, there is little to be gained for the monopolist by seeking regulation.)

The major stated purpose of medical licensure is certainly one of quality control—i.e., to limit entry into the medical profession to practitioners of at least a minimum level of competency. Whether or not licensure has (or could) serve this function is a testable proposition, and licensure as a QA mechanism could be subjected to a benefit/cost study just as any other QA program.

Prima facie evidence on the subject is not conclusive. There certainly has been a substantial restriction, at least historically, in the number of persons who graduated from medical school. This was the stated intent and acknowledged result of the famous Flexner report.[28] If admissions standards for medical schools are positively correlated with skill in medical practice, then the quality argument would be considerably buttressed, but at least within the range of personal skills admitted to medical schools, no demonstrable effect has ever been identified.

There is also the argument that personal medical skills may vary (or decay) over time, so that periodic recertification would be a more direct method of guaranteeing quality. The operational difficulties of such a procedure seem overwhelming to me at present and, given the lack of success of other tests and licensure procedures in identifying good and bad doctors, would seem to be, at best, discriminatory

Licensure itself is seldom revoked for physicians in practice. Virtually all of those doctors who are defrocked in fact are alleged to have been of bad moral character, rather than to have been medically incompetent. Thus, either one must argue that licenses originally granted were only to competent doctors, and that none of those doctors' skills decayed over time, or else one must argue that present licensure laws are ineffective as a quality control mechanism.

Some recent evidence shows the extent of action brought by medical licensure boards to preserve medical competence in the state of California. In 1974, the State Board of Medical Examiners had approximately 72,000 licensed physicians in their jurisdiction, approximately 46,000 of whom were actively practicing medicine. During 1974, the board took disciplinary action against 58 licensees, including 50 physicians (0.1 percent of all active physicians). The actions which led to licensure revocation hearings were:[29]

Narcotic offenses	28
Theft, bribery, embezzlement and tax evasion	5
Fraudulent billings	4
Mental incompetence	4
Sex offenses	3
Criminal medical activities	3
Alcoholism	2
Incompetence and gross negligence	1

The report of the Board of Medical Examiners in California goes into extensive detail on why they have not been able to pursue incompetent physicians more actively. For our purposes, however, it is sufficient to note that as a quality control device monitoring active physicians (activities beyond initial quality screening), licensure cannot be thought of as exerting any effective control on quality of care in California. (Chapter 9 presents other evidence supporting this point as well.)

Local vs. Federal Monopoly

The argument initially proposed by Friedman and Kuznets,[24] and detailed by Kessel,[25] suggests that physicians gain "monopoly rent" through restriction of entry into their profession. However, local (hospital-level) quality control mechanisms have the same possibility for introducing unseen or indirect costs while attempting to achieve quality control. A primary example is hospital control of hospital privileges, a control feature which has been exercised in the name of quality control for many years (and is essentially a legal requirement of hospitals now following the Darling case[30]). As with licensure, however, this form of quality control has the possible outcome of reducing competition among physicians in the community, and thus the possible increase in prices. The long history of arguments about "open" and "closed" hospitals bears some evidence that this is a real issue, and the use of hospital privilege denial as a method of combatting the early introduction of prepaid group practices has been well documented.[31] Thus, even hospital-specific quality control mechanisms appear to have at least the possibility of inducing some indirect costs on patients that should indeed be counted in a cost/benefit study of any such program.

Inappropriate Populations Subjected to Quality Control— The Case of Compulsory Mass Screening

Mass screening for certain diseases has been widely touted as an efficacious procedure, and has been made mandatory in certain cases (VDRL before marriage, PKU in infants, sickle-cell trait for blacks in some states) and has been so widely recommended as to have nearly the same effect for other methods (Pap smear). Only recently has the theory behind such mass screenings been analyzed carefully, and the results are often startling. With careful analysis, one often concludes that the costs are higher than the benefits.* The reason, almost universally, is that much of the true cost of these screening programs is ignored in earlier studies.[32,33,34] The "casual" benefit/cost study of a screening program would study the probability of obtaining a positive result, assess the value of early treatment of the disease (typically later medical costs that do not have to be made, plus the value of the sick time saved for the patients if the study is more sophisticated), and assess the costs of the program as the actual laboratory and technician time necessary to undertake the screening.[33] The missing element of cost is revealed by a simple example.

Suppose that you have a test for Disease X with a high probability of detecting a person who truly has the disease (say, 99 percent), and with a false-positive rate also quite good (say the false-positive rate is only one percent). Suppose the true incidence of the disease in your population is $\frac{1}{10,000}$, and you apply the screening test against 100,000 persons. The test is

---

* Conflicting views are presented in Dickerson et al. and Webster.[35,36]

highly likely to identify accurately the 10 truly sick persons. Unfortunately, it will also identify 1,000 persons as being sick who are actually well, because of the false-positive probability of one percent. Thus, 99 percent of the persons who are identified as being sick are indeed healthy.

Continuing, let us suppose that there is a backup test, completely independent of the first test, which is used to confirm the results of the first test. Let us again assign the same generous capabilities to this test as the first—99 percent specificity, one percent false-positive rate. Of the 1,010 persons who are positive, we almost certainly retain the correct identification of the 10 truly sick persons, and they receive the benefit of being correctly screened for the disease. Suppose they are now treated with a $100 procedure which saves a later procedure with a $500 present value that would have arisen had the disease gone unchecked. Net benefits are 10 X $400 = $4,000. But, we still have 1,000 persons with false positives, 10 of whom will be identified by the backup test as being sick, and who will each have a $100 procedure performed on them. If the actual cost of doing the test is $.04, a casual benefit/cost analysis would suggest that screening should be undertaken because total program costs are 100,000 X .04 = $4,000, and the benefits are at least that high. Correct computation of the costs also would add $1,000 for the unnecessary procedures performed on the 10 truly healthy patients, and would also impute a cost for the pain and anxiety incurred by them and their families because they felt they had Disease X. Note also that a casual analysis would probably also presume that all 20 persons on whom the $100 treatment had been performed were truly sick, so that a likely estimate of the benefits of the program would be overstated by a factor of two!

Analysis of this sort can be applied to many types of activities besides screening examinations. In that application, however, it may be particularly difficult to find correct statistics on the true incidence of the disease, because existing data may rely upon the results of an identical test to determine prevalence.

The concept of false-positive treatment affects many more programs than mass screening. It is inherent, of course, in any diagnostic procedure in medical care, and must be recognized as a fact of life by physicians and patients alike. What is particularly important to recognize is that the problem is more pervasive, the lower the true probability of the disease in the population being diagnosed.[37] In some cases, assignment or estimation of costs becomes quite difficult because the costs (and benefits) may be primarily psychic, rather than physical or monetary. Screening for genetic disorders is probably an important case in point. Sometimes (e.g., PKU, Tay Sachs disease), the identification of a person as a carrier of the disease may have profound psychological implications for the person. While the value of

PKU screening is obviously high to those with the disease (who would otherwise be undetected until subsequent mental retardation had irreversibly set in), false-positive identification of persons as PKU victims enforces a stringent dietary regimen for many years, and seriously affects the lifestyle of entire families. Other conditions affecting the child (and even those affecting only the mother) will cause elevation of serum phenylalanine, thus falsely identifying the patient as a PKU victim. These costs should be carefully identified in a correct benefit/cost analysis. Since a large number of these types of screening programs are undertaken at the local or hospital level, rather than at a state or national level, this means that the decision is often undertaken to do (or not to do) these types of screening programs within a hospital staff committee. My current beliefs are that a large number of screening tests now being applied throughout the country's hospitals are inappropriate, and probably have much higher costs than are currently recognized. This type of error is likely to be common at the hospital level of decision making as well as at higher levels.

The Hidden Cost of Inappropriate Decision Rules

A common methodology employed by QA programs, and indeed by physicians analyzing the results of a laboratory test, is to assess the distribution of results for a large (and presumably relevant) group of persons, and then to arbitrarily define some given percentage (usually 5 percent) as abnormal or low quality. I call this methodology the "5 percent-worship" syndrome because it has no more and no less logic behind it than the worship of any other object, person, or deity. I shall illustrate this problem with the case of reading a laboratory test, although similar applications can be drawn for a large variety of QA programs.

The "true" state of the world is characterized by the condition that "sick" people have an average score of 8.0 on diagnostic test A. "Well" people, on the average, have an average score of 5.0 on this test. The standard deviation of scores on this test for either population is 1.0, and the scores are normally distributed so that 97.5 percent of the healthy population has a score of 7 or less. The two distributions obviously overlap to some extent, as shown in Figure 14-12. Suppose also that for the patients being tested, one half of them have the disease and the other half are healthy. The 95 percent worshipers will assign a person to the "sick" state if his score is 2 standard deviations or more above the mean score of 5.0—i.e., if his score is 7 or more. This rule has some unfortunate implications for both healthy and sick persons in this situation. First of all, by definition, 2.5 percent of the persons who are truly healthy will be called "sick." Further, since a score of 7 is one standard deviation to the left of the mean of the distribution of the truly sick people, roughly 17 percent of the sick population (the double-cross-hatched area) will be declared healthy. What is the optimal cutoff rule? It obviously must depend upon what the costs are of making each type of error. Suppose the costs of declaring a healthy person "sick" are $100 worth of procedures done unnecessarily, and the costs of declaring a sick person "well" are $1,000 (present value) in later medical bills to restore the cumulated damage. The decision rule is to minimize expected costs. (The methodology is derived in Exhibit 14-1.) The solution for the optimal decision point is $D = 5.73$. Because of the higher cost of misclassifying sick people, the correct cutoff decision rule will classify over one-quarter (27 percent) of the healthy people as "sick," but only 1.2 percent of the sick population as "well."

Clearly, the decision rule changes with the relative costs of the two types of mistakes. For example, if the second type of error really costs $10,000 rather than $1,000, then the decision rule is to declare the person sick with a score of 4.96 or higher. (In this case, slightly over half of the healthy persons would be declared "sick.") As counterintuitive as this might seem, it would minimize expected losses in this circumstance.

On the other hand, suppose that (with costs of $100 and $1,000) the probability of being truly "sick" in the population being tested is only 10 percent. In that case, the expected loss formula replaces the values of one-half (the prior probabilities of being in each state) with 0.9 and 0.1 (see Exhibit 14-1) and the expected-loss-minimizing decision rule is to declare the person "sick" if his score is above 6.46. Thus, the decision rule also varies with the true frequency of sick and well persons in the population.

To complete the argument in the benefit/cost analysis, one can compute the cost of the incorrect decision rule by assessing the expected loss using the "95 percent worship rule" and the optimal rule. The 95 percent rule would declare every person with a score of 7 or greater "sick," and would thus encounter an expected loss of $100 for 2.5 percent of the truly healthy population (who were inappropriately treated) and a loss of $1,000 for 34 percent of the truly sick population (who will not be treated until their disease is worse and more difficult to treat). Under the assumption that half of the population being tested is truly sick, expected loss from the 95 percent worship rule is $(0.25 \times \$100 \times .05) + (0.5 \times \$1,000 \times .34) = \$171.25$. Under the correct decision rule for this case (using a cutoff of 5.73), 27 percent of the healthy population will incur a cost of $100, and 1.2 percent of the sick population will incur a cost of $1,000. Thus, the expected loss is $(0.5 \times \$100 \times .27) + (0.5 \times \$1,000 \times .012) = \$19.50$. The hidden cost from using the inappropriate decision rule is $\$171.25 - \$19.50 = \$151.75$.

The important inference to be drawn from this exercise is that simple decision rules used to classify persons as being in one or another group can often lead to error. The correct procedure depends in large part on what the

Figure 14-12: Distribution of Test Scores for Truly Healthy and Truly Sick Populations

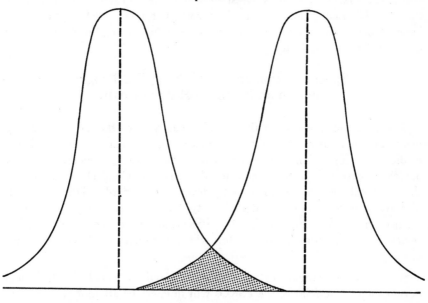

relative costs are of making mistakes of one type or another in misclassification.

A particularly important application of this concept occurs in the hospital where, upon admission of a patient, it is routine and mandatory in almost every hospital to run a battery of automated laboratory blood tests, commonly known as the SMA-12 (or SMA-20) series, which compile a set of measurements on certain characteristics of the blood chemistry of each patient. The 95 percent worship rule is also frequently found in this domain, so that a patient is now subjected simultaneously to 12 or 20 tests for which an inappropriate decision mechanism may be used. If the 95 percent rule is applied independently to each test, the betting odds are nearly 2 to 1 that a person receiving the SMA-20 will have *at least one* test score declared "abnormal," and the odds are nearly even that the same result will occur for a person receiving the SMA-12. These tests are dealt with differently by different physicians. Some realize that these anomalies occur commonly, and do nothing, particularly in the absence of other corroborative clinical data pointing to a problem. Others, however, will follow up the test with a repeat test, or other more expensive, invasive, and painful tests, and problems are almost certain to be generated.

It is interesting to note that hospital mass screening via the SMA-20 or

SMA-12 is a double problem—it is a test not applied to the (necessarily) correct population, and it is a test in which the incorrect decision rule is likely to be used. Both can lead to costs not recognized by the casual benefit/cost analyst of this QA procedure commonly employed in virtually every hospital in the country.

A Specific Examination of the PSRO Program and Some Potential Hidden Costs

The 1972 amendments to the Social Security Act (the Bennett Amendment) create a nationwide system of monitoring the quantity and quality of medical care for patients receiving medical care under any federal programs paying for care (Medicare, Medicaid, Maternal and Child Health Services), through local application of regionally developed standards relating to length of stay, appropriateness of admission, type of care received, and type of facility employed. Through this law, PSROs are permitted (potentially) to review every hospital admission for which national standards have been developed.

Several important features of this program should be noted. First, through development of standards, the PSROs will in effect be attempting to classify patients with a given disease as being in one of two categories—appropriately treated, or not appropriately treated. The mechanisms by which these standards will be developed over time, and the methods by which exceptions will be allowed, are not fully known yet. Yet this classification system is conceptually identical to the problem described earlier as a simple laboratory analysis—i.e., an attempt to classify a person in one of two categories (there, "well" or "sick") on the basis of certain data. In effect, PSROs will set cutoff decision rules that classify patients. Thus, the possibility exists (with high probability) that at least for some diseases, the wrong cutoffs will be established, and costs will not be minimized in appropriate fashion. Thus some hidden costs of the PSRO programs may be developed.

Second, because the acknowledged goal of PSROs is to reduce hospitalization, it seems likely that analysts of the PSRO program itself will attribute to the program as a benefit the entire cost-saving of each day eliminated from use. Such an imputation is incorrect, except in the extremely unlikely case that demand for care is totally inelastic to price. Indeed, the whole concept of unnecessary care upon which the amendments are predicted seems to be based on an implicit demand curve that is totally inelastic to price, and this is known to be incorrect empirically.

Finally, the PSRO amendment specifies particularly that persons carrying out the review process, and physicians who conform to PSRO standards in their treatment of particular patients, are to be held immune from malpractice action so long as due care is exercised. Thus, at least nominally, the PSRO mechanism will override and eliminate malpractice liability of the physician as a mechanism (however faulty) for controlling quality of care. PSRO-established norms are intended to replace expert testimony in malpractice cases as a reference of acceptable standards, *but only in those dimensions of care to which the PSRO norms apply.* It appears at least to some observers that the blanket immunity established for those administering the PSRO program may be effectively circumvented since the due care clause also apparently extends to PSRO administration itself, so that before care could be denied (and blanket immunity retained), the PSRO administrators would have to undertake, in effect, a sufficient medical examination to determine what treatment was unnecessary. Thus, the PSRO law may eventually only transfer liability from individual physicians to PSRO administrators.[38]

CONCLUSION AND SUMMARY

QA programs are being promoted as devices capable of improving the quality of medical care, reducing malpractice and malpractice law suits, and reducing the costs of medical care through elimination of unnecessary treatment. The efficacy of these programs in achieving any of these goals has not been tested yet in any systematic fashion. In this chapter, I have set forth some general considerations that should apply to such testing when it is undertaken. Benefit measurement from QA can be derived from observable changes in consumer behavior in the medical market. While some may argue that consumer behavior is an inappropriate place to seek benefit measurements from QA programs (on grounds that consumers are ignorant—indeed, the very grounds justifying introduction of some of the programs), I would respond that the proposed consumer surplus measures are the only logical choice for measurement in any but the most paternalistic society. While such measures are at least conceptually available when the QA program alters the amount of information held by consumers, the problem is unfortunately much more difficult when the effect of the QA program is to reduce variance (uncertainty) about medical outcomes. This is certainly an area deserving further research efforts.

Costs of QA programs, while superficially straightforward, often are increased by indirect costs imposed by the programs. Such costs can arise out of changes in market power (e.g., through licensure), through inappropriate application of QA mechanisms to the wrong populations, or through mistaken statistical classification techniques used by the QA program. Not only will such indirect effects raise the true costs of the QA programs, but they are likely also to increase the calculated benefits of the programs by introducing error into those calculations as well.

Exhibit 14-1: Optimal Decision Rules
for Selecting the Category Into Which
a Person Should Be Placed

The problem formulated is to categorize a person into one of two classes based upon prior (i.e., before-test) information and upon the results of a specific test. In the problem in the text, persons were divided into the two classes of "healthy" and "sick," and the distributions of test scores for each class of persons were assumed to be normal, with standard deviation of 1.0 and means of 5.0 and 8.0, respectively. Losses in the event of inappropriate classification are L_1 for false positives, and L_2 for false negatives. In the example in the text, $L_1 = 100$, and $L_2 = 1,000$. The prior probabilities of being in each class (i.e., the probabilities you would assign if the test were unavailable) reflect the true prevalence of the disease in the population; these are designated as p_1 and p_2. In the example, these were set each at 0.5. Then the formula for expected loss is

$$E(L) = p_1 \times L_1 \times p(\text{"S"}|H,D) + p_2 \times L_2 \times p(\text{"H"}|S,D)$$

where $p(\text{"S"}|H,D)$ is the probability of being declared "sick" when truly healthy, and similarly for $p(\text{"H"}|S,D)$ when the decision cutoff is D. Thus,

$$p(\text{"S"}|H,D) = \frac{1}{\sqrt{2\pi}} \int_D^\infty e^{-1/2 \left(\frac{D-5}{1} \right)^2}$$

and

$$p(\text{"H"}|S,D) = \frac{1}{\sqrt{2\pi}} \int_{-\infty}^D e^{-1/2 \left(\frac{D-8}{1} \right)^2}$$

Expected loss is minimized by setting the first derivative of $E(L)$ to zero:

$$\frac{\partial E(L)}{\partial D} = \frac{\partial}{\partial D} \left[p_1 \times L_1 \times \frac{1}{\sqrt{2\pi}} \int_D^\infty e^{-1/2\,(D-5)^2} + \right.$$
$$\left. p_2 \times L_2 \times \frac{1}{\sqrt{2\pi}} \int_{-\infty}^D e^{-1/2\,(D-8)^2} \right]$$

which, using the Leibnitz rule for differentiation of integrals, is:

$$\frac{\partial E(L)}{\partial D} = -p_1 L_1 \ e^{-1/2 \ (D-5)^2} + p_2 L_2 \ e^{-1/2 \ (D-8)^2} = 0$$

Taking logarithms,

$$-\ln (p_1 L_1) + \frac{1}{2} (D-5)^2 + \ln (p_2 L_2) - \frac{1}{2} (D-8)^2 = 0$$

Solving for D gives

$$D = \frac{39 - 2 \ln \left(\dfrac{p_2 L_2}{p_1 L_1} \right)}{6}$$

which is the optimal decision rule.

The ratio of the *prior expected losses* $p_2 L_2 / p_1 L_1 = R$ drives the decision rule completely, and this is of course made up of the losses for each type of mistake and the inherent probabilities in the population of each class of person (sick or healthy). If both the probabilities and the losses are identical for both states, so that the ratio R is unity, then $\ln(1) = 0$ is used in the decision formula, and $D = 39/6 = 6.5$, which is exactly half way between the two means for the healthy and sick populations. As either the loss L_2 or the probability of being sick p_2 rises, the decision cutoff point shrinks towards zero. In the first case of the example, $p_2 L_2 / p_1 L_1 = (0.5 \times 1,000)/(0.5 \times 100) = 10$, and the decision cutoff point is $D = (39 - 2 \times \ln(10))/6 = (39 - 2 \times 2.30)/6 = 5.73$. If the loss L_2 rises to 10,000, the decision point is $D = (39 - 2 \times \ln(100))/6 = 4.965$, which is slightly under the mean score of the healthy group, a result that seems counterintuitive to some, but which accurately reflects the relative costs of mistakes.

NOTES

1. Hanke, Steve H., Phillip H. Carver and Paul Bugg, "Project Evaluation During Inflation," in *Benefit-Cost and Policy Analysis,* Richard Zeckhauser, et al., eds. (Chicago: Aldine Publishing Co., 1975). Reprinted from Water Resources Research, 1974.

2. Grossman, Michael, *The Demand for Health: A Theoretical and Empirical Investigation* (New York: Columbia University Press, 1972).

3. Phelps, Charles E., *Demand for Health Insurance: A Theoretical and Empirical Investigation* (Santa Monica, California: The Rand Corporation, 1973).

4. Phelps, Charles E. and Joseph P. Newhouse, "Coinsurance, the Price of Time, and the Demand for Medical Services," *Review of Economics and Statistics,* 56, No. 3 (August 1974).

5. Acton, Jan Paul, "Nonmonetary Factors in the Demand for Medical Services: Some Empirical Evidence," *Journal of Political Economy,* 83, No. 3 (June 1975).

6. Monsma, George, "Marginal Revenue and the Demand for Physician Services," in *Empirical Studies in Health Economics,* Herbert Klarman, ed. (Baltimore: Johns Hopkins Press, 1970).

7. Pauly, Mark V., "The Role of Demand Creation in the Provision of Health Services," mimeo, Northwestern University Department of Economics (1975).

8. White, Kerr L., "An Examination of the PSRO 'Prescription'," *The Hospital Medical Staff* (March 1975).

9. Wallace, Robert F. and Michael Donnelly, "Computing Quality Assurance Costs," *Hospital Progress* (May 1975).

10. Pauly, Mark V., "The Economics of Moral Hazard: Comment," *American Economic Review*, 58, No. 3 (1968).

11. Arrow, Kenneth J., "Uncertainty and the Welfare Economics of Medical Care," *American Economic Review*, 53 (1963), pp. 941-973.

12. Marshall, John M., "Moral Hazard," University of California, Santa Barbara, Working Paper in Economics #18 (November 1974).

13. Peltzman, Sam, "An Evaluation of Consumer Protection: The 1962 Drug Amendments," *Journal of Political Economy*, 81, No. 5 (1973).

14. McGuire, Thomas; Richard Nelson; and Thomas Spavins, "An Evaluation of Consumer Protection Legislation: The 1962 Drug Amendments—A Comment," *Journal of Political Economy*, 83, No. 3 (June 1975).

15. Peltzman, Sam, "An Evaluation of Consumer Protection Legislation: The 1962 Drug Amendments—A Reply," *Journal of Political Economy*, 83, No. 3, (June 1975).

16. Calabrisi, Guido and J. Hirshoff, *Toward a Test for Strict Liability In Torts*, 81 YALE L. J. (1972).

17. Coase, Ronald, "The Problem of Social Cost," *Journal of Law and Economics*, 3 (October 1960).

18. Posner, Richard A., "A Theory of Negligence," *Journal of Legal Studies*, 1, No. 1 (January 1972).

19. *Comparative Approaches to Liability for Medical Maloccurences*, 84 YALE L. J. 1141-1163. (1975).

20. Beham, Lee, "The Effect of Advertising on the Price of Eyeglasses," *Journal of Law and Economics*, 15, No. 2, (October 1972).

21. Alchian, Armen A. and William R. Allen, *Exchange and Production Theory in Use* (Belmont, California: Wadsworth Publishing Co., Inc., 1969).

22. Henderson, J. M. and R. E. Quandt, *Microeconomic Theory* (New York: McGraw-Hill and Co., 1958).

23. Frech, H. E., "Regulation Reform: The Case of the Medical Care Industry," University of California, Santa Barbara, Working Paper in Economics #35 (August 1975).

24. Friedman, Milton and Simon S. Kuznets, *Income from Independent Professional Practice* (New York: Columbia University Press, 1972).

25. Kessel, Reuben, "Price Discrimination in Medicine," *Journal of Law and Economics*, 1 (October 1958).

26. Jordan, William, "Producer Protection, Prior Market Structure and the Effects of Government Regulation," *Journal of Law and Economics*, 15, No. 1 (April 1972).

27. Crew, Michael, "Coinsurance and the Welfare Economics of Medical Care," *American Economic Review*, 59, No. 5 (December 1969).

28. Flexner, Abraham, *Medical Education in the U.S. and Canada,* Carnegie Foundation for the Advancement of Teaching, Bulletin No. 4 (1910).

29. "Disciplining of Physicians by the Board of Medical Examiners," Report of the Office of the Auditor General to the Joint Legislative Audit Committee, State of California (August 1975).

30. *Darling vs. Charleston Community Memorial Hospital,* 33 Ill.2d 326, 211 N.E.2d 253

(1965), *cert. denied,* 383 U.S. 946 (1966). See also *Purcell vs. Zimbelman,* Ariz. App. 75,500 P.2d 335 (1972), relating to the duty of a hospital to review the competence of its attending staff physicians.

31. MacColl, William A., *Group Practice and the Prepayment of Medical Care* (Washington, D.C.: Public Affairs Press, 1966).

32. Weil, Roman, "Benefits from Screening for Cervical Cancer do not Appear to Justify Its Cost," undated mimeo, University of Chicago.

33. Collen, Morris F., et al., "Dollar Cost Per Positive Test for Automated Multiphasic Screening," *New England Journal of Medicine,* 283, No. 9 (August 27, 1970).

34. Bates, Barbara and Joel A. Yellin, "The Yield of Multiphasic Screening," *Journal of the American Medical Association,* 222, No. 1 (October 2, 1972).

35. Dickinson, Louis, et al., "Evaluation of the Effectiveness of Cytologic Screening for Cervical Cancer," *Mayo Clinic Proceedings,* 47 (August 1972).

36. Webster, Ian W., "A Preliminary Report of the Operation of a Multiple Screening Centre in Sydney," *The Medical Journal of Australia,* (August 26, 1972).

37. Vecchio, Thomas J., "Predictive Value of a Single Diagnostic Test in Unselected Populations," *New England Journal of Medicine* 2734, No. 21 (May 26, 1966).

38. Crothers, Leah S., "Professional Standards Review and the Limitation of Health Services: An Interpretation of the Effect of Statutory Immunity on Medical Malpractice Liability." 54 BOSTON UNIV. L. R., 54 (November 1974).

Chapter 15
Policy Recommendations

1. COST CONTROL

The Department of Health, Education, and Welfare and the Congress must accept that the PSRO program has only limited potential as a cost-containment vehicle. A realistic assessment is that the program can:

   (a) produce cost-savings only where gross over-utilization of medical procedures is found to be present;

   (b) provide safeguards during implementation of other cost-control measures (e.g., prospective reimbursement, HMO encouragement) with respect to inappropriate diagnostic or treatment regimens;

Greater emphasis should be given to the area where the program can make its most significant contribution: defining the components of cost-effective, quality health care. Critical assessment and understanding of these components in the health delivery system as it *currently* operates is needed before major initiatives are taken to modify or restructure the existing system.

2. TRANSITIONAL PERIOD: RESEARCH AND DEVELOPMENT

The PSRO program is in a "transitional" startup period which requires "front-end" investment. Priority should be given to providing sufficient funds, first, to developing the structure and staff of local PSROs, and second, to a vigorous R&D effort. In the latter area, funding should be targeted during the next three to five years for study and applied research so that data will be available at the end of this transitional period: (a) on the components of cost-effective, quality health care; and (b) on the potential of PSRO and other quality assurance systems to foster this kind of care. We do not have the detailed information needed to assess either the management structures of

331

PSROs or the results to be expected from the activation of PSROs under different local circumstances. Concurrent with this intensive quality *assessment* effort the PSRO program should be focused on eliminating gross deficiencies in health services utilization and incompetent practice. Stringent criteria-setting and sanctioning should be delayed until the necessary knowledge is generated about quality-assurance methodologies and the real components of cost-effective, quality health care.

3. EXPANSION OF PSRO MANDATE

The Secretary of DHEW should activate a series of meetings, between the third-party carriers and DHEW, to work out implementation procedures for expanding PSRO review to cover *all* hospitalized patients. It is clear that the potential advantage of the PSRO process will be incompletely realized unless "private" patients covered by Blue Cross and commercial health insurance are included in the process. This change will help clarify the respective roles of PSRO and institutional providers with respect to the monitoring and financing of review activities.

4. UNIFORM DATA COLLECTION
AND ANALYSIS SYSTEMS

The development of a uniform hospital data collection and analysis system, its implementation in the PSRO and HSA programs, and its acceptance and utilization by private sector providers and insurers are *vital*. This will require real compromises by all concerned parties and aggressive leadership by the Secretary of DHEW. Particular attention should be given to developing independent public-private data consortia that will cooperate in both generating and sharing essential health care data.

5. DATA CONFIDENTIALITY

DHEW should institute a series of seminars to ensure an active dialogue between health care providers and consumer groups on the question of access to health care data. Regulations in this sensitive area of data confidentiality must be based on as much public consensus as possible. Policy for dissemination of data should be based not on the desires of any single group, but on optimal protection of everyone's rights. Toward that end, a considerable degree of leadership and thoughtful analysis and discussion involving individuals and groups with differing viewpoints will be necessary, as a prelude to acceptable regulation of health care data.

6. RESOURCE ALLOCATION DECISION MAKING

The Department of DHEW should institute a series of policy discussions at the national level to clarify the dichotomy between "health" and "medical care." Full exploration of the issue will require broad representation from both the public and private sectors, both in the discussions and in the development of the cost-benefit analyses needed for optimal decision making about future resource allocations.

Selected Bibliography[*]

QUALITY OF MEDICAL CARE

Albert, Jack; Hegarty, M.; Robertson, L., Kosa, J., and Haggerty, R. "Effective Use of Comprehensive Pediatric Care: Utilization of Health Resources." *American Journal of Diseases of Children* 116 (1968): 529-533.

Ament, Richard F., and Luttman, Roger. "P.A.S. Finds the Elderly Are Staying Longer in Smaller Hospitals." *Modern Hospital* 109 (1967): 106-107.

American Medical Association, Division of Medical Practice. *PSRO: Program Information and Resources.* Chicago: American Medical Association, 1975.

Bellin, S.; Geiger, J. J.; and Gibson, C. "Impact of Ambulatory Health Care Services on the Demand for Hospital Beds." *New England Journal of Medicine* 280 (1969): 808-812.

Bentley, Herschel P., Jr. "Neonatal Mortality." *Journal of the Medical Association of Alabama* 36 (1966): 377-381.

Best, W. R. "Automatic Auditing." *Medical Record News* 35 (1964): 53-66.

Blum, Henrik L. "Evaluating Health Care." *Medical Care* 12 (1974): 999-1011.

Blumstein, James F., and Zubkoff, Michael. "Perspectives on Government Policy in the Health Section." *Milbank Memorial Fund Quarterly* 51 (1973): 395-426.

Brook, R. "An Audit of the Quality of Care in Social Medicine." *Milbank Memorial Fund Quarterly* 46 (1968): 351-374.

[*] Prepared, in part, by the Health Care Research Section, Division of Medicine, Boston University School of Medicine, under a subcontract from the Institute for Professional Standards, No. IPS-N.T. 74-1.

Brook, R. "Effectiveness of Patient Care in an Emergency Room." *New England Journal of Medicine* 283 (1970): 904-907.

Brook, R. H. "Effectiveness of Inpatient Follow-Up Care." *New England Journal of Medicine* 285 (1971): 1509-1514.

Brook, R. H., and Appel, F. A. "Quality of Care Assessment: Choosing A Method for Peer Review." *New England Journal of Medicine* 288 (1973): 1323-1329.

Bubeck, Roy. G., Jr.; Mathhews, James G.; Reimann, Martin L.; and Orth, Harvey C., Jr. "Maternal Mortality: Report of Ten Year Study of Patients under Osteopathic Care." *Journal of the American Osteopathic Association* 67 (1967): 379-395.

Buck, Charles R., Jr. "Terms and Trends in Quality Assurance." *Trustee* 28 (September 1975): 32-34.

Buck, Charles R., Jr., and White, Kerr L. "Peer Review: Impact of a System Based on Billing Claims." *New England Journal of Medicine* 291 (1974): 877-883.

Bussman, John. *Outcome Evaluation: Experimental Medical Care Review Organization, Multnomah Medical Care Review Organization.* Washington, D.C.: National Center for Health Service Research, Department of HEW, 1975.

Cammarn, M. "Computerized Records Provide Audit of Clinic Patient Care." *Hospital* 42 (1968): 74-79.

Caron, Herbert S., and Roth, Harold, P. "Patients' Cooperation with a Medical Regimen: Difficulties in Identifying the Noncooperator." *JAMA* 203 (1968): 922-926.

Cohen, Harris S. "Professional Licensure, Organizational Behavior and the Public Interest." *Milbank Memorial Fund Quarterly* 51 (1973): 73-94.

Colwell, A. R., and Fern., G. K. "Standards of Practice of Internal Medicine: Methods of Judging its Quality in Hospitals." *Annals of Internal Medicine* 51 (1959): 821-832.

Commission on Professional and Hospital Activities. *Length of Stay in Short-Term General Hospitals* (1963-64). New York: McGraw-Hill Co., 1966.

Cottrell, J. D. "The Consumption of Medical Care and the Evaluation of Efficiency." *Medical Care* 4 (1966): 214-236.

Decker, B., and Bonner, P. *Criteria in Peer Review.* Cambridge, Mass.: Arthur D. Little, Inc., 1974.

Densen, Paul M., and Shapiro, Sam. "Opportunities and Responsibilities for Evaluation and Research in Professional Standards Review Organizations." Presented to the Association of American Medical Colleges meeting, November 1974, Chicago, Ill.

Donabedian, A. "An Evaluation of Prepaid Group Practice." *Inquiry* 6 (1) (1969): 3-27

Donabedian, Avedis. *Aspects of Medical Care Administration.* Cambridge, Mass.: Harvard University Press, 1973.

Donabedian, Avedis. "Evaluating the Quality of Medical Care." *Milbank Memorial Fund Quarterly* 44 (1966): 166-206.

Donabedian, Avedis. "Promoting Quality Through Evaluating the Process of Patient Care." *Medical Care* 6 (1968): 181-202.

Donabedian, A., and Rosenfeld, L. S. "Follow-Up Study of Chronically Ill Patients Discharged from Hospital. *Journal of Chronic Diseases* 17 (1964): 847-862.

Doyle, J. C. "Unnecessary Hysterectomies: Study of 6,248 Operations in Thirty-Five Hospitals During 1948." *JAMA* 151 (1953): 360-365.

Doyle, J. C. "Unnecessary Ovariectomies: Study Based on Removal of 704 Normal Ovaries from 546 Patients." *JAMA* 148 (1952): 1105-1111.

Eisele, C. W. *The Medical Staff in the Modern Hospital.* New York: McGraw-Hill Co., 1967.

Eisele, C. W.; Slee, V. N.; and Hoffman, R. G. "Can the Practice of Internal Medicine be Evaluated?" *Annals of Internal Medicine* 44 (1956): 144-161.

Ellwood, Paul M., Jr. "Quantitative Measurement of Patient Care Quality: Part 1—Measures of Care." *Hospitals* 40: (1966): 42-45.

Ellwood, Paul M., Jr. "Quantitative Measurement of Patient Care Quality: Part 2—A System for Identifying Meaningful Factors." *Hospitals* 40 (1966): 59-63.

Ellwood, Paul M. et al. *Assuring the Quality of Health Care.* Minneapolis: Interstudy, 1973.

Elmendorf, T. "PSRO: An Opportunity for True Professionalism." *Hospital Medical Staffs* 4 (April 1975): 16-19.

Falk, I. S. "Medical Care in the U.S.A.: 1932-1972." *Milbank Memorial Fund Quarterly* 51 (1973): 1-40.

Falk, I. S. et al. "The Development of Standards for the Audit and Planning of Medical Care, I: Concepts, Research Design, and the Content of Primary Physician's Care." *American Journal of Public Health* 57 (1967): 1118-1136.

Flook, E. Evelyn, and Sanazaro, Paul J., eds. *Health Services Research and R&D in Perspective.* Ann Arbor, Mich.: University of Michigan Press, 1973.

Ford, A. B., Katz, S. "Prognosis After Strokes, I: A Critical Review." *Medicine* 45 (1966): 223-246.

Frederick, Larry. "PSROs: How the First Ones Are Working." *Medical World News,* October 25, 1974. pp. 53-69.

Garwin, Richard L. "Impact of Information-Handling Systems on Quality and Access to Health Care." *Public Health Reports* 83 (1968): 345-351.

Gersten, Jerome W.; Cenkovich, Frank; Dinken, Harold; and Miller, Barry. "Evaluation of Rehabilitation in Home or Clinic Setting: Problems in Methodology." *Archives of Physical Medicine* 47 (1966): 199-203.

Goldberg, George A., and Holloway, Don C. "Emphasizing 'Level of Care' Over 'Length of Stay' in Hospital Utilization Review." *Medical Care* 13 (1975): 474-485.

Gonnella, Joseph S., and Goran, Michael J. "Quality of Patient Care—A Measurement of Change: The Staging Concept." *Medical Care* 13 (1975): 467-473.

Gonnella, Joseph S. and Zeleznik, Carter. "Factors Involved in Comprehensive Patient Care Evaluation." *Medical Care* 12 (1974): 928-934.

Goodman, Raymond D., ed. *The Proceedings from PSRO, An Educational Symposium.* Los Angeles: University of California Extension, 1975.

Grier, George S., III, and McClellan, Jason E. "Effectiveness of a Large Community Coronary Care Unit." *Southern Medical Journal* 61 (1968): 429-433.

Gruenberg, E., ed. "Evaluating the Effectiveness of Mental Health Services." *Milbank Memorial Fund Quarterly* 41 (1966): 1-39.

Hagner, Samuel B.; LoCicero, Victor J.; and Steiger, William A. "Patient Outcome in a Comprehensive Medicine Clinic: Its Retrospective Assesment and Related Variables." *Medical Care* 6 (1968): 144-156.

Hare, Robert L. *American Society of Internal Medicine Study of Evaluation of Quality of Medical Care.* San Francisco: American Society of Internal Medicine, 1973.

Havighurst, Clark C., and Blumstein, James F. "Coping with Quality-Cost Tradeoffs in Medical Care; The Role of PSROs." 70 *Northeastern Law Review* (1975): 6-68.

Havighurst, Clark C., and Tancredi, Laurence R. "Medical Adversity Insurance—A No-Fault Approach to Medical Malpractice and Quality Assurance." *Milbank Memorial Fund Quarterly* 51 (1973): 125-168.

Helfer, R. "Estimating the Quality of Care in a Pediatric Emergency Room." *Journal of Medical Education* 42 (1967): 244-248.

Hopkins, Carl E. *Outcomes Conference I-II: Methodology of Identifying, Measuring and Evaluating Outcomes of Health Service Programs, Systems and Subsystems.* Washington, D.C.: National Center for Health Services Research and Development, Department of HEW, 1970.

Huntley, R. R. et al. "The Quality of Medical Care: Techniques and Investigation in the Outpatient Clinic." *Journal of Chronic Diseases* 14 (1961): 630-642.

Institute of Medicine. *Advancing the Quality of Health Care; A Policy Statement.* Washington, D.C.: National Academy of Sciences, August 1974.

Institute of Medicine. *A Strategy for Evaluating Health Services.* Washington, D.C.: National Academy of Sciences, 1973.

Jessee, William F. et al. "PSRO: An Educational Force for Improving Quality of Care." *New England Journal of Medicine* 292 (1975): 668-671.

Jones, Ellen W.; McNitt, Barbara J.; and McKnight, Eleanor M. *Patient Classification for Long-Term Care: Users Manual.* Washington, D.C.: HEW Bureau of Health Services Research, December 1973.

Katz, S. et al. "Long Term Course of 147 Patients with Fracture of the Hip." *Surgery, Gynecology and Obstetrics* 124 (1967): 1219-1230.

Katz, Sidney; Jackson, Beverly A.; Jaffee, Marjorie W.; Littell, Arthur; and Turk, Charles E. "Multidisciplinary Studies of Illness in Aged Persons— IV: Comparison Study of Rehabilitated and Nonrehabilitated Patients with Fracture of the Hip." *Journal of Chronic Diseases* 15 (1962): 979-984.

Kelman, H. et al. "Monitoring Patient Care." *Medical Care* 7 (1969): 1-13.

Kessner, David. *Development of Methodology for Evaluation of Neighborhood Health Centers.* Washington, D.C.: Institute of Medicine, National Academy of Sciences, 1972.

Klein, Bonnie Winters. *Evaluating Outcomes of Health Services, An Annotated Bibliography.* Los Angeles: University of California, 1970.

Kutner, Bernard. *Modes of Treating the Chronically Ill,* Proceedings of a Symposium on Research in Long-Term Care. St. Louis: Jewish Hospital of St. Louis, 1963.

Lambertsen, Eleanor C. "Evaluating the Quality of Nursing Care." Hospitals 39 (1965): 61-66.

Lambertsen, E. C. "Planning and Evaluating Patient Care on Interdisciplinary Health Team." *Journal of the Arkansas Medical Society* 62 (1965): 129-130.

Last, J. M. "The Measurement of Medical Care in General Practice." *Medical Journal of Australia* 1 (1965): 280-282.

Last J., and White, K. "The Content of Medical Care in Primary Practice." *Medical Care* 7 (1969): 40-47.

Lawton, M. Powell; Ward, Morton; and Yaffe, Silvia. "Indices of Health in an Aging Population. *Journal of Gerontology* 22 (1967): 334-342.

Le Maitre, George D. "The Council of Medical Staffs." *Massachusetts Physician* (October 1975): 34-37.

Lembcke, P. A. "A Scientific Method for Medical Auditing." *Hospitals* 33 (1959): 65-71.

Lembcke, P. A. "Evolution of the Medical Audit." *JAMA* 199 (1967): 543-550.

Lembcke, P. A. "Measuring the Quality of Medical Care Through Vital Statistics Based on Hospital Service Areas: 1. Comparative Study of Appendectomy Rates." *American Journal of Public Health* 42 (1952): 276-286.

Lembcke, P. A. "Medical Auditing." *Journal of the American Association of Medical Record Librarians* 30 (1959): 324-327, 346.

Lembcke, P. A. "Medical Auditing by Scientific Methods: Illustrated by Major Female Pelvic Surgery." *JAMA* 162 (1956): 646-655.

Leonard, Robert C.; Skipper, James. J., Jr.; and Wooldrige, Powhatten J. "Small Sample Field Experiments for Evaluating Patient Care." *Health Services Research* 2 (1967): 46-60.

Levin, Arthur L. "Cost Effectiveness in Maternal and Child Health: Implications for Program Planning and Evaluation." *New England Journal of Medicine* 278 (1968): 1041-1047.

Lipworth, L.; Lee, J. A. H.; and Morris, J. N. "Case-Fatality in Teaching and Non-Teaching Hospitals 1956-1959." *Medical Care* 1 (1963): 71-76.

Makeover, H. B. "The Quality of Medical Care; Methodology of Survey of the Medical Groups Associated with the Health Insurance Plan of New York." *American Journal of Public Health* 41 (1951): 824-832.

McKinlay, John B., ed. *Economic Aspects of Health Care.* New York: Milbank Memorial Fund, 1973.

McKinlay, John B., ed. *Politics and Law in Health Care Policy.* New York: Milbank Memorial Fund, 1973.

McKinlay, John B., ed. *Research Methods in Health Care.* New York: Milbank Memorial Fund, 1973.

McMahon, John Alexander. "PSROs: Implications for Hospitals" *Hospitals* 48 (1974): 53-55.

Medalie, Jack H., and Mann, Kalman J. "Evaluation of Medical Care: Methodological Problems in a 6-Year Follow-Up of a Family and Community Health Center." *Journal of Chronic Diseases* 19 (1966): 17-33.

Muller, Jonas N.; Tobis, Jerome S.; and Kelman, Howard R. "The Rehabilitation Potential of Nursing Home Residents." *American Journal of Public Health* 53 (1963): 243-247.

Murnaghan, Jane H. *Ambulatory Medical Care Data.* Baltimore: Johns Hopkins University Press, 1973.

Murnaghan, Jane H. "Health-Services Information Systems in the United States Today." *New England Journal of Medicine* 290 (1974): 603-610.

Murnaghan, Jane H., and White, Kerr L., eds. "Hospital Discharge Data." *Medical Care* 8 (1970 Supp.): 1-215.

Myers, R. S. "Justification for Surgery." *Bulletin of the American College of Surgeons* 41 (1956): 173-174.

Myers, R. S. "Quality of Patient Care—Measurable or Immeasurable?" *Journal of Medical Education* 36 (1961): 776-784.

Myers, R. S. "Statistical Audits Prove Effective in Improving Medical Standards." *Modern Hospital* 103 (1964): 124.

Navarro, Vincente. "National Health Insurance and the Strategy for Change." *Milbank Memorial Fund Quarterly* 51 (1973): 223-252.

Nelson, Alan R. "Relation Between Quality Assessment and Utilization Review in a Functioning PSRO." *New England Journal of Medicine* 292 (1975): 671-675.

O'Donnell, W. E. "Who's Guilty of Overhospitalization? Me—and Probably You." *Medical Economics,* October 13, 1975, pp. 80-85.

Payne, B. C. "Continued Evolution of a System of Medical Care Appraisal." *JAMA* 201 (1967): 536-540.

Payne, B. C. "Function of the Audit Committee in the General Hospital." *Hospitals* 37 (1963): 66-73.

Payne, B. C. "Use of the Criteria Approach to Measurement of Effectiveness of Hospital Utilization." *JAMA* 196 (1966): 1066-1068.

Payne, B. C. *Use of the Criteria Approach to Measurement of Effectiveness of Hospital Utilization Review: A Handbook for the Medical Staff.* Chicago: American Medical Association, 1965.

Peterson, O. L. "Medical Care: Its Social and Organizational Aspects—Evaluation of the Quality of Medical Care." *New England Journal of Medicine* 269 (1963): 1238-1245.

Peterson, O. L.; Andrews, L. P.; Spain, R. S.; and Greenberg, B. G. "An Analytical Study of North Carolina General Practice, 1953-54." *Journal of Medical Education* 31 (1965): 1-165.

Pratt, Louis; Seligmann, Arthur; and Reader, George. "Physicians' Views on the Level of Medical Information Among Patients." *American Journal of Public Health* 47 (1957): 1277-1283.

Preuss, Hans, and Soloman, Philip. "The Patient's Reaction to Bedside Teaching." *New England Journal of Medicine* 259 (1958): 520-525.

Reinert, H. V. "Effectiveness of Hospital Tissue Committee in Raising Surgical Standards." *JAMA* 150 (1952): 992-996.

Respess, James. *Albemarle County, Virginia Medical Care Foundation: Outcome Evaluation.*

Rider, Rowland V.; Harper, Paul A.; Knobloch, Hilda; and Fetter, Sara E "An Evaluation of Standards for the Hospital Care of Premature Infants." *JAMA* 165 (1957): 1233-1236.

Riedel, D. C., and Fitzpatrick, T. B. *Patterns of Patient Care.* Ann Arbor: University of Michigan Press, 1964.

Ringholtz, Sharon, and Morris, Miriam. "A Test of Some Assumptions About Rooming-In." *Nursing Research* 10 (1961): 196-199.

Roemer, Milton I. "Is Surgery Safer in Larger Hospitals?" *Hospital Management* 87 (1959): 35-37.

Roemer, Milton I. *The Organization of Medical Care under Social Security.* Geneva: International Labor Office Studies and Reports, New Series No. 73, 1969.

Roemer, Milton I.; Moustafa, A. Taher; and Hopkins, Carl E. "A Proposed Hospital Quality Index: Hospital Death Rates Adjusted for Case Severity." *Health Services Research* 3 (1968): 96-118.

Rosenberg, Charlotte L. "How Close are They to Evaluating Your Office Care?" *Medical Economics,* June 23, 1975, pp. 132 ff.

Sanazaro, Paul J. "The Evaluation of Medical Care Under Public Law 89-239." *Medical Care* 5 (1967): 162-168.

Sanazaro, Paul J.; et al. "Research and Development in Quality Assurance: The Experimental Medical Care Review Organization Program." *New England Journal of Medicine* 287 (1972): 1125-1131.

Sanazaro, Paul J., and Williamson, John W. "End Results of Patient Care: A Provisional Classification Based on Reports by Internists." *Medical Care* 6 (1968): 123-130.

Sanders, Barkev S. "Completeness and Reliability of Diagnoses in Therapeutic Practice." *Journal of Health and Human Behavior* 5 (1964): 84-94.

Sanders, Barkev S. "Measuring Community Health Levels." *American Journal of Public Health* 54 (1964): 1063-1070.

Shapiro, Sam. "End-Result Measurements of Quality of Medical Care." *Milbank Memorial Fund Quarterly* 45 (1967): 7-30.

Shapiro, Sam; Jacobziner, Harold; Densen, Paul M.; and Weiner, Louis. "Further Observations on Prematurity and Perinatal Mortality in a General Population and in the Population of a Prepaid Group Practice Medical Care Plan." *American Journal of Public Health* 50 (1960): 1304-1317.

Shapiro, Sam; Weiner, Louis; and Densen, Paul M. "Comparison of Prematurity and Perinatal Mortality in a General Population and in the Population of a Prepaid Group Practice Medical Care Plan." *American Journal of Public Health* 48 (1958): 170-187.

Shapiro, Sam; Williams, Josephine J.; Yerby, Alonzo S.; Densen, Paul M.; and Rosner, Henry. "Patterns of Medical Use by the Indigent Aged Under Two Systems of Medical Care. *American Journal of Public Health* 57 (1967): 784-790.

Sheps, M. C. "Approaches to the Quality of Hospital Care." *Public Health Reports* 70 (1955): 877-886.

Sheps, M. C. *Assessing Effectiveness of Programs in Operation. Transactions of the Fourth Macy Conference 1955.* New York: Josiah Macy, Jr., Foundation, 1956.

Sheps, M. C., and Sheps, C. G. *Assessing the Effectiveness of Programs in Operation Study Group Reports,* Committee IV on Research, National Conference on Care of the Long-Term Patient. Baltimore: Commission on Chronic Illness, 1954, pp. 93-104.

Sheridan, Bart. "What Happens When Doctors Say 'No' to PSRO." *Medical Economics,* October 27, 1975, pp. 19-29.

Sidel, Victor W. "Evaluation of the Quality of Medical Practice." *JAMA* 198 (1966): 763-764.

Simmons, Henry E. "PSRO Today: The Program's Viewpoint." *New England Journal of Medicine* 292 (1975): 365-366.

Schlesinger, Edward. "The Impact of Federal Legislation of Maternal and Child Health Services in the United States." *Milbank Memorial Fund Quarterly* 52 (1974): 1-14.

Somers, Herman M., and Somers, Anne R. *Medicare and Hospitals: Issues and Prospects.* Washington, D. C.: The Brookings Institute, 1967.

Sparling, J. Frederick. "Measuring Medical Care Quality: A Comparative Study." *Hospitals* 36 (1962): 56-61; 62-68.

Stapleton, John F., and Zwerneman, James A. "The Influence of an Intern-Resident Staff on the Quality of Private Patient Care." *JAMA* 194 (1965): 877-882.

Starfield, Barbara. "Measurement of Outcome: A Proposed Scheme." *Milbank Memorial Fund Quarterly* 52 (1974): 1-14.

Stuart, Bruce, and Stockton, Ronald. "Control Over the Utilization of Medical Services." *Milbank Memorial Fund Quarterly* 51 (1973): 341-394.

Taylor, E. Steward, and Walker, Louise C. "Premature Infant Deaths: A Ten-Year Study of Causes and Prevention." *Obstetrics and Gynecology* 13 (1959): 555-562.

Thompson, John D.; Marquis, Don B.; Woodward, Robert L.; and Yeomans, Richard C. "End-Result Measurements of the Quality of Obstetrical Care in Two U. S. Air Force Hospitals." *Medical Care* 6 (1968): 131-143.

U. S., HEW, National Center for Health Statistics. *Ambulatory Medical Care Records: Uniform Minimum Basic Data Set.* Rockville, Md.: HEW, 1974.

U. S., HEW, National Center for Health Statistics. *Inpatient Utilization of Short Stay Hospitals by Diagnosis.* Rockville, Md.: Vital and Health Statistics, Series 13, No. 6, 1974.

U. S., HEW, National Center for Health Statistics. *Uniform Hospital Abstract: Minimum Basic Data Set.* Rockville, Md.: Vital and Health Statistics, Series 4, No. 14, 1972.

U. S., HEW, Regional Medical Programs Service. *Quality Assurance of Medical Care,* monograph. Rockville, Md.: HEW, 1973.

U. S., Social Security Administration, Office of Research and Statistics. *Health Insurance for the Aged, 1970: Length of Stay by Diagnosis.* Washington, D. C. 1973.

Vail, D. J. "Strategy in Evaluating the Effectiveness of Community Mental Health Programs." Public Health Reports 76 (1961): 975-978.

Weed, Lawrence L. *Medical Records, Medical Education, and Patient Care.* Cleveland: Case Western Reserve University Press, 1969.

Weinerman, E. Richard. "Patients' Perceptions of Group Medical Care: A Review and Analysis of Studies on Choice and Utilization of Prepaid Group Practice Plans." *American Journal of Public Health* 54 (1964): 880-889.

Wenberg, John, and Gittelsohn, Alan. "Small Area Variations in Health Care Delivery." *Science* 182 (1973): 1102-1108.

Williamson, J. W. "Evaluating Quality of Patient Care: A Strategy Relating Outcome and Process Assessment." *JAMA* 218 (1971): 564-569.

Wylie, C., and White, B. "A Measure of Disability." *Archives of Environmental Health* 8 (1964): 834-839.

Zeleznik, Carter. "Patient Care Evaluation: 10 Basic Principles." *Hospital Medical Staff* 2 (1973): 2-9.

Zola, Irving K., and McKinlay, John B. *Organizational Issues in the Delivery of Health Services.* New York: Milbank Memorial Fund, 1974.

PEER REVIEW

American Medical Association. *Peer Review Manual.* Chicago: Council on Medical Service, 1971.

American Society of Internal Medicine. *PSRO: A Guide to Implementation Through Peer Review.* San Francisco, 1973.

Boisseree, V. R. "A Case Study in Peer Review." *Journal of the American Pharmaceutical Association* 12 (1972): 171-172.

Brook, Robert H. *Quality of Care Assessment: A Comparison of Five Methods of Peer Review.* Rockville, Md.: HEW, 1973.

Costilow, M. S. "Peer Review: Inevitable Evolution of Our Quest for Quality of Care." *Journal of the Mississippi State Medical Association* 12 (1971): 577-585.

Decker, Barry, and Bonner, Paul, eds. *PSRO: Organization for Regional Peer Review.* Cambridge, Mass.: Ballinger Publishing Co., 1973.

Goran, Michael J., et al. "The PSRO Hospital Review System." *Medical Care* 13 (1975 Supp.): 1-33.

Grenedier, I. "Peer Review and the Medicaid Program." *New York State Dental Journal* 39 (1969): 168-169.

Holbrook, Fred K. "Computerization Aids Utilization Review." *Hospitals*

49 (September 1975): 53-55.

Ingelfinger, F. J. "Peer Review of Obstetric Mishaps." *New England Journal of Medicine* 285 (1971): 858.

Kincaid, W. H. "The Professional Activity Study." *Inquiry 2* (1965): 30-38.

Kuehm, H. "Peer Review: An Introduction to its Purpose, Scope, and Function." *Bulletin of the American College of Surgeons* 56 (1971): 54-57.

Orme, June Y., and Lindbeck, Rosemary S. "Nurse Participation Medical Peer Review." *Nursing Outlook* 22 (1974): 27-30.

Puiger, S. "Peer Review: Cost Contol or Quality Control?" *California Medicine* 113 (1970): 75-80.

Richardson, F. M. "Peer Review and Medical Care." *Medical Care* (1972): 29-39.

Sheridan, Bart. "We Get Postgraduate Credits for Peer Review." *Medical Economics,* July 21, 1975, pp. 77 ff.

Slee, V. N. "Professional Activity Study." *Medical Care* 8 (1970 Supp): 34-40.

Stroud, H. H. "Peer Review and Professional Evaluation." *Delaware Medicine* 42 (1970): 46-47.

Task Force on Peer Review in Psychiatry. "Position Statement on Peer Review in Psychiatry." *American Journal of Psychiatry* 130 (1973): 381-385.

Watson, C. G. "Peer Review." *Journal of the American College of Dentistry* 38 (1971): 103-111.

Welch, C. "Professional Standards Review Organizations—Problems and Prospects." *New England Journal of Medicine* 289 (1973): 291-295.

Welch, C. "Professional Standards Review Organizations." *New England Journal of Medicine* 290 (1974): 1318-1322.

Wilbur, R. S. "Peer Review." *Rhode Island Medical Journal* 53 (1970): 38-42.

MEDICAL AUDIT

Albert Einstein College of Medicine. *The Baseline Medical Audit-Evaluation Unit.* New York: Department of Community Health, 1970.

Dague, James, and Johenning, Paul W. "Simplified Method Costs Only 23 Cents Per Patient Day." *Hospitals* 49 (October 1975): 51-55.

Devitt, James E., and Ironside, Mary. "Difficulties in Applying Patient Care Audit to Surgeons." *Bulletin of the American College of Surgeons* 60 (May 1975): 18-21.

Dreyfus, E. G., et al. "Internal Chart Audits in a Neighborhood Health Program: A Problem-Oriented Approach." *Medical Care* 9 (1971): 449-454.

Eisele, C. W. "The Medical Audit in Continuing Education." *Journal of Medical Education* 44 (1967): 263-265.

Goldberg, George A., et al. "Medical Care Evaluation Studies." *JAMA* 220 (1972): 383-387.

Goldberg, W. M. "Medical Audit." *Journal of the Canadian Medical Association* 108 (1972): 671-674.

Healy, F. M., and Healy, J. J. "Computers and Privacy: The Medical Records Case." *Journal of the Irish Medical Association* 68 (1975): 211-216.

Holloway, Don C., et al. "Evaluating an Information System for Medical Care Evaluation Studies." *Medical Care* 13 (1975): 320-340.

Joint Commission on Accreditation of Hospitals. *The PEP Primer.* Chicago: Joint Commission on Accreditation of Hospitals, 1974.

Rosenberg, Charlotte L. "What Those New JCAH Quality Audits Mean to You." *Medical Economics,* September 1, 1975, pp. 23-33.

Sanazaro, Paul J. "Medical Audit: Experience in the USA." *British Medical Journal* 1 (1974): 271-274.

Schonfeld, H. K. *The Development of Standards for the Audit and Planning of Medical Care: Audit of Hospital Outpatient Care.* Edited by G. Geaumont, B. McCollum, and L. Fish. Minneapolis: University of Minnesota Health Sciences Center, 1968.

Schonfeld, H. K. "Standards for the Audit and Planning of Medical Care: A Method for Preparing Audit Standards for Mixtures of Patients." *Medical Care* 8 (1970): 287-298.

Schonfeld, H. K. "Standards for the Audit and Planning of Medical Care With Regard for Pathways of Good Care." Paper presented at the 19th Annual Southern Conference on Gerontology, 1970, Gainesville, Fla.

Slee, V. N. "Automation in the Management of Hospital Records." *Circulation Research* 11 (1962): 637-645.

Slee, V. N. "How Can You Audit All the Care?" *Modern Hospital* 97 (1961): 1-7.

Slee, V. N. "Streamlining the Tissue Committee." *Bulletin of the American College of Surgeons* 44 (1959): 1-4.

Streichy, A. J. "Auditing of Physician's Records." *Connecticut Medicine* 34 (1970): 516-526.

Winwick, W. "An Automated System for Review of Medical Care." *Hospital and Community Psychiatry* 23 (1972): 27-29.

LEGAL ISSUES

"ACP Speaks Out on PSRO Legislation." *Bulletin of the American College of Physicians* 15 (1974): 10-12.

Blum, John D. " 'Due Process' in Hospital Peer Review." *New England Journal of Medicine* 294 (1976): 29-30.

Boikess, Olga, and Winsten, Jay A. "Can PSRO Procedures be Both Fair and Workable?" *Catholic University Law Review* 24 (1975): 407-447.

Bulger, Roger J. "Let's Think for Ourselves About National Health Policy." *Prism* 2 (1974): 35-37.

Consumers Union. "A Proposal for Regulations by the Secretary, DHEW, for PSRO Data Confidentiality and Disclosure." Mimeographed. Washington, D.C.: Consumers Union of the U.S., Inc. 1975.

Flynn, Paul F. "Physicians, Do You Really Know the Medicare Law?" *Hospital Medical Staff* 3 (1974): 17-24.

Gosfield, Alice. *PSROs: The Law and the Health Consumer.* Cambridge Mass: Ballinger Publishing Co., 1975.

Greenberg, Daniel S. "Medicare and Public Affairs: DHEW's Long-Term Plan for the Federal Role in Health." *New England Journal of Medicine* (1974): 291.

Greenfield, Jesse L. "Government Versus Health: 1974." *Annals of Internal Medicine* 81 (1974): 541-544.

Jacobs, Charles M., and Weagly, Susan. *The Liability Myth Exposed: Hospital Review Activities Pose No Risk.* Revised Edition. Chicago: Joint Commission on Accreditation of Hospitals, Quality Review Center, 1975.

"PSRO: Answers to Questions for Internists." *Bulletin of the American College of Physicians* 15 (1974): 6-10.

Willett, David E. "PSRO Today: A Lawyers Assessment." *New England Journal of Medicine* 292 (1975): 340-343.

INDEX

The Editors

Paul M. Gertman, chief of the Health Care Research Section, Boston University School of Medicine (BUSM), also serves as director of the Health Service Research and Development Program of Boston University Medical Center and director of the Quality Assurance Unit of University Hospital, Boston. He is an assistant professor of medicine and surgery at BUSM. Among Dr. Gertman's principal current research interests are the economic costs to society of various approaches to cancer management; the tradeoffs between preventive and primary-care medicine; and the concept of preventable hospital admissions. He received his A.B. and M.D. degrees from Johns Hopkins University and was a Carnegie-Commonwealth Clinical Scholar there. While on duty with the U.S. Public Health Service, Dr. Gertman was research director of the President's Advisory Council on Management Improvement, a staff member of the Office of Science and Technology, and special assistant to the director of the National Center for Health Services Research and Development.

Richard H. Egdahl is academic vice president for health affairs at Boston University, director of Boston University Medical Center, and executive vice president of University Hospital, Boston. An active surgeon specializing in endocrine surgery, he also directs the Health Policy Center of Boston University. In the latter role, Dr. Egdahl is director of the Program on Public Policy for Quality Health Care, sponsored by the Robert Wood Johnson Foundation, and coordinates and moderates Administrator's Seminars for the senior staff of the Health Resources Administration of the Department of Health, Education, and Welfare. Among his principal interests in the fields of health planning and health policy are problems of access, cost and quality; manpower and facility distribution; the role of the private sector in financing and organization of primary-care models; and the development of appropriate mechanisms for regulation of the quality of health care. Dr. Egdahl was senior health consultant to the President's Advisory Council on Management Improvement. He studied at Dartmouth College and received his M.D. from Harvard Medical School and his Ph.D. from the University of Minnesota.